Surgical Techniques in Trauma

Surgical Techniques in Trauma

Editor: Eliana Copeland

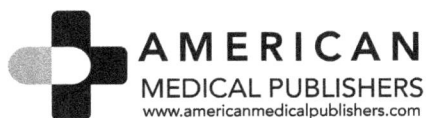

AMERICAN
MEDICAL PUBLISHERS
www.americanmedicalpublishers.com

AMERICAN
MEDICAL PUBLISHERS
www.americanmedicalpublishers.com

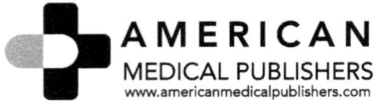

Cataloging-in-Publication Data

Surgical techniques in trauma / edited by Eliana Copeland.
  p. cm.
Includes bibliographical references and index.
ISBN 978-1-63927-501-4
1. Wounds and injuries--Surgery. 2. Surgery, Operative. 3. Surgical technology. I. Copeland, Eliana.
RD93 .S87 2022
617.1--dc23

American Medical Publishers,
41 Flatbush Avenue,
1st Floor, New York,
NY 11217, USA

ISBN 978-1-63927-501-4 (Hardback)

Contents

Preface

Trauma can cause prolonged disability or death. Its management requires quick medical action and often surgery. Surgical techniques can also be part of the diagnostic procedure to assess the condition of the patient. A tube or catheter may be placed to drain fluid from the peritoneum, the pericardium or the chest, especially when there is severe blunt trauma to the chest or abdomen. In cases where the patient is exhibiting dropping blood-pressure levels, possibly due to bleeding in the abdominal cavity, surgically cutting through the abdominal wall is vital. The assessment of the injury is made with the aid of imaging and physical examination. This allows the understanding of the severity of the injury and the location of the damage. A majority of trauma-related deaths occur from unrecognized intra-abdominal bleeding. These could be prevented if prompt surgical intervention takes place. Therefore, exploratory surgeries are often conducted to determine the extent of abdominal injuries. Damage control surgery can save life and limb. This book elucidates new surgical procedures for the management of trauma in a comprehensive manner. It strives to provide a fair idea about clinical trauma and its manifestations as well as develop a better understanding of the surgical interventions applied in trauma care. A number of latest researches have been included to keep the readers up-to-date with the global concepts in this area of study.

This book unites the global concepts and researches in an organized manner for a comprehensive understanding of the subject. It is a ripe text for all researchers, students, scientists or anyone else who is interested in acquiring a better knowledge of this dynamic field.

I extend my sincere thanks to the contributors for such eloquent research chapters. Finally, I thank my family for being a source of support and help.

Editor

Management of blunt extracranial traumatic cerebrovascular injury

Mark R Harrigan[1]*, Jordan A Weinberg[2], Ya-Sin Peaks[3], Steven M Taylor[4], Luis P Cava[5], Joshua Richman[6] and Beverly C Walters[1]

Abstract

Background: Extracranial traumatic cerebrovascular injury (TCVI) is present in 1-3% of all blunt force trauma patients. Although options for the management of patients with these lesions include anticoagulation, antiplatelet agents, and endovascular treatment, the optimal management strategy for patients with these lesions is not yet established.

Objective: Multidisciplinary survey of clinicians about current management of TCVI.

Methods: A six-item multiple-choice survey was sent by electronic mail to a total of 11,784 neurosurgeons, trauma surgeons, stroke neurologists, and interventional radiologists. The survey included questions about their choice of imaging, medical management, and the use of endovascular techniques. Survey responses were analyzed according to stated specialty.

Results: Seven hundred eighty-five (6.7%) responses were received. Overall, a total of 325 (42.8%) respondents favored anticoagulation (heparin and/or warfarin), 247 (32.5%) favored antiplatelet drugs, 130 (17.1%) preferred both anticoagulation and antiplatelet drugs, and 57 (7.5%) preferred stenting and/or embolization. Anticoagulation was the most commonly preferred treatment among vascular surgeons (56.9%), neurologists (50.2%) and neurosurgeons (40.7%), whereas antiplatelet agents were the most common preferred treatment among trauma surgeons (41.5%). Overall, 158 (20.7%) of respondents recommended treatment of asymptomatic dissections and traumatic aneurysms, 211 (27.7%) did not recommend it, and 39.4% recommended endovascular treatment only if there is worsening of the lesion on follow-up imaging.

Conclusions: These data demonstrate the wide variability of physicians' management of traumatic cerebrovascular injury, both on an individual basis, and between specialties. These findings underscore the need for multicenter, randomized trials in this field.

Background

Blunt extracranial traumatic cerebrovascular injury (TCVI) is found in some 1-3% of all blunt force trauma patients [1-15]. Estimates of overall neurological morbidity associated with TCVI range as high as 31% [2,14,16]. Ischemic stroke appears to be the greatest source of neurological morbidity in this setting. A recent report of 147 patients with TCVI found an ischemic stroke rate of 12% attributable to carotid injuries and 8% due to vertebral artery injuries [2]. Although antithrombotic therapy to prevent ischemic stroke has been widely reported, several different options exist, including anticoagulation[2,7,9,17-19] and antiplatelet therapy [2,16,20-22]. Furthermore, the use of endovascular techniques in patients with TCVI appears to be gaining in popularity [23-26].

The optimal management strategy for patients with TCVI has not yet been established. No randomized trials in the management of patients with TCVI have yet been published. The issue is complicated by the complex

* Correspondence: mharrigan@uabmc.edu
[1]Division of Neurosurgery, University of Alabama, Birmingham, Birmingham, Alabama, USA
Full list of author information is available at the end of the article

nature of many patients with TCVI, such as the variety of cerebrovascular injuries as well as the presence of polytrauma. Furthermore, cerebrovascular injury in trauma patients frequently involves the participation of numerous specialists, such as neurosurgeons, trauma surgeons, stroke neurologists, and interventional neuroradiologists. Differing disciplines may have different perspectives and practices in the management of patients with TCVI.

The purpose of the current investigation was to assess the current management of patients with TCVI across the United States and also across the various medical specialties involved with the management of patients with TCVI.

Methods

A six-item multiple-choice survey was sent by electronic mail to 11,784 members of the American Association for the Surgery of Trauma, the American Association of Neurological Surgeons, the American Heart Association Stroke Council, and the Society for Clinical Vascular Surgery. Email addresses were obtained from published membership lists. The authors attempted to exclude email addresses that overlapped between organizations. This project was approved by the Institutional Review Board.

Results were collected on a commercial survey website (http://www.surveymonkey.com). Only a single mass emailing was completed, and the survey was closed after one month. No follow-up emails or repeat email solicitations were used. All responses were kept completely confidential.

Standard two-sided chi-square tests were used to test for significant associations between specialty and survey responses. Because some expected cell counts were less than 5, results were confirmed using Monte-Carlo approximations of Fisher's exact test with one million repetitions. Testing was done using R version 2.10.1.

Results

A total of 785 responses were received, representing an overall response rate of 6.7%. Members of the American Association for the Surgery of Trauma had the highest response rate, at 15.7% (Table 1). Several emails were received from recipients of the survey, explaining that they were not clinicians, not physicians, or did not take care of patients with TCVI.

Overall survey results

The total responses to the survey questions are listed in Table 2. The largest number of respondents were neurosurgeons (342, 45.2%) and the next largest responding specialty was neurology (205, 27.1%). Only 46 of the respondents (6.0%) reported seeing no TCVI cases each

Table 1 Responses according to professional society

	Number of survey requests sent	Number of responses
American Association of Neurological Surgeons	5,481	335 (6.1%)
American Association for the Surgery of Trauma	923	145 (15.7%)
American Heart Association Stroke Council	4,638	263 (5.7%)
Society for Clinical Vascular Surgery	742	42 (5.7%)

year; the most common frequency was 1-5 per year, which was reported by 442 (57.4%) of the respondents. A conservative estimate of the total number of TCVI cases seen by the respondents can be estimated by multiplying number of respondents reporting each range of cases per year by the lowest number in each range. Thus, as a group, the respondents estimated that they see at least 2,680 TCVI cases each year.

The most common preferred method of imaging was computed tomographic angiography (CTA, 22.8%), followed by MRI/MRA (22.8%) and catheter angiography (15.0%). The most common preferred treatment was anticoagulation (42.8%) and antiplatelet drugs (32.5%). Regarding management of a patient with intraluminal thrombus and no related symptoms, the most common choice was heparin and/or warfarin (65.7%), followed by antiplatelet drugs (22.9%) and thrombolytics (6.2%). Some 20.7% of the respondents recommend treatment of asymptomatic dissections and traumatic aneurysms with endovascular techniques, while 2.7% would not and 51.6% would do so only if there were worsening of the lesion on follow-up imaging.

Analysis by specialty

For each question there was a statistically significant association between response and medical specialty (all $P < 0.00005$ for both chi-square test and Fisher's exact test). The medical specialties with the greatest annual number of TCVI cases seen per respondent were interventional radiologists, followed by trauma surgeons and neurologists (Table 3). Regarding imaging, CTA was favored by a majority of respondents in each specialty, although 39.0% of neurologists preferred MRI/MRA (Table 4). Some 26.7% of interventional radiologists and 21.8% of neurosurgeons preferred catheter angiography. Anticoagulation was the most common preferred treatment among neurosurgeons, vascular surgeons, and neurologists, whereas antiplatelet agents were most commonly favored among trauma surgeons and general surgeons (Table 5). A minority of respondents in each specialty, ranging from 3.0% to 10.7%, preferred stenting and/or embolization. Responses to questions about

Table 2 Overall responses to the questionnaire

1. What is your specialty?

   - Trauma surgeon = 137 (18.1%)
   - General surgeon = 19 (2.5%)
   - Neurosurgeon = 342 (45.2%)
   - Vascular surgeon = 52 (6.9%)
   - Neurologist = 205 (27.1%)
   - Interventional radiologist = 30 (4.0%)

2. What is the approximate number of traumatic carotid or vertebral artery dissections or other injuries that you see per year?

   - None = 46 (6.0%)
   - 1-5 = 442 (57.4%)
   - 5-10 = 144 (18.7%)
   - > 10 = 138 (17.9%)

3. What is your preferred method of imaging?

   - MRI/MRA = 175 (22.8%)
   - CTA = 464 (60.5%)
   - Doppler = 13 (1.7%)
   - Catheter angiography = 115 (15.0%)

4. In most cases which treatment do you prefer?

   - Anticoagulation (heparin and/or warfarin) = 325 (42.8%)
   - Antiplatelet drugs = 247 (32.5%)
   - Both anticoagulation and antiplatelet drugs = 130 (17.1%)
   - Stent and/or embolization = 57 (7.5%)

5. How would you manage a patient with intraluminal thrombus and no related neurological symptoms?

   - Thrombolytics = 47 (6.2%)
   - Heparin and/or warfarin = 500 (65.7%)
   - Antiplatelet drugs = 174 (22.9%)
   - None of the above = 40 (5.3%)

6. Should asymptomatic traumatic dissections and traumatic aneurysms be treated with endovascular techniques, such as stenting and/or embolization?

   - Yes = 158 (20.7%)
   - No = 211 (27.7%)
   - Only if there is worsening of the lesion on follow-up imaging = 394 (51.6%)

treatment of asymptomatic lesions are listed in Table 6. For patients with an asymptomatic intraluminal thrombus, the majority of respondents in all specialties preferred heparin and/or warfarin; antiplatelet agents were the next most commonly favored treatment, followed by

thrombolytics. Regarding asymptomatic dissections and traumatic aneurysms, the most common opinion among all specialties was that endovascular techniques should either not be used or they should be reserved for lesions that are found to worsen on follow-up imaging. However, neurosurgeons, trauma surgeons, and general surgeons were significantly more likely than vascular surgeons, neurologists and interventional radiologists to recommend endovascular treatment of asymptomatic lesions.

Discussion

The overall response rate in this study, 6.7%, is lower than the response rates reported in other published neurosurgical and trauma email surveys, which have ranged from 11.4% to 56% [27-31]. However, a significant number of the recipients of this email survey were either not clinicians or are clinicians who do not see patients with TCVI. The authors received several emails from recipients of the survey explaining this. For instance, many members of the AANS are neurosurgeons who do not see trauma patients, and a number of members of the AHA Stroke Council are Ph.D.s or nurses who also do not participate in the care of patients with traumatic injury. Furthermore, the recipients of the survey who did respond may account for a significant percentage of the clinicians who actually do take care of patients with TCVI in the United States. The lowest estimated total number of TCVI cases per year seen by the respondents is 2,680. The average annual number of blunt trauma admissions from 2000 to 2004 in the United States, as tabulated by the National Trauma Data Bank, was 162,306 [32]. Therefore, the lowest estimate of TCVI cases seen annually by the survey respondents represent approximately 1.7% of the total number of blunt trauma admissions in the United States, which is within the range of the overall incidence of TCVI (1-3%) among blunt trauma patients [1-15]. Thus, despite the seemingly low survey response rate, the respondents of this survey may represent a sizable fraction of the clinicians managing TCVI in the United States.

This survey demonstrates considerable variability in all aspects of the management of patients with TCVI, from

Table 3 Case volume by specialty

Question: What is the approximate number of traumatic carotid or vertebral artery dissections or other injuries that you see per year?				
	None	1 to 5	5 to 10	> 10
Neurosurgeon n = 342	28 (8.2%)	237 (69.5%)	35 (10.3%)	41 (12.0%)
Trauma surgeon n = 136	2 (1.5%)	58 (42.6%)	29 (21.3%)	47 (34.6%)
General surgeon n = 19	4 (21.1%)	6 (31.6%)	4 (21.1%)	5 (26.3%)
Vascular surgeon n = 52	4 (7.7%)	36 (69.2%)	9 (17.3%)	3 (5.8%)
Neurologist n = 204	6 (2.9%)	102 (50.0%)	61 (29.9%)	35 (17.2%)
Interventional radiologist n = 30	0	6 (20.0%)	8 (26.7%)	16 (53.3%)

Table 4 Preferred imaging by specialty

Question: What is your preferred method of imaging?

	MRI/MRA	CTA	Doppler	Catheter angiography
Neurosurgeon n = 339	72 (21.1%)	189 (55.8%)	4 (1.2%)	74 (21.8%)
Trauma surgeon n = 137	6 (4.4%)	127 (92.7%)	0	4 (2.9%)
General surgeon n = 19	6 (31.6%)	12 (63.2%)	0	1 (5.3%)
Vascular surgeon n = 52	7 (13.5%)	40 (76.9%)	3 (5.8%)	2 (3.8%)
Neurologist n = 205	80 (39.0%)	87 (42.4%)	6 (2.9%)	32 (15.6%)
Interventional radiologist n = 30	2 (6.7%)	20 (66.7%)	0	8 (26.7%)

imaging to medical therapy and the use of endovascular techniques. The most commonly preferred method of imaging was CTA, which likely reflects the ubiquity of CT scanning in the work-up of trauma patients, the widespread use of CTA for screening of trauma patients who are at risk of having a TCVI, and numerous published studies of CTA in this setting [14,33-37]. However, a significant subset of respondents (22.8%) favored MRI/MRA. This modality was most popular among neurologists, of whom 39.0% favored MRI/MRA. This may reflect current practice in the management of patients with spontaneous cervical artery dissection as expressed in a recent survey of members of the British Association of Stroke Physicians, 90% of whom indicated MRI/MRA as their preferred method of imaging in that setting. Overall, only 15% in the present survey preferred catheter angiography. Recently published guidelines for the management of blunt cerebrovascular injury by the Eastern Association for the Surgery of Trauma concluded that four-vessel cerebral angiography remains the gold standard for diagnosis, that duplex ultrasonography is not adequate for screening, and that multislice (eight or greater) CTA may be considered as a screening modality in place of catheter angiography[38] The authors of the guidelines also recommended that follow-up catheter angiography be done for grades I to III injuries. Grade I injuries include intimal irregularities with < 25% narrowing; grade II injuries consist of dissections or intramural hematomas with > 25% narrowing; and grade III injuries are dissecting aneurysms [39].

With respect to management, the most commonly preferred treatments overall were anticoagulation (42.8%) and antiplatelet agents (32.5%). These results are

virtually identical to the findings of the British survey about spontaneous cervical artery dissection; those respondents were also divided between preferring anticoagulation (50%) or antiplatelet agents (30%) [40]. A number of studies of TCVI have found an association between antithrombotic therapy and lower ischemic stroke rates [2,7,9,14,17-19,41], although a cause and effect relationship has not been demonstrated in a controlled study. Treatment of patients with TCVI with anticoagulation using heparin and warfarin has been more widely reported than treatment with antiplatelet agents [2,7,9,17-19]. However, systemic anticoagulation is associated with bleeding complication rates up to 16% [7,14,17,42] and up to 36% of patients with TCVI are not candidates for systemic anticoagulation due to coexistent injuries [2,20]. Antiplatelet therapy (single agent treatment with aspirin is the most commonly reported regimen) may have a lower risk of complications and several retrospective studies have indicated that antiplatelet therapy is equal to or superior to anticoagulation in terms of neurological outcomes [2,16,20-22].

The Eastern Association for the Surgery of Trauma blunt TCVI guidelines made treatment recommendations according to the type of lesion [38]. Barring contraindications, antithrombotic medications such as aspirin or heparin were recommended for grade I and II TCVIs. The authors of the guidelines concluded that either heparin or antiplatelet therapy may be used with seemingly equivalent results. Although they stated that they could not make any recommendations about how long antithrombotic therapy should be administered for patients receiving anticoagulation, the authors

Table 5 Preferred treatment by specialty

Question: In most cases which treatment do you prefer?

	Anticoagulation	Antiplatelet drugs	Both	Stent/embolization
Neurosurgeon n = 337	137 (40.7%)	105 (31.2%)	59 (17.5%)	36 (10.7%)
Trauma surgeon n = 135	39 (28.9%)	56 (41.5%)	34 (25.2%)	6 (4.4%)
General surgeon n = 19	7 (36.8%)	8 (42.1%)	2 (10.5%)	2 (10.5%)
Vascular surgeon n = 51	29 (56.9%)	8 (15.7%)	9 (17.6%)	5 (9.8%)
Neurologist n = 202	101 (50.0%)	71 (35.1%)	24 (11.9%)	6 (3.0%)
Interventional radiologist n = 30	13 (43.3%)	13 (43.3%)	2 (6.7%)	2 (6.7%)

Table 6 Management of asymptomatic lesions by specialty

Question: How would you manage a patient with intraluminal thrombus and no related neurological symptoms?

	Thrombolytics	Heparin and/or warfarin	Antiplatelets	None of the above
Neurosurgeon n = 339	35 (10.3%)	205 (60.5%)	85 (25.1%)	14 (4.1%)
Trauma surgeon n = 135	7 (5.2%)	82 (60.7%)	34 (25.2%)	12 (8.9%)
General surgeon n = 19	2 (10.5%)	12 (63.2%)	3 (15.8%)	2 (10.5%)
Vascular surgeon n = 52	2 (3.8%)	39 (75.0%)	4 (7.7%)	7 (13.5%)
Neurologist n = 202	1 (0.5%)	148 (73.3%)	46 (22.8%)	7 (3.5%)
Interventional radiologist n = 29	0	22 (75.9%)	6 (20.7%)	1 (3.4%)

Question: Should asymptomatic traumatic dissections and traumatic aneurysms be treated with endovascular techniques, such as stenting and/or embolization?

	Yes	No	Only if there is worsening on follow-up imaging
Neurosurgeon n = 339	85 (25.1%)	66 (19.5%)	188 (55.5%)
Trauma surgeon n = 134	37 (27.6%)	33 (24.6%)	64 (47.8%)
General surgeon n = 19	5 (26.3%)	7 (36.8%)	7 (36.8%)
Vascular surgeon n = 52	8 (15.4%)	20 (38.5%)	24 (46.2%)
Neurologist n = 202	25 (12.4%)	86 (42.6%)	91 (45.0%)
Interventional radiologist n = 30	4 (13.3%)	7 (23.3%)	19 (63.3%)

recommended treatment with warfarin for 3 to 6 months. They recommended consideration of surgery or endovascular treatment of grade III lesions (dissecting aneurysms), and surgical or endovascular repair of carotid lesions associated with an early neurological deficit.

Regarding the management of asymptomatic lesions, the majority of respondents overall (65.7%) would manage a patient with a clinically silent intraluminal thrombus with heparin and/or warfarin, whereas 22.9% would use antiplatelet drugs and 6.2% would use thrombolytics. Additionally, 20.7% would use stenting and/or embolization to treat asymptomatic dissections and traumatic aneurysms, while a slim majority (51.6%) would use these techniques only if there were worsening of the lesion on follow-up imaging. The question of the management of asymptomatic TCVI lesions is important because of the widespread use of CTA screening protocols. Screening protocols call for CTA imaging of blunt trauma patients with risk factors for TCVI, such as cervical spine injuries and skull base fractures. Screening of asymptomatic patients is somewhat controversial [38], as some data indicates that a significant number of ischemic strokes due to TCVI occur prior to diagnosis [2,43], and that asymptomatic TCVI lesions may carry a relatively low risk of subsequent stroke, particularly when some variety of antithrombotic therapy is used. Thus, the situation with extracranial TCVI may be analogous to extracranial atherosclerotic disease, in that asymptomatic lesions carry a much more benign prognosis than symptomatic lesions. Differentiation in outcomes and management options between symptomatic and asymptomatic TCVI lesions is fertile ground for future investigation.

Endovascular treatment with stenting and/or embolization was the preferred method of treatment for 7.5% of the respondents overall, and was most popular among neurosurgeons (10.7%), compared to other specialists. The use of endovascular techniques in the management of patients with TCVI has been reported with increasing frequency in recent years [16,23-26,44-49]. However, compared to the other issues surrounding TCVI, the actual clinical benefit of endovascular treatment remains the least well defined, underscoring the need for prospective clinical investigation.

Responses to the survey questions varied considerably by specialty. Differences in opinion between specialties were significant for estimated case volume, preferred imaging, preferred treatment, and the management of asymptomatic lesions. These differences likely reflect standards of training within each field, clinical perspectives, experience, and philosophies within individual disciplines. It is not surprising that trauma surgeons see a large volume of TCVI cases and that CTA is their preferred method of imaging, since CT is currently widely used for imaging of trauma patients. Similarly, the observation that the majority (56.9%) of vascular surgeons prefer anticoagulation for treatment - more than any other specialty - may parallel practice guidelines for the treatment of other problems commonly encountered by vascular surgeons, such as peripheral arterial disease [50]. It is less clear why neurosurgeons, trauma surgeons, and general surgeons are more likely to use endovascular techniques to treat clinically silent TCVI lesions than vascular surgeons, neurologists, and interventional radiologists. The care of TCVI patients, particularly those with polytrauma, does typically involve the participation of multiple specialists. The large practice variation found by this survey highlights the utility of involving multiple specialties in future clinical trials of TCVI, and to include multiple specialties in the formulation of future practice guidelines.

Limitations of this study include the modest overall response rate and the variability in the numbers of respondents representing the different medical disciplines. However, as mentioned above, the respondents to this survey may represent a significant proportion of clinicians who actively participate in the management of TCVI in the United States. Another limitation concerns the restricted format of this survey. This single-page six-question format, without a large number of answer options for each question and without space to type out comments, was intended to keep the email survey brief to maximize recipient participation. In the view of some of the recipients of this survey, however, the brevity of the survey over-simplified the issues associated with TCVI management. The survey was meant to focus on the core questions without taxing the respondents' time and effort to an unreasonable degree.

Conclusions

The results of this survey show that there is poor agreement on the management of patients with TCVI, from the method of imaging to medical and endovascular treatment and the handling of patients with asymptomatic lesions. These differing views reflect the absence of randomized trial data and well-defined treatment algorithms. Practice differences between medical disciplines underscores the need for and the value of multidisciplinary clinical trials and guidelines.

Author details
[1]Division of Neurosurgery, University of Alabama, Birmingham, Birmingham, Alabama, USA. [2]Division of Trauma and Critical Care Surgery, University of Tennessee Health Science Center, Memphis, Tennessee, USA. [3]University of Alabama, Birmingham School of Medicine, Birmingham, Alabama, USA. [4]Division of Vascular Surgery, University of Alabama, Birmingham, Birmingham, Alabama, USA. [5]Department of Neurology, University of Alabama, Birmingham, Birmingham, Alabama, USA. [6]Division of Preventative Medicine, University of Alabama, Birmingham, Alabama, USA.

Authors' contributions
MRH participated in and contributed to all phases of the study. JAW participated in and contributed to all phases of the study. YSP, SMT, LPC, and BCW participated in designing, organizing, and implementing the survey. JR did the statistical analysis. All authors read and approved the final manuscript.

Competing interests
The authors declare that they have no competing interests (political, personal, religious, ideological, academic, intellectual, commercial or any other) in relation to this manuscript.

References
1. Hughes KM, Collier B, Greene KA, Kurek S: Traumatic carotid artery dissection: a significant incidental finding. *Am Surg* 2000, 66:1023-1027.
2. Stein DM, Boswell S, Sliker CW, Lui FY, Scalea TM: Blunt cerebrovascular injuries: does treatment always matter? *J Trauma* 2009, 66:132-143, discussion 143-134.
3. Sliker CW: Blunt Cerebrovascular Injuries: Imaging with Multidetector CT Angiography. *Radiographics* 2008, 28:1689-1710.
4. Davis JW, Holbrook TL, Hoyt DB, Mackersie RC, Field TO Jr, Shackford SR: Blunt carotid artery dissection: incidence, associated injuries, screening, and treatment. *J Trauma* 1990, 30:1514-1517.
5. Cogbill TH, Moore EE, Meissner M, Fischer RP, Hoyt DB, Morris JA, Shackford SR, Wallace JR, Ross SE, Ochsner MG, *et al*: The spectrum of blunt injury to the carotid artery: a multicenter perspective. *J Trauma* 1994, 37:473-479.
6. Rogers FB, Baker EF, Osler TM, Shackford SR, Wald SL, Vieco P: Computed tomographic angiography as a screening modality for blunt cervical arterial injuries: preliminary results. *J Trauma* 1999, 46:380-385.
7. Miller PR, Fabian TC, Bee TK, Timmons S, Chamsuddin A, Finkle R, Croce MA: Blunt cerebrovascular injuries: diagnosis and treatment. *J Trauma* 2001, 51:279-285, discussion 285-276.
8. Kerwin AJ, Bynoe RP, Murray J, Hudson ER, Close TP, Gifford RR, Carson KW, Smith LP, Bell RM: Liberalized screening for blunt carotid and vertebral artery injuries is justified. *J Trauma* 2001, 51:308-314.
9. Biffl WL, Ray CE Jr, Moore EE, Franciose RJ, Aly S, Heyrosa MG, Johnson JL, Burch JM: Treatment-related outcomes from blunt cerebrovascular injuries: importance of routine follow-up arteriography. *Ann Surg* 2002, 235:699-706, discussion 706-697.
10. Biffl WL, Moore EE, Ryu RK, Offner PJ, Novak Z, Coldwell DM, Franciose RJ, Burch JM: The unrecognized epidemic of blunt carotid arterial injuries: early diagnosis improves neurologic outcome. *Ann Surg* 1998, 228:462-470.
11. Berne JD, Norwood SH, McAuley CE, Vallina VL, Creath RG, McLarty J: The high morbidity of blunt cerebrovascular injury in an unscreened population: more evidence of the need for mandatory screening protocols. *J Am Coll Surg* 2001, 192:314-321.
12. Berne JD, Norwood SH, McAuley CE, Villareal DH: Helical computed tomographic angiography: an excellent screening test for blunt cerebrovascular injury. *J Trauma* 2004, 57:11-17, discussion 17-19.
13. Cothren CC, Moore EE, Biffl WL, Ciesla DJ, Ray CE Jr, Johnson JL, Moore JB, Burch JM: Cervical spine fracture patterns predictive of blunt vertebral artery injury. *J Trauma* 2003, 55:811-813.
14. Miller PR, Fabian TC, Croce MA, Cagiannos C, Williams JS, Vang M, Qaisi WG, Felker RE, Timmons SD: Prospective screening for blunt cerebrovascular injuries: analysis of diagnostic modalities and outcomes. *Ann Surg* 2002, 236:386-393, discussion 393-385.
15. Thibodeaux LC, Hearn AT, Peschiera JL, Deshmukh RM, Kerlakian GM, Welling RE, Nyswonger GD: Extracranial vertebral artery dissection after trauma: a 5-year review. *Br J Surg* 1997, 84:94.
16. Edwards NM, Fabian TC, Claridge JA, Timmons SD, Fischer PE, Croce MA: Antithrombotic therapy and endovascular stents are effective treatment for blunt carotid injuries: results from longterm followup. *J Am Coll Surg* 2007, 204:1007-1013, discussion 1014-1005.
17. Fabian TC, Patton JH Jr, Croce MA, Minard G, Kudsk KA, Pritchard FE: Blunt carotid injury. Importance of early diagnosis and anticoagulant therapy. *Ann Surg* 1996, 223:513-522, discussion 522-515.
18. Cothren CC, Moore EE, Biffl WL, Ciesla DJ, Ray CE Jr, Johnson JL, Moore JB, Burch JM: Anticoagulation is the gold standard therapy for blunt carotid injuries to reduce stroke rate. *Arch Surg* 2004, 139:540-545, discussion 545-546.
19. Cothren CC, Moore EE, Ray CE Jr, Ciesla DJ, Johnson JL, Moore JB, Burch JM: Screening for blunt cerebrovascular injuries is cost-effective. *Am J Surg* 2005, 190:845-849.
20. Wahl WL, Brandt MM, Thompson BG, Taheri PA, Greenfield LJ: Antiplatelet therapy: an alternative to heparin for blunt carotid injury. *J Trauma* 2002, 52:896-901.
21. Cothren CC, Biffl WL, Moore EE, Kashuk JL, Johnson JL: Treatment for blunt cerebrovascular injuries: Equivalence of anticoagulation and antiplatelet agents. *Arch Surg* 2009, 144:685-690.

22. Beletsky V, Nadareishvili Z, Lynch J, Shuaib A, Woolfenden A, Norris JW: Cervical arterial dissection: time for a therapeutic trial? *Stroke* 2003, 34:2856-2860.

23. Donas KP, Mayer D, Guber I, Baumgartner R, Genoni M, Lachat M: Endovascular repair of extracranial carotid artery dissection: current status and level of evidence. *J Vasc Interv Radiol* 2008, 19:1693-1698.

24. Fava M, Meneses L, Loyola S, Tevah J, Bertoni H, Huete I, Mellado P: Carotid artery dissection: endovascular treatment. Report of 12 patients. *Catheter Cardiovasc Interv* 2008, 71:694-700.

25. Schulte S, Donas KP, Pitoulias GA, Horsch S: Endovascular treatment of iatrogenic and traumatic carotid artery dissection. *Cardiovasc Intervent Radiol* 2008, 31:870-874.

26. DuBose J, Recinos G, Teixeira PG, Inaba K, Demetriades D: Endovascular stenting for the treatment of traumatic internal carotid injuries: expanding experience. *J Trauma* 2008, 65:1561-1566.

27. Siomin V, Angelov L, Li L, Vogelbaum MA: Results of a survey of neurosurgical practice patterns regarding the prophylactic use of anti-epilepsy drugs in patients with brain tumors. *J Neurooncol* 2005, 74:211-215.

28. Kim YJ, Xiao Y, Mackenzie CF, Gardner SD: Availability of trauma specialists in level I and II trauma centers: a national survey. *J Trauma* 2007, 63:676-683.

29. Berry C, Sandberg DI, Hoh DJ, Krieger MD, McComb JG: Use of cranial fixation pins in pediatric neurosurgery. *Neurosurgery* 2008, 62:913-918, discussion 918-919.

30. Lebude B, Yadla S, Albert T, Anderson DG, Harrop JS, Hilibrand A, Maltenfort M, Sharan A, Vaccaro AR, Ratliff JK: Defining "Complications" in Spine Surgery: Neurosurgery and Orthopedic Spine Surgeons' Survey. *J Spinal Disord Tech* 2010, 23(8):493-500.

31. Glotzbecker MP, Bono CM, Harris MB, Brick G, Heary RF, Wood KB: Surgeon practices regarding postoperative thromboembolic prophylaxis after high-risk spinal surgery. *Spine (Phila Pa 1976)* 2008, 33:2915-2921.

32. American College of Surgeons Committee on Trauma: National Trauma Data Bank. Chicago, IL; 2010.

33. Hollingworth W, Nathens AB, Kanne JP, Crandall ML, Crummy TA, Hallam DK, Wang MC, Jarvik JG: The diagnostic accuracy of computed tomography angiography for traumatic or atherosclerotic lesions of the carotid and vertebral arteries: a systematic review. *Eur J Radiol* 2003, 48:88-102.

34. Hoit DA, Schirmer CM, Weller SJ, Lisbon A, Edlow JA, Malek AM: Angiographic detection of carotid and vertebral arterial injury in the high-energy blunt trauma patient. *J Spinal Disord Tech* 2008, 21:259-266.

35. Biffl WL, Egglin T, Benedetto B, Gibbs F, Cioffi WG: Sixteen-slice computed tomographic angiography is a reliable noninvasive screening test for clinically significant blunt cerebrovascular injuries. *J Trauma* 2006, 60:745-751, discussion 751-742.

36. Bub LD, Hollingworth W, Jarvik JG, Hallam DK: Screening for blunt cerebrovascular injury: evaluating the accuracy of multidetector computed tomographic angiography. *J Trauma* 2005, 59:691-697.

37. Berne JD, Reuland KS, Villarreal DH, McGovern TM, Rowe SA, Norwood SH: Sixteen-slice multi-detector computed tomographic angiography improves the accuracy of screening for blunt cerebrovascular injury. *J Trauma* 2006, 60:1204-1209, discussion 1209-1210.

38. Bromberg WJ, Collier BC, Diebel LN, Dwyer KM, Holevar MR, Jacobs DG, Kurek SJ, Schreiber MA, Shapiro ML, Vogel TR: Blunt cerebrovascular injury practice management guidelines: the Eastern Association for the Surgery of Trauma. *J Trauma* 2010, 68:471-477.

39. Biffl WL, Moore EE, Offner PJ, Brega KE, Franciose RJ, Burch JM: Blunt carotid arterial injuries: implications of a new grading scale. *J Trauma* 1999, 47:845-853.

40. Menon RK, Markus HS, Norris JW: Results of a UK questionnaire of diagnosis and treatment in cervical artery dissection. *J Neurol Neurosurg Psychiatry* 2008, 79:612.

41. Bassi P, Lattuada P, Gomitoni A: Cervical cerebral artery dissection: a multicenter prospective study (preliminary report). *Neurol Sci* 2003, 24(Suppl 1):S4-7.

42. Eachempati SR, Vaslef SN, Sebastian MW, Reed RL: Blunt vascular injuries of the head and neck: is heparinization necessary? *J Trauma* 1998, 45:997-1004.

43. Mayberry JC, Brown CV, Mullins RJ, Velmahos GC: Blunt carotid artery injury: the futility of aggressive screening and diagnosis. *Arch Surg* 2004, 139:609-612, discussion 612-603.

44. Cox MW, Whittaker DR, Martinez C, Fox CJ, Feuerstein IM, Gillespie DL: Traumatic pseudoaneurysms of the head and neck: early endovascular intervention. *J Vasc Surg* 2007, 46:1227-1233.

45. Diaz-Daza O, Arraiza FJ, Barkley JM, Whigham CJ: Endovascular therapy of traumatic vascular lesions of the head and neck. *Cardiovasc Intervent Radiol* 2003, 26:213-221.

46. Fassett DR, Dailey AT, Vaccaro AR: Vertebral artery injuries associated with cervical spine injuries: a review of the literature. *J Spinal Disord Tech* 2008, 21:252-258.

47. Higashida RT, Halbach VV, Tsai FY, Norman D, Pribram HF, Mehringer CM, Hieshima GB: Interventional neurovascular treatment of traumatic carotid and vertebral artery lesions: results in 234 cases. *AJR Am J Roentgenol* 1989, 153:577-582.

48. Joo JY, Ahn JY, Chung YS, Chung SS, Kim SH, Yoon PH, Kim OJ: Therapeutic endovascular treatments for traumatic carotid artery injuries. *J Trauma* 2005, 58:1159-1166.

49. Maras D, Lioupis C, Magoufis G, Tsamopoulos N, Moulakakis K, Andrikopoulos V: Covered stent-graft treatment of traumatic internal carotid artery pseudoaneurysms: a review. *Cardiovasc Intervent Radiol* 2006, 29:958-968.

50. Hirsch AT, Haskal ZJ, Hertzer NR, Bakal CW, Creager MA, Halperin JL, Hiratzka LF, Murphy WR, Olin JW, Puschett JB, *et al*: ACC/AHA 2005 Practice Guidelines for the management of patients with peripheral arterial disease (lower extremity, renal, mesenteric, and abdominal aortic): a collaborative report from the American Association for Vascular Surgery/Society for Vascular Surgery, Society for Cardiovascular Angiography and Interventions, Society for Vascular Medicine and Biology, Society of Interventional Radiology, and the ACC/AHA Task Force on Practice Guidelines (Writing Committee to Develop Guidelines for the Management of Patients With Peripheral Arterial Disease): endorsed by the American Association of Cardiovascular and Pulmonary Rehabilitation; National Heart, Lung, and Blood Institute; Society for Vascular Nursing; TransAtlantic Inter-Society Consensus; and Vascular Disease Foundation. *Circulation* 2006, 113:e463-654.

2

GCS as a predictor of mortality in patients with traumatic inferior vena cava injuries

Michael Cudworth[1*], Angelo Fulle[1], Juan P Ramos[1] and Ivette Arriagada[2]

Abstract

Introduction: Recent research has determined Glasgow Coma Scale (GCS) to be an independent predictor of mortality in patients with traumatic inferior vena cava (IVC) injuries. The aim of this study was to evaluate the use of GCS, as well as other factors previously described as determinants of mortality, in a cohort of patients presenting with traumatic IVC lesions.

Methods: A 7-year retrospective review was undertaken of all trauma patients presenting to a tertiary care trauma center with trauma related IVC lesions. Factors described in the literature as associated with mortality were assessed with univariate analysis. ANOVA analysis of variance was used to compare means for continuous variables; dichotomous variables were assessed with Fischer's exact test. Logistic regression was performed on significant variables to assess determinants of mortality.

Results: Sixteen patients with traumatic IVC injuries were identified, from January 2005 to December 2011. Six patients died (mortality, 37.5%); the mechanism of injury was blunt in one case (6.2%) and penetrating in the 15 others (93.7%). Seven patients underwent thoracotomy in the operating room (OR) to obtain vascular control (43.7%). Upon univariate analysis, non-survivors were significantly more likely than survivors to have lower mean arterial pressures (MAP) in the emergency room (ER) (45.6 +/− 8.6 vs. 76.5 +/− 25.4, p = 0.013), a lower GCS (8.1 +/− 4.1 vs. 14 +/− 2.8, p = 0.004), more severe injuries (ISS 60.3 +/− 3.5 vs 28.7 +/− 22.9, p = 0.0006), have undergone thoracotomy (83.3% vs. 16.6%, p = 0.024), and have a shorter operative time (105 +/− 59.8 min vs 189 +/− 65.3 min, p = 0.022). Logistic regression analysis revealed GCS as a significant inverse determinant of mortality (OR = 0.6, 0.46-0.95, p = 0.026). Other determinants of mortality by logistic regression were thoracotomy (OR = 20, 1.4-282.4, p = 0.027), and caval ligation as operative management (OR = 45, 2.28-885.6, p = 0.012).

Conclusions: GCS, the need to undergo thoracotomy, and caval ligation as operative management are significant predictors of mortality in patients with traumatic IVC injuries.

Keywords: Vascular, Trauma, Inferior vena cava, Glasgow, Injury

Introduction

Traumatic inferior vena cava (IVC) lesions represent 30% to 40% of trauma related abdominal vascular injuries [1-4]. In spite of significant advances in pre-hospital care, surgical technique, and surgical critical care, traumatic IVC lesions continue to carry a high overall mortality of 43% [1,5-11]. Roughly 30% to 50% of patients sustaining traumatic IVC injuries will die of their injuries before

reaching a hospital [1,5-7,9,11,12]. Of those patients that survive long enough to be hospitalized, another 30% to 50% will decease in spite of surgical therapy and resuscitation efforts [13-15]. Penetrating trauma is the cause of 86% of IVC injuries, with blunt trauma causing only 14% of IVC injuries [1,5,7-10,14,16-18]. The IVC is anatomically divided into five segments: infra-renal (IRIVC), para-renal (PRIVC), supra-renal (SRIVC), retro-hepatic (RHIVC), and supra-hepatic (SHIVC). Overall, the most frequently injured segment is the IRIVC (39%), followed by the RHIVC (19%), SRIVC (18%), PRIVC (17%), and the

* Correspondence: mcudworth@gmail.com
[1]Adult Emergency Services, Surgery, Hospital Dr. Sotero del Rio, Concha y Toro, 3459 Puente Alto, Santiago, Chile
Full list of author information is available at the end of the article

SHIVC (7%) [1,5,7-10,14,16-18]. Numerous studies have analyzed factors associated with mortality in IVC lesions. Factors predictive of mortality reported include level of the IVC injury, hemodynamic status on arrival, number of associated injuries, blood loss and transfusional requirements, among others [1,5,7-10,14,16-18]. Recent work by Huerta el al described Glasgow Coma Scale (GCS) as an independent predictor of mortality in IVC trauma [5]. The aim of this study was to assess GCS, as well as other factors previously described as determinants of mortality, in a cohort of patients presenting with traumatic IVC lesions at an urban tertiary care trauma center.

Methods

Approval for this study was obtained from the Hospital's ethics committee. A retrospective chart review was performed from January 2005 to December 2011, of all abdominal vascular trauma patients presenting to the tertiary care trauma center at Hospital Dr. Sotero del Rio. Patients that died before operative intervention or pronounced dead on arrival were excluded. All patient charts were individually reviewed for the following parameters: demographic data, Injury Severity Score (ISS), initial systolic blood pressure in the ED (SBP), initial diastolic blood pressure in the ED (DBP), initial heart rate in the ED, admission base deficit expressed as base excess (BE), time in the ED prior to operative intervention, and GCS as determined by a chief resident or the most senior attending trauma surgeon in the trauma bay. Operative records were reviewed for mechanism and location of IVC injury, the number of associated injuries encountered, the method of vascular control and repair, the need for thoracotomy for vascular control, transfusional

Table 1 Distribution of associated injuries between groups

	Survivors (n = 10)	Non-survivors (n = 6)	P value*
Gastric	1 (10%)	1 (16%)	NS
Duodenum	2 (20%)	1 (16%)	NS
Small bowel	4 (40%)	2 (33%)	NS
Large bowel	1 (10%)	1 (16%)	NS
Spleen	1 (10%)	1 (16%)	NS
Kidney	3 (30%)	2 (33%)	NS
Liver	2 (20%)	1 (16%)	NS
Pancreas	1 (10%)	1 (16%)	NS
Lung	1 (10%)	1 (16%)	NS
Diaphragm	0 (0%)	1 (16%)	NS
Cardiac	2 (20%)	0 (0%)	NS
Aorta	0 (0%)	3 (50%)	NS
Superior mesenteric artery	0 (0%)	1 (16%)	NS
Splenic or iliac vein	1 (10%)	1 (16%)	NS

*NS, not significant.

Table 2 Significant differences between groups

	Survivors (n = 10)	Nonsurvivors (n = 6)	P value
ER MAP (mmHg)	76.5 +/− 25.4	45.6 +/− 8.6	0.013*
GCS	14 +/− 2.8	8.17 +/− 4.1	0.004*
Operative time (min)	189 +/− 65.3	105 +/− 59.8	0.022*
ISS	28.7 +/− 3.5	60.3 +/− 22.9	0.0006*
OR thoracotomy	20%	83.3%	0.024 +

*Oneway ANOVA analysis of variance.
+ Fischer's exact test.

requirements, and operative time. Other data assessed included length of hospital stay. Statistical analysis was performed with STATA 12.1 (Stata Corp LP, College Station, TX). Data is represented as means +/− SE for univariate and logistic regression analysis, and means +/− SD for one-way ANOVA analysis of variance. P values of less than 0.05 were considered significant. Univariate analysis was performed using either Student's T-test or one-way ANOVA analysis of variance for continuous variables and Fischer's exact test for dichotomous variables. Outcome association with mechanism of injury, and level of injury were assessed using Kruskal–Wallis rank test. Variables achieving statistical significance on univariate analysis were included in a logistic regression model to assess variables predictive of survival. A receiver operating characteristic curve was determined to assess model fit of the regression model.

Results

During the 7-year period from January 2005 to December 2011, sixteen traumatic IVC injuries were identified at the Hospital Dr. Sotero del Rio, Santiago, Chile (mean age = 25.6 +/− 1.9 years; ISS = 40.5 +/− 5.19; 87% male and 12% female). The mortality rate was 37.5% (6 patients). The mechanism of IVC injury was 56.2% gun shot wound (GSW) (9 patients), 37.5% stab wound (SW) (6 patients), and 6.3% blunt injury (1 patient). In our series, the initial GCS was 11.8 +/− 1.1. The number of associated injuries was 2.3 +/− 0.3, including one or more of the following: superior mesenteric vasculature, gastric, duodenum, small bowel, large bowel, splenic, pancreatic, liver, lung, diaphragm, and cardiac. Univariate analysis did not show a significant increase in mortality with any associated injury (Table 1). Non-survivors were significantly more likely to be hypotensive in the

Table 3 Mortality by operative management (caval ligation versus simple repair)

Operative management	Number of patients	Number of deaths	ISS +	Mortality rate*
IVC ligation	6 (37.5%)	5	59 +/− 10.1	83.3%
Simple repair	10 (62.5%)	1	29.5 +/− 1.2	16.6%

+P value = 0.002, Student's T-test.
*P value = 0.008, Fischer's exact test.

Table 4 Significant predictors of mortality by logistic regression

	OR	P value	Confidence interval	Area under ROC curve*
Thoracotomy	20	0.027	1.4-282.4	0.81
IVC ligation	45	0.012	2.28-885.6	0.86

Significant inverse predictors of mortality by logistic regression

	OR	P value	Confidence interval	Area under ROC curve*
GCS	0.6	0.026	0.46-0.95	0.85

*Area under ROC curve as a measure of model fit.

ER (ER MAP, 45.6 +/- 8.6 mmHg vs. 76.5 +/- 25.4 mmHg, p = 0.013), have a lower GCS (8.1 +/- 4.1 vs. 14 +/- 2.8, p = 0.004), have undergone thoracotomy in the OR (83.3% vs. 16.6%, p = 0.024), have a shorter operative time (105 +/- 59.8 min vs 189 +/- 65.3 min, p = 0.022), and have more severe injuries (ISS 60.3 +/- 3.5 vs 28.7 +/- 22.9, p = 0.0006) (Table 2).

Six patients (37.5%) were managed with IVC ligation due to difficulty in obtaining adequate exposure and intraoperative hemodynamic instability, and ten patients (62.5%) were managed with simple primary repair.

Caval ligation was significantly associated with increased mortality, with five out of the six patients managed with IVC ligation deceasing (mortality: 83.3%) as opposed to one patient out of ten managed with primary repair (mortality: 16.67%, p = 0.008) (Table 3). Upon logistic regression analysis, significantly increased odds of mortality were seen with the need to undergo thoracotomy for vascular control (OR = 20, 1.4-282.4, p = 0.027), and the use of caval ligation as operative management (OR = 45, 2.28-885.6, p = 0.012) (Table 4). GCS as a linear scale displayed an inverse relation with the risk of mortality expressed as a binary outcome. Upon linear regression analysis, GCS was a significant inverse predictor of mortality, (p = 0.005) (Table 5). Upon logistic regression, a higher GCS was associated with significantly lower odds of mortality (OR = 0.6, 0.46-0.95, p = 0.026). ROC curves after logistic regression as a measure of model fit were 0.85 for GCS, 0.86 for caval ligation as operative management, and 0.81 for thoracotomy. In our cohort of patients, neither the mechanism of injury, nor the level of the IVC injury were significantly associated with an increase in mortality (Tables 6 and 7). No statistically significant differences existed among non-survivors

Table 5 GCS as a determinant of mortality by linear regression

	Beta coefficient	P value*	R² +
GCS	−0.07	0.005	0.44
Intercept	1.27		

*Inverse relation between GCS and mortality by linear regression.
+ R-squared as a measure of model fit.

Table 6 Mortality by mechanism of injury

Mechanism	Number	Mortality rate*
Blunt	1 (6.25%)	0%
GSW	9 (56.25%)	44.4%
SW	6 (37.5%)	33.3%
Total	16	37.5%

*P = 0.6 (NS), Kruskal–Wallis analysis of variance rank test.

and survivors for BE on admission (−19.4 +/- 8.3 vs. -12.7 +/- 6.1, p = 0.08), total number of associated injuries (2.8 +/- 1.4 vs. 1.9 +/- 0.9, p = 0.15), transfusional requirements expressed as packed red blood cells (PRBC) (7.09 +/- 2.5 vs. 7.23 +/- 2.7, p = 0.9), or time to surgical treatment (19.5 +/- 6.9 min vs. 32.3 +/- 18.5 min, p = 0.13). Non-survivors mainly died on the operating table due to massive hemorrhage that was impossible to control operatively, with subsequent cardiac arrest. The mean hospital stay of survivors was 24.5 +/- 14.2 days.

Discussion

Traumatic IVC injuries are a relatively rare event, occurring in only up to 5% of penetrating injuries and only up to 1% of blunt abdominal trauma [8]. Nonetheless, IVC trauma continues to present a formidable challenge to trauma surgeons, carrying an overall high mortality rate in spite of recent improvements in pre-hospital care, resuscitation upon arrival at a trauma center, diagnostic imaging, and timely surgical care. Our overall mortality rate for IVC trauma (37.5%) is consistent with previous reports of IVC trauma mortality ranging from 21% to 56%, with an overall mortality rate of 43% [1,5,7-10,14,16-18]. Previous reports have described predictors of mortality to be level of injury, shock on admission, timing of diagnosis to definitive management, blood loss, requirements for blood transfusions, associated injuries, ED thoracotomy, preoperative lactate and base deficits, ISS, and GCS [1,5,7-10,16-18]. In our cohort, we found statistically significant associations with the risk of mortality with hypotension upon arrival at the ER, thoracotomy,

Table 7 Mortality by number of injuries and IVC level of injury

Level of injury	Number of injuries	Number of deaths	Mortality rate
Infrarenal	4 (25%)	1	25%
Pararenal	4 (25%)	1	25%
Suprarenal	5 (31.2%)	3	60%
Retrohepatic	1 (6.25%)	1	100%
Intrapericardial	2 (12.5%)	0	0%
	P value = 0.8 (NS)*		P value = 0.3 (NS)*

*Kruskal–Wallis analysis of variance rank test.

operative time, injury severity expressed as ISS, and GCS. There was a trend towards ascending mortality as the level of injury approached the heart, however we were unable to find a statistically significant relation between level of injury and mortality. This is likely due to the small size of our cohort, and the fact that the two patients in our series with intra-perdicardial lesions, both survived. Upon regression analysis, significant predictors of mortality were thoracotomy, IVC ligation as operative management, and GCS.

GCS as an independent predictor of mortality in IVC trauma has been previously described in a patient population with a higher incidence of blunt trauma (28%) than our patient cohort (6.3%) [5]. Nonetheless, in our patient cohort presenting with a high incidence of penetrating IVC trauma (93.7%), logistic regression confirmed GCS is significantly associated with mortality. In our cohort, patients did not sustain major head injuries, thus the significant association GCS demonstrated with mortality likely reflects substantial hemodynamic compromise, as has been previously proposed [5].

The other determinants of mortality in our regression model were thoracotomy and to have undergone IVC ligation instead of simple suture repair. The use of thoracotomy to obtain vascular control likely suggests more extensive vascular injuries, which is consistent with the fact non-survivors had significantly more severe injuries as expressed by a higher ISS. Significantly better survival has been previously described in IVC injuries treated with IVC ligation [1], and thus our results must be interpreted with caution. However, in our cohort IVC ligation was utilized as a salvage method to treat vascular injuries not amenable to primary repair or when the surgical team faced difficulty in obtaining adequate exposure in a patient at risk of exsanguination. Patients treated with IVC ligation had more severe injuries as reflected by a significantly higher ISS (Table 3).

Our study has several limitations, including our small sample size and its retrospective nature. However our results are relevant as we confirm GCS as a predictor of mortality in patients with traumatic IVC injuries. This study, along with others, point to the relevance of GCS as a predictor of mortality in patients with IVC trauma, of both blunt and penetrating etiology. Further prospective studies are needed to confirm the validity of GCS along with other previously described determinants of mortality in IVC trauma. Likewise, management protocols need be established to decrease the high mortality rate that is still seen with traumatic IVC injuries, which has not improved in spite of improved resuscitation and pre-hospital care.

Conclusions

In spite of being a relatively rare event, trauma related IVC injuries present a formidable challenge to the trauma surgeon, with a high overall mortality rate of 43%, which has not changed in recent years despite vast improvements in pre-hospital transport time and care, hospital resuscitation and surgical critical care. Our results confirm GCS is an independent predictor of mortality in IVC trauma. Other significant determinants of mortality in our cohort were the use of thoracotomy, and the use of IVC ligation as operative management. Further prospective studies are needed to confirm the validity of the described determinants of mortality in IVC trauma. Management protocols need be established to decrease the high mortality rate still carried by traumatic IVC injuries.

Abbreviations
IVC: Inferior vena cava; GCS: Glasgow coma scale; ISS: Injury severity score; ED: Emergency department; OR: Operating room; BE: Base excess; MAP: Mean arterial pressure; SBP: Systolic blood pressure; DBP: Diastolic blood pressure; IRIVC: Infra-renal vena cava; PRIVC: Para-renal vena cava; SRIVC: Supra-renal vena cava; RHIVC: Retro-hepatic vena cava; SHIVC: Supra-hepatic vena cava; ROC: Receiver operator curve; NS: Not significant.

Competing interests
The author's declare that they have no competing interests.

Authors' contributions
All authors: 1) have made substantial contributions to conception and design, or acquisition of data, or analysis and interpretation of data; 2) have been involved in drafting the manuscript or revising it critically for important intellectual content; 3) have given final approval of the version to be published. MC: Study conception and design, acquisition of data, analysis and interpretation of data, drafting of manuscript. JR: Study conception and design, acquisition of data, analysis and interpretation of data, drafting of manuscript. AF: Study conception and design, acquisition of data, critical revision of manuscript. IA: Study conception and design, acquisition of data, analysis and interpretation of data, critical revision of manuscript. All authors have read and approved the final manuscript.

Author details
[1]Adult Emergency Services, Surgery, Hospital Dr. Sotero del Rio, Concha y Toro, 3459 Puente Alto, Santiago, Chile. [2]Vascular Surgery, Hospital Dr. Sotero del Rio, Concha y Toro, 3459 Puente Alto, Santiago, Chile.

References
1. Kuehne J, Frankhouse J, Modrall G, Golshani S, Aziz I, Demetriades D: Determinants of survival after inferior vena cava trauma. Am Surg 1999, 65(10):976–981.
2. Jackson MR, Olson DW, Beckett WC Jr: Abdominal vascular trauma: a review of 106 injuries. Am Surg 1992, 58:622–626.
3. Ombrellaro MP, Freeman MB, Stevens SL, et al: Predictors of survival after inferior vena cava injuries. Am Surg 1997, 63:178–183.
4. Leppaniemi AK, Savolainen HO, Salo JA: Traumatic inferior vena caval injuries. Scand J Thorac 1994, 28:103–108.
5. Huerta S, Bui T, Nguyen T, Banimahd F, Porral D: Predictors of mortality and management of patients with traumatic inferior vena cava injuries. Am Surg 2006, 72(4):290–296.
6. Burch JM, Feliciano DV, Mattox KL: The atriocaval shunt. Facts and fiction. Ann Surg 1988, 207:555–568.
7. Klein SR, Baumgartner FJ, Bongard FS: Contemporary management strategy for major inferior vena caval injuries. J Trauma 1994, 37:35–41.
8. Kudsk KA, Bongard F, Lim RX Jr: Determinants of survival after vena caval injury. Analysis of a 14year experience. Arch Surg 1984, 119:1009–1012.

9. Rosengart M, Smith D, Melton S, May A: **Prognostic factors in patients with inferior vena cava injuries.** *Am Surg* 1999, **65**(9):849–856.
10. Turpin I, State D, Schwartz A: **Injuries to the inferior vena cava and their management.** *Am J Surg* 1977, **134**:25–32.
11. Wilson RF, Wiencek RG, Balog M: **Factors affecting mortality rate with iliac vein injuries.** *J Trauma* 1990, **30**:320–323.
12. Buckman RF, Pathak AS, Badellino MM, *et al*: **Injuries of the inferior vena cava.** *Surg Clin North Am* 2001, **81**:1431–1447.
13. Blaisdell FW, Lim RC Jr: **Liver resection.** *Major Probl Clin Surg* 1971, **3**:131–145.
14. Bricker DL, Morton JR, Okies JE, *et al*: **Surgical management of injuries to the vena cava: changing patterns of injury and newer techniques of repair.** *J Trauma* 1971, **11**:722–735.
15. Brown RS, Boyd DR, Matsuda T, *et al*: **Temporary internal vascular shunt for retrohepatic vena cava injury.** *J Trauma* 1971, **11**:736–737.
16. Byrne DE, Pass HI, Crawford FA Jr: **Traumatic vena caval injuries.** *Am J Surg* 1980, **140**:600–602.
17. Graham JM, Mattox KL, Beall AC Jr, *et al*: **Traumatic injuries of the inferior vena cava.** *Arch Surg* 1978, **113**:413–418.
18. Millikan JS, Moore EE, Cogbill TH, *et al*: **Inferior vena cava injuries: a continuing challenge.** *J Trauma* 1983, **23**:207–212.

3

Surgical telepresence: the usability of a robotic communication platform

Antonio Marttos[1], Fernanda M Kuchkarian[1*], Emmanouil Palaios[1], Daniel Rojas[1], Phillipe Abreu-Reis[2], Carl Schulman[1]

Abstract

Introduction: The benefits of telepresence in trauma and acute surgical care exist, yet its use in a live, operating room (OR) setting with real surgical cases remains limited.

Methods: We tested the use of a robotic telepresence system in the OR of a busy, level 1 trauma center. After each case, both the local and remote physicians completed questionnaires regarding the use of the system using a five point Likert scale. For trauma cases, physicians were asked to grade injury severity according to the American Association for the Surgery of Trauma (AAST) Scaling System.

Results: We collected prospective, observational data on 50 emergent and elective cases. 64% of cases were emergency surgery on trauma patients, almost evenly distributed between penetrating (49%) and blunt injuries (51%). 40% of non-trauma cases were hernia-related. A varied distribution of injuries was observed to the abdomen, chest, extremities, small bowel, kidneys, spleen, and colon. Physicians gave the system high ratings for its audio and visual capabilities, but identified internet connectivity and crowding in the operating room as potential challenges. The loccal clinician classified injuries according to the AAST injury grading system in 63% (n=22) of trauma cases, compared to 54% (n=19) of cases by the remote physicians. The remote physician cited obstruction of view as the main reason for the discrepancy. 94% of remote physicians and 74% of local physicians felt comfortable communicating via the telepresence system. For 90% of cases, both the remote and local physicians strongly agreed that a telepresence system for consultations in the OR is more effective than a telephone conversation.

Conclusions: A telepresence system was tested on a variety of surgical cases and demonstrated that it can be an appropriate solution for use in the operating room. Future research should determine its impact on processes of care and surgical outcomes.

Introduction

Telemedicine extends the reach of trauma and surgical care specialists in real-time and regardless of distance, yet its widespread adoption remains elusive. Currently healthcare and market forces are driving the demand for innovative solutions to address the discrepancies in access to quality care and patient outcomes. Trauma remains a leading cause of death worldwide; nevertheless the number of trauma specialists continues to decline. Researchers estimate that there will be a 7% deficit in general surgeons by 2020, and close to 20% by 2050 [1]. It is estimated that two billion people have no access to even basic surgical care [2]. Moreover many parts of the world lack access to trauma care, such as in rural areas and austere environments [3]. Simultaneously, rapid evolution of new surgical techniques and procedures has created the necessity for physicians to maintain their knowledge base current and quickly access training and continuing education opportunities. However, travel and logistics can become an

* Correspondence: fkuchkarian@med.miami.edu
[1]University of Miami Miller School of Medicine Surgery Department (D40), PO Box 016960 Miami, FL 33101, USA
Full list of author information is available at the end of the article

impediment, and other cost-effective solutions may be a better option.

Due to technological advances and declines in cost, telemedicine for trauma and surgical care is becoming increasingly a viable option to address these current challenges and demands.

Telemedicine is generally thought of as the utilization of telecommunications and information technologies in providing health care at a distance. Not a novel concept, examples can be dated back to the 1960s when the first surgical case was broadcasted overseas through videoconferencing for educational purposes [4]. Today, telemedicine can facilitate the mentoring of less experienced surgeons remotely, known as telementoring, as well as transfer information between clinicians for consultation purposes. Teleconsultation can be particularly useful for physicians needing to obtain a second opinion from remote medical specialists. Access to remote specialists may also help in patient transfer decision-making, helping distant hospitals treat patients locally when possible by bringing the specialist to the patient. This potentially can improve patient outcomes and safety; while reducing the need for costly, unnecessary transfers.

Although promising, before implementing new technologies it is crucial that the chosen system be appropriately evaluated. For the past two years, the University of Miami Miller School of Medicine has been testing different mobile telemedicine solutions in the operating room of a large, urban level 1 trauma center. The Ryder Trauma Center at Jackson Memorial Hospital is the only level 1 trauma center serving all residents of Miami-Dade County. The primary objective of this study is to ascertain the usability and feasibility of a remote presence robot for use in the operating room during real surgical cases. The goal is to determine the strengths and weaknesses to its implementation for future telementoring and consultation purposes.

Materials and methods
Study design
We collected prospective, observational data regarding the usability of a telepresence robot in the operating room (Figure 1). Data was collected on 50 surgical cases over a 4 month period from December 2010 to March 2011. We included both trauma and non-trauma surgical cases. Once notified of a case, the robot was wheeled into the operating room by a member of the research team. From a remote location in the hospital - an office on the second floor- the remote physician connected to the robot to see the activities in the operating room and communicate with local clinicians. From the remote location the physician can control the camera (pan, tilt and zoom) to get the best angle of the procedure. At the end of the surgical procedure, both the remote and local

physicians are surveyed on their perceptions of using the telepresence robot.

Participants
Participants included trauma center attending physicians and fellows. Prior to the study, physicians were notified about the telemedicine robot and the study via a study memo. Physicians who were interested in participating received a briefing from the research team and gave consent verbally to participate. Survey data was collected anonymously. No patient data was collected. Physicians received a short training on how to maneuver the robot prior and a member of the research team was present at all times to ensure that the research did not interfere with standard clinical activities.

Technology
The Karl Storz-InTouch VISITOR1™ system is an intraoperative, spring arm mounted communications platform comprised of a ControlStation and Robot. The ControlStation and Robot are linked via the Internet over a secure broadband connection. Through the ControlStation, either installed on a laptop or desktop, a remote physician can gain access to the OR from home or office (Figure 2). The system communicates bi-directionally using TCP and/or UDP, and requires outbound HTTP access to connect to the In Touch Health servers. The VISITOR1 System incorporates encryption methodology utilizing a combination of RSA public/private key and 128-bit AES symmetric encryption.

Survey
The survey consisted of mainly usability and technical questions, as well as some descriptive questions about the surgical procedure. Responses were rated using a 5-point Likert scale. Survey questions were pretested among a similar study population in a previous pilot study. Examples of technical questions include audio/visual capabilities as well as ease of operation of the robot. An independent observer was present in the operating room to ensure the robot did not interfere with the OR activities. In addition to the usability and technical information of the equipment, we also added some questions regarding the ability of the remote physician to grade the injuries observed. Clinicians were given a copy of the American Association for the Surgery of Trauma (AAST) Scaling System for Organ Specific Injuries [5] Tables as a guide. Grading scales exist for the following organ systems: Cervical Vascular Injury, Chest Wall Injury, Heart Injury, Lung Injury, Thoracic Vascular Injury, Diaphragm Injury, Spleen Injury, Liver Injury, Extrahepatic Billiary Tree Injury, Pancreas Injury, Esophagus Injury, Stomach Injury, Duodenum Injury, Small Bowel Injury, Colon Injury, Rectum

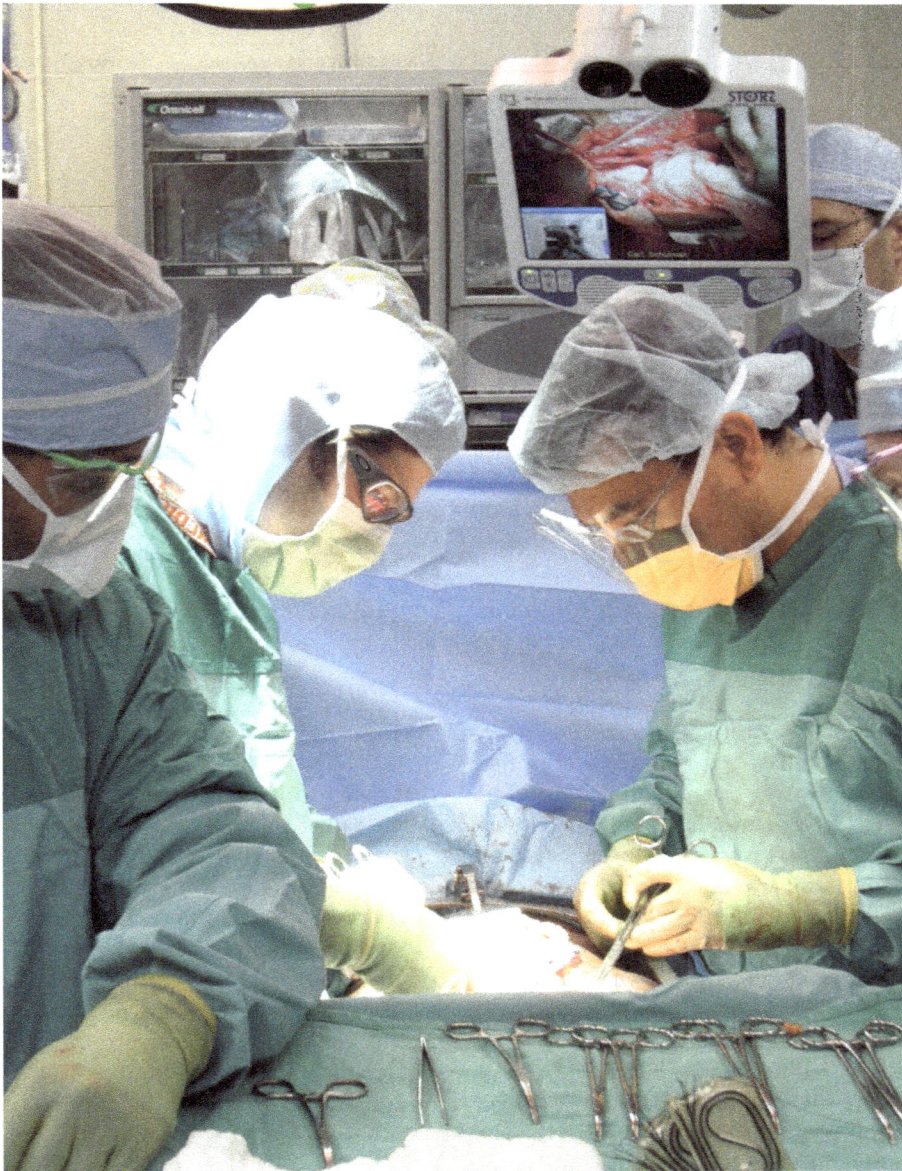

Figure 1 The VisitOR1™ adjustable height gives the remote specialist a view of the surgical field, allowing for consultation and interactive mentoring in real-time with the local on-site surgeons.

Injury, Abdominal Vascular Injury, Adrenal Organ Injury, Kidney Injury, Ureteral Injury, Bladder Injury, Urethra Injury, Uterus (non-pregnant) Injury, Uterus (pregnant) Injury, Fallopian Tube Injury, Ovary Injury, Vagina Injury, Vulva Injury, Testis Injury, Scrotum Injury, Penis Injury, Peripheral Vascular Organ Injury.

During the procedure, the remote physician asked the on-site surgeon to expose the injury and was able to ask questions in order to determine the grade of injury for each damaged system. The grade determined by the remote physician was not communicated to the on-site

physician, who was then asked to grade all the injuries at the end of the operative procedure. The two grades were compared to determine the accuracy of the remote physician in grading traumatic injuries through the telepresence robot. Descriptive statistics was used to analyze all survey results.

Institutional Review Board
The study was reviewed and approved by the University of Miami Institutional Review Board, the Jackson Memorial Hospital Clinical Research Review Committee and

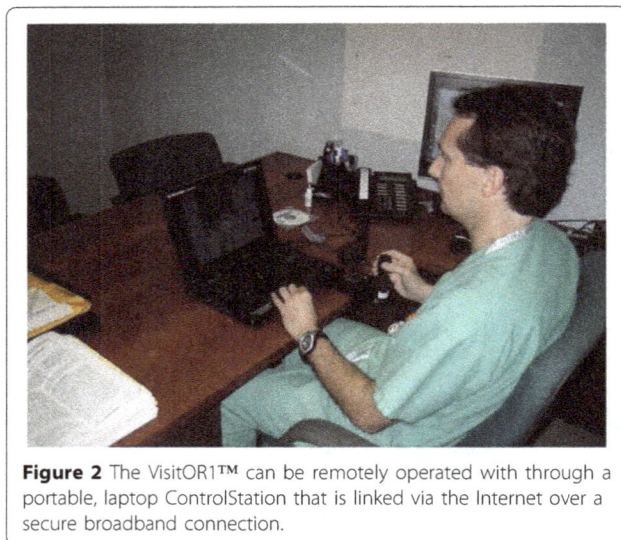

Figure 2 The VisitOR1™ can be remotely operated with through a portable, laptop ControlStation that is linked via the Internet over a secure broadband connection.

Table 1 Injury location distribution

	# of cases		# of cases
Trauma Patients		**Non-Trauma Patients**	
Head	1		
Neck		Abdomen	
Larynx	1	Wall	2
		Inguinal Hernia	5
Chest		Ventral Hernia	2
Wall	4	Small bowel	3
Rib	1	Spleen	1
Vena Cava	1		
Subclavian Artery/Vein	2	Inguinal Lymph Node	1
Abdomen		Unspecified	1
Wall	3		
Stomach	1		
Spleen	4		
Bladder	1		
Kidney	1		
Small Bowel	4		
Colon	5		
Unspecified	2		
Extremities	3		
Miscellaneous			
Skin graft	1		

the Department of Defense Human Research Protection Office.

Results

Data was collected on 50 surgical cases, both emergency (80%) and elective cases (20%). Patients were classified as trauma (70%) and non-trauma patients (30%). The majority of cases (64%) were emergency surgery on trauma patients, almost evenly distributed between penetrating (49%) and blunt trauma (51%). 40% of non-trauma cases were hernia-related Participants included 13 attending physicians and 9 fellows. There was a varied distribution of injuries and operative anatomical structures (Table 1)

Remote physicians reported a high level of satisfaction with the use of the telepresence robot (Figure 3). Almost all remote participants (94%) agreed or strongly agreed being able to see the procedure well (Figure 4). The only times the remote clinician noted having difficulties visualizing the procedure occurred when the operating table was surrounded by a team of clinicians. Internet connectivity was an issue in 24% of the cases, ranging from minimal interruption to slow connection speeds. Crowding in the operating room obstructed the view for the remote physician in less than 20% of the cases; however, due to the slim design of the robot it could be moved to either the foot or head of the bed without interference. 94% of remote physicians and 74% of local physicians felt comfortable communicating via the telepresence system (Figures 5 and 6). To measure the value of the telepresence robot, we compared its use to that of the telephone. The most significant finding from the study is that all the local clinicians agreed that having access to a remote expert would be beneficial, and

that to do so it would be more effective through telemedicine rather than just the telephone (Figures 7 and 8).

When appropriate, the local clinician used the AAST injury grading system to classify injuries in 63% (n=22) of trauma cases, compared to 54% (n=19) of cases by the remote physicians. In one case, the remote physician reported not being able to differentiate structures such as nerves, arteries or veins due to the amount of blood in the field. In two cases, the remote physician could not grade the injuries due to the overcrowding in the operating room. There was only one case that the

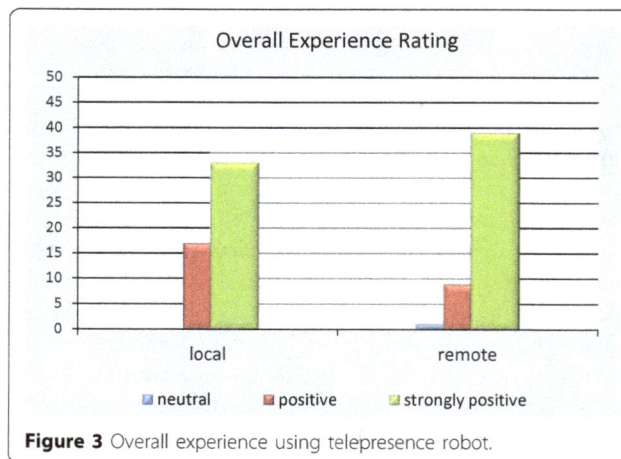

Figure 3 Overall experience using telepresence robot.

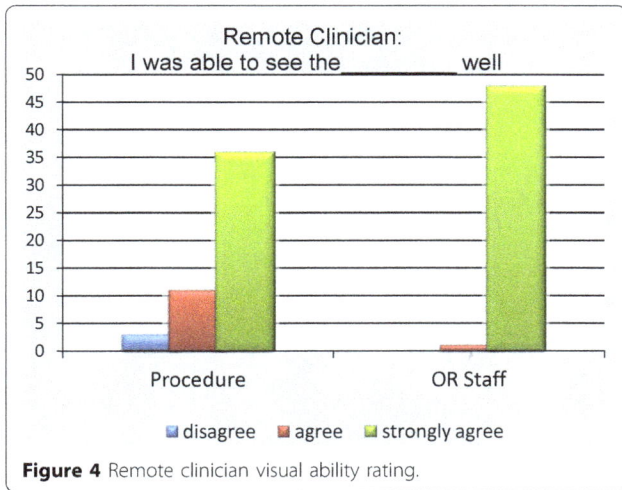

Figure 4 Remote clinician visual ability rating.

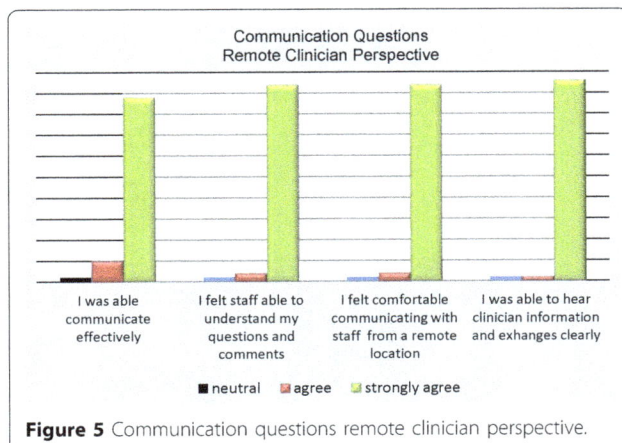

Figure 6 Communication questions local clinician perspective.

remote physician graded one of the injuries, but missed a level III small bowel injury, but the reason was not recorded.

Discussion

In this observational study, descriptive data was obtained on the use of a robotic telepresence system and its usability inside the operating rooms of a level 1 trauma center. We collected data on 50 surgical cases with the robotic telemedicine system. The majority of the cases were trauma surgical cases, with a few elective general surgery cases. Participants as well as OR staff found the system to be compact and easy to maneuver, which made it more readily acceptable by the operating room staff. The majority of the responses regarding the audio and visual capabilities of the system were highly positive. The only times the remote clinician noted having difficulties visualizing the procedure occurred when the patient was surrounded by a team of clinicians. However, due to the slim design, the cart could be moved to either the foot or head of the bed without interference. Both the local and remote clinicians

positively rated the communication abilities and level of comfort using the system. Moreover, the use of a telemedicine system was seen as more beneficial than the traditional phone for consultation purposes. The ability to have the remote expert connect using audio/visual capabilities enhances the experience. We also found that the robot used in this study has sufficient video qualities to allow remote clinicians to see the wounds and organs clearly enough to identify the injury severity.

This study has important limitations. First, a convenience sample was used for the surgical cases. This was done due to several factors, but mainly because the main objective of this study was only to understand the system's functions, strengths and weaknesses. The main purpose of testing a novel technology is to understand the system's capabilities as well as how its acceptance can affect the integration of new technology. However, we were able to engage a good number of attendings

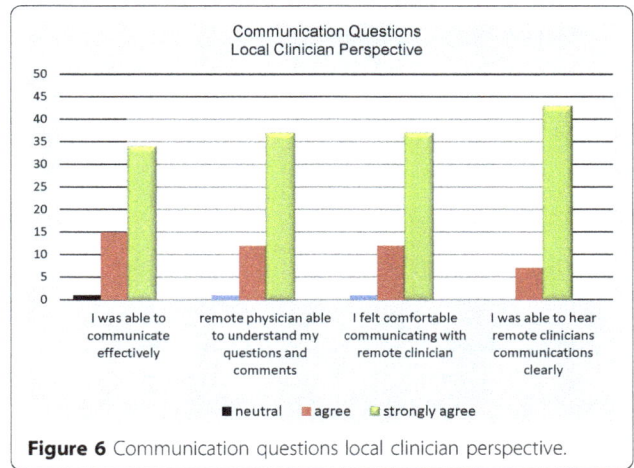

Figure 5 Communication questions remote clinician perspective.

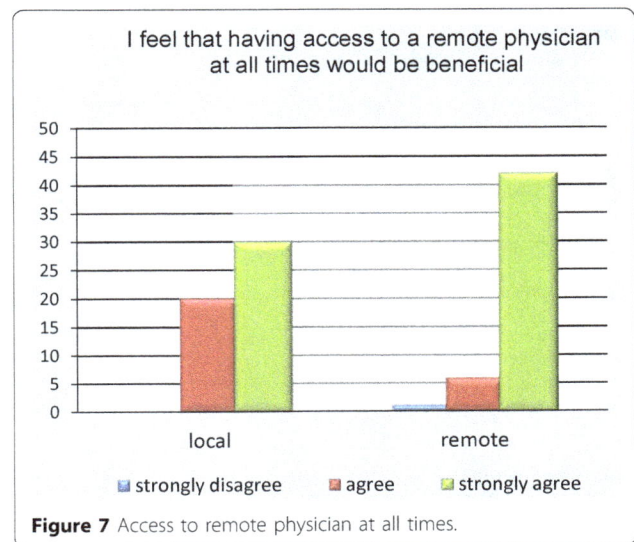

Figure 7 Access to remote physician at all times.

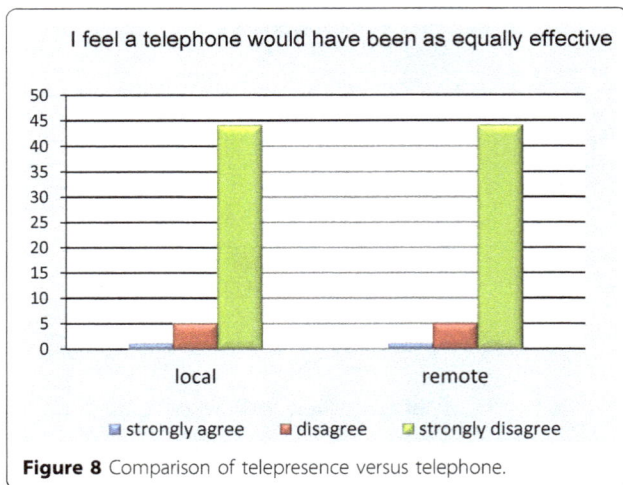

Figure 8 Comparison of telepresence versus telephone.

References
1. Williams TE, Ellison EC: **Population analysis predicts a future critical shortage of general surgeons.** *Surgery* 2008, **144**:548-556.
2. Harvard School of Public Health: **More than 2 billion people worldwide lack access to surgical services.** *ScienceDaily* 2010.
3. Ereso AQ, Garchia P, Tseng E, *et al*: **Live transference of surgical subspecialty skills using telerobotic proctoring to remote general surgeons.** *J Am Coll Surg* 2010, **211(3)**:400-411.
4. Jarvis-Selinger S, *et al*: **Clinical telehealth across the disciplines: lessons learned.** *Telemed J E Health* 2008, **14**:720-725.
5. Moore EE, Cogbill TH, Malangoni M, Jurkovich GJ, Champion HR: **Scaling System for organ specific injuries.**.

and fellows to participate to reduce the number of repeat times for any one participant. We were able to capture a variety of injuries and anatomical locations. The results of our study may not be applicable to other hospitals or trauma centers. The results from this study will, however, help guide future efforts. Future directions are to determine if the use of a telepresence system for mentoring and consultation purposes impacts the process and outcomes of care.

Conclusion

In conclusion, a robotic telepresence system that is mobile and compact in size was readily accepted by the staff in the operating room and physicians. Physicians were able to use the ControlStation with little training or experience. We were able to test the system's functionalities on a variety of trauma and surgical cases. The potential applications of this system for military and civilian purposes should be further evaluated.

Acknowledgements
This article has been published as part of *World Journal of Emergency Surgery* Volume 7 Supplement 1, 2012: Proceedings of the World Trauma Congress 2012. The full contents of the supplement are available online at http://www.wjes.org/supplements/7/S1.

Author details
[1]University of Miami Miller School of Medicine Surgery Department (D40), PO Box 016960 Miami, FL 33101, USA. [2]Universidade Federal do Parana, Rua XV de Novembro, 1299, CEP 80.060-000 .Curitiba, PR Brasil.

Authors' contributions
AM provided the direction and guidance to the research conception and design. FK was involved with the data management and analysis, and drafted the manuscript. EP and DR assisted with the data collection and entry. PA-R assisted with the data interpretation and draft of manuscript. CS assisted with study concept and design, and data interpretation. All authors read and approved the final manuscript.

Competing interests
The authors declare that they have no competing interests.

4

Does trauma team activation associate with the time to CT scan for those suspected of serious head injuries?

Alma Rados[1], Corina Tiruta[1], Zhengwen Xiao[1], John B Kortbeek[1,2,3], Paul Tourigny[4,5], Chad G Ball[1,2] and Andrew W Kirkpatrick[1,2,3]*

Abstract

Background: Traumatic brain injury (TBI) constitutes the leading cause of posttraumatic mortality. Practically, the major interventions required to treat TBI predicate expedited transfer to CT after excluding other immediately life-threatening conditions. At our center, trauma responses variably consist of either full trauma activation (FTA) including an attending trauma surgeon or a non-trauma team response (NTTR). We sought to explore whether FTAs expedited the time to CT head (TTCTH).

Methods: Retrospective review of augmented demographics of 88 serious head injuries identified from a Regional Trauma Registry within one year at a level I trauma center. The inclusion criteria consisted of a diagnosis of head injury recorded as intubated or GCS < 13; and CT-head scanning after arriving the emergency department. Data was analyzed using STATA.

Results: There were 58 FTAs and 30 NTTRs; 86% of FTAs and 17% of NTTRs were intubated prehospital out of 101 charts reviewed in detail; 13 were excluded due to missing data. Although FTAs were more seriously injured (median ISS 29, MAIS head 19, GCS score at scene 6.0), NTTRs were also severely injured (median ISS 25, MAIS head 21, GCS at scene 10) and older (median 54 vs. 26 years). Median TTCTH was double without dedicated FTA (median 50 vs. 26 minutes, p < 0.001), despite similar justifiable delays (53% NTTR, 52% FTA). Without FTA, most delays (69%) were for emergency intubation. TTCTH after securing the airway was longer for NTTR group (median 38 vs. 26 minutes, p =0.0013). Even with no requirements for ED interventions, TTCTH for FTA was less than half versus NTTR (25 vs. 61 minutes, p =0.0013). Multivariate regression analysis indicated age and FTA with an attending surgeon as significant predictors of TTCTH, although the majority of variability in TTCTH was not explained by these two variables ($R^2 = 0.33$).

Conclusion: Full trauma activations involving attending trauma surgeons were quicker at transferring serious head injury patients to CT. Patients with FTA were younger and more seriously injured. Discerning the reasons for delays to CT should be used to refine protocols aimed at minimizing unnecessary delays and enhancing workforce efficiency and clinical outcome.

Keywords: Trauma triage, Trauma activation, Trauma human factors, Traumatic brain injury, Diagnostic imaging

* Correspondence: Andrew.kirkpatrick@albertahealthservices.ca
[1]Regional Trauma Services, Foothills Medical Centre, University of Calgary, 29 Street, Calgary, NW 1403, Alberta
[2]Departments of Surgery, Foothills Medical Centre, University of Calgary, Calgary, Alberta
Full list of author information is available at the end of the article

Background

All trauma systems need to define the optimal criteria with which to activate full trauma responses in order to respond to the immediate clinical needs of the critically injured. Thus, the American College of Surgeons Committee on Trauma (ACS COT) has defined guidelines to guide prehospital triage to trauma centers [1]. Building on these guidelines, many centers recognize the need for two or three tiered activation criteria to more efficiently manage hospital and human resources [2-8]. Many systems including our own, require the immediate or urgent presence of attending trauma surgeons as their "highest level" response. Of the various criteria used to initiate full trauma activations, severe head injuries denoted by a depressed Glasgow Coma Scale (GCS) have long been the most controversial at our institution and the most problematic in terms of adherence to protocols and standards. Routine trauma quality assurance (QA) activities in our center note that this criterion represents the majority of failures to activate the trauma team [9]. While trauma surgeons from a general surgery specialty practically do not operate on severe head injuries it is perceived that they both contribute to resuscitative care and expedite the work-up. However, there is limited information regarding the time factors and efficiency of different trauma systems in triaging and optimizing the prompt attainment of CT imaging in the critically injured [10]. This prompted us to review the association between the type of trauma response and the efficiency of obtaining a CT scan in seriously head injured patients.

Methods

The Alberta Health Services Calgary Region (AHSCR) is a fully integrated, publicly funded health system that provides virtually all medical and surgical care to the residents of the city of Calgary and a large surrounding area including smaller towns and communities (population ~ 1.2 million). In the AHSCR, adult trauma services are regionalized to the Foothills Medical Centre (FMC), and pediatric trauma services (age mandate ≤14 years) to the Alberta Children's Hospital. These are the only accredited tertiary trauma care centers providing trauma services for Southern Alberta, Canada (~35% of the population of the Province of Alberta). Patients may also be transported to Calgary from trauma care services in neighboring provinces.

At FMC, full trauma activations (FTAs) involve an expedited response by an attending trauma surgeon and trauma team (TT), residents from critical care medicine, respiratory therapists, and other dedicated trauma resources including anesthesia and the operating room, in addition to emergency physicians and nurses who are the typical responders to initial non-trauma team responses (NTTR) (Table 1). Patients with an initial NTTR

Table 1 Alberta health services - Calgary Region trauma activation criteria

1.	Shock defined by BP systolic < 90 mmHg or Temperature ≤ 30°C
2.	Patient intubated for respiratory compromise/airway obstruction
3.	Patient with GCS ≤ 8
4.	Gunshot wound to the head, neck, or torso
5.	Need for blood transfusion *en route* to hospital or in the ED

are often seen after the initial assessment by the emergency medicine team in the format of a trauma consult by the TT if admission or ongoing care is required. A FTA may be initiated by the emergency physician based on changing patient status, updated prehospital information, or clinical judgment. The response performance of trauma personnel is a trauma quality assurance audit filter and is assessed and reported annually in the Trauma Services Annual Report noting that recent audit revealed the attending trauma surgeons are typically always present within 20 minutes at a FTA [9].

In order to assess the efficiencies and human resource implications of trauma activations not focusing on traditional thoracoabdominal injuries, a retrospective review of trauma patient resuscitations with head injuries requiring intubation or with a GCS < 13 in whom a CT scan was obtained. Patients were identified from the FMC Trauma Registry as having been admitted between April 01 2008 and March 31, 2009. To qualify for the trauma registry a patient must have an Injury Severity Score (ISS) ≥ 12 and be admitted to the trauma centre or die in the emergency department of the trauma centre.

From the eligible cohort (186 TBI patients who met the inclusion criteria), a convenience sample of 101 charts was selected by medical records for review. Demographic data reviewed included age, gender, emergency department (ED) admission date, ED admission time, injury description, Maximum Abbreviated Injury Scale (MAIS) Head, Injury Severity Score (ISS), scene GCS, trauma centre GCS, patient intubation status at the time of the GCS was calculated, whether FTA was activated, time of trauma team activation, trauma surgeon, intensive care unit (ICU) admission, ICU length of stay (LOS), and discharge status. The following data was collected directly from the charts: whether patient had a CT done at previous hospital, arrival time of trauma surgeon at FTA, CT head date and time, picture archiving and communication (PACS) time of CT head, electronic medical record time of CT Head, whether there was a reason for CT delay, and if there was a reason for delay then which interventions were done, interventions date, interventions time, and any comments about the patient. We initially sought to study the times until completion of the CT head. However review of the time imprints embedded with the CT images in

PACS was found to be non-sensical clinically, and a subsequent review of the electronic clocks in the CT scanners found them to be significantly inaccurate. Thus, the charted time the patient left the trauma bay for the CT scanner was used instead. The "Time from ED admission to CT head (TTCTH-unqualified)" was defined as the unqualified number of minutes from ED admission until the patient left for the CT scan. The "Time in ED after airways were secure (TTCT-after airways secure)" was defined as either the time in the ED until leaving for CT head if intubated pre-hospital or never intubated, or as the time in the ED after ED intubation until leaving for CT head. For those re-intubated in ED, the time from re-intubation until leaving for CT was used for this designation. The "Time in the ED after intubation or procedure (TTCTH-after any procedure)" was defined as the time in the ED after any required procedure was performed including any of ED intubation, chest tube insertion, or arterial or central venous line insertion, and Focused Assessment with Sonography (FAST). If the time of the procedure was unavailable, or if no procedure was required, this time was measured from arriving in the ED until leaving for CT head. We also separately examined the TTCTH in patients who had no interventions of any type in the ED (TTCTH-no interventions), the TTCTH excluding patients who required intubation or re-intubation for misplaced endotracheal tubes in the ED (TTCTH-exclude intubation), and the TTCTH including only patients intubated (pre-hospital or in the ED) (TTCTH-intubation only).

The data were analyzed using STATA (version 9.2, College Station, Texas) and presented as medians with interquartile ranges (IQR) for non-normally distributed variables. Medians were compared using the Mann-Whitney U test, categorical data were analyzed by Fisher's exact test. To identify independent factors associated with the time to CT Head a multiple linear regression model was developed, using backward stepwise variable elimination. Statistically significant differences were defined as a *p* value < 0.05.

Results

One hundred and one (101) eligible patients' charts were reviewed. Thirteen (13) patients were excluded from the final analysis as seven patients had CT head done at a referring hospital, four had missing times to CT, one was not trauma patient and one did not have a TBI leaving 88 records for analysis. Fifty-eight (58) patients had a FTA, and 30 had a NTTR. Patients in the FTA group were younger (median age 26 vs 54 years), higher median ISS (29 vs 25, p = 0.007), and lower scene GCS score (6 vs 10, p = 0.08) than the NTTR patients, with the majority being intubated prehospital. Table 2 shows the characteristics of the two groups. The actual time of

the trauma team activation was recorded in only 21 (36%) of activations, but all had ER admission time recorded. In 11 cases the FTA was prior to emergency department (ED) admission, in 8 it was coincident with ED admission, and in 2 after admission. Thus the median time to FTA was 1 minute before ED admission with an average time of 5.5 minutes noting one outlying activation 164 minutes after ED admission.

Patients who presented during FTA (n = 58) had a significant shorter time to CT head compared with patients evaluated with a NTTR (n = 30) (TTCTH-unqualified 26 min [IQR = 19.5-36.5] vs 49.5 min [IQR = 32-80.5]; p <0.0001) (Table 2). As expected, there was an association between trauma team activation and pre-hospital intubation, with a coefficient of correlation r =0.6. Using CT head as the dependant variable, a multiple linear regression analysis with age, ISS, MAIS head, ED intubation, trauma team activation designation, pre-hospital intubation, and requirement for any ED intervention as predictors was performed (Table 3). Backward stepwise variable elimination identified age and trauma team activation as significant predictive factors influencing reduced time to CT head. Time to CT Head was predicted to be 1.8 minutes lower per one unit increase in FTA; however, this group of variables does not fully explain the variability in time to CT Head (R^2 = 0.33).

Although the majority of cases were intubated prehospital, 11 (37%) of the NTTR pts vs. 5 (9%) FTA pts were intubated after arriving in ED. The TTCTH was shorter for FTA (median 25 vs. 45 minutes for NTTR) but limited by the few patients intubated in ED. With intubation after arriving in ED being the top cause of delays to CT for NTTRs, we examined only those patients without any need for ED intubation to ensure more similarity between the two groups. The TTCTH-exclude intubation was 27 versus 55 minutes (p =0.0015) favoring FTA (Table 4). For the whole group of patients (intubated pre-hospital, intubated in ED, or never intubated) the TTCTH-after airways secure was 26 minutes versus 38 minutes (p =0.0013) in favor of FTA (Table 2). Just over half of each group had documented resuscitative procedures before being taken to CT (FTA = 47%, NTTR = 47%). For all patients, the TTCTH-after any procedures was 23 versus 35 minutes (p =0.0007) favoring FTA (Table 2), and the TTCTH-no interventions was 25 versus 61 minutes (p =0.0013) favoring FTA as well (Table 5). For patients intubated pre-hospital or in ED the time from arriving in the ED until CT was also shorter for FTA group (median 26 versus 45 minutes, p =0.002). Although a specific review of TTCTH-unqualified for all patients with pre-hospital intubation was limited by the few patients in NTTR (n = 5), this group took 33 minutes compared to 26 minutes in FTA (n = 50). All comparison of times is summarized in Table 6.

Table 2 Patient characteristics in resuscitative groups (FTA and NTTR)

No. of patients		FTA	NTTR	p value
N = 88		(n = 58)	(n = 30)	
Age (y)	median (IQR)	26 (21–46.5)	54 (25.5-76.5)	0.0017
	mean ± SD	35 ± 18	51 ± 24	
Male gender		46 (79%)	22 (73%)	0.6
ISS	median (IQR)	29 (23.5-41.5)	25 (17–29)	0.0071
	mean ± SD	32 ± 11	25 ± 7.5	
MAIS Head,	median (IQR)	16 (16-25)	20.5 (16-25)	0.5
	mean ± SD	19 ± 6	20 ± 6	
GCS at scence,	median (IQR)	6.0 (3.0-12.0)	10.0 (5.75-13)	0.08
Intubated prehospital		50 (86%)	5 (17%)	<0.0001
Intubated in ED[1]		5 (8.6%)	11 (37%)	0.0026
No. pts with reason for delay to CT[2]		30 (52%)	16 (53%)	1
No. pts with ED Interventions[3]		27 (47%)	14 (47%)	0.9
TTCTH-unqualified				
Time from ED adm to CT (min), median (IQR)		26 (19.5-36.5)	49.5 (32–80.5)	<0.001
TTCTH-after airways secure (min)[4]		25.5 (17.5-35)	38 (27.5-78)	0.0013
TTCTH-after any procedure (min)[5]		22.5 (16–32)	34.5 (24–78)	0.0007
ICU Admissions		43 (74%)	13 (43%)	0.006
ICU LOS[6], median (IQR)		3 (1–10.5)	3 (1-9)	0.7
In-hospital death, n (%)		16 (27.5)	12 (40)	0.334

[1] one FTA pt and 2 NTTR pts were reintubated in ED.
[2] delay to CT could be caused by an intervention in ED or by non-procedure factors.
[3] interventions in ED include: intubation,chest tube,FAST, arterial line,resuscitation,etc.
[4] Time in the ED after intubation until CT or from ED admission until CT if intubated prehospital or never intubated (includes prehospital intubated, intubated in ED, never intubated).
[5] Time of intervention done in ED was not found in all cases, thus time from ED admission to CT was used.
[6] LOS, length of stay in days.

Discussion

Many combinations of mechanistic, anatomic, physiologic, and demographic criteria, generally adapted from the Field Triage Decision scheme of the ACS COT [1], have been adopted by numerous investigators and organizations to guide the field triage of the trauma patient [1,4-7]. The ideal triage system to manage competing clinical needs with practical resource management remains elusive. Such an ideal system would equally match the severity of injury and resources required for optimal care with the optimal facilities, personnel, and response criteria [1.5]. One of the most limited resources

Table 3 Multiple linear regression: predictors of time to CT Head

Initial independent Variables	Coefficients	Std. Err	t	p > |t|	[95% Conf. interval]	
Age	0.0070221	0.0028789	2.44	0.017	0.0012917	0.0127525
MAIS Head	-0.0156356	0.0100677	-1.55	0.124	-0.0356748	0.0044067
ISS	-0.0000174	0.0066377	-0.00	0.998	-0.0132293	0.0131945
Pre-hospital intubation	-0.2816034	0.1642582	-1.71	0.090	-0.6085512	0.0453443
Trauma team activation	-0.4942918	0.1754433	-2.82	0.006	-0.8435029	-0.1450807
ED intubation	-0.2740521	0.1862904	-1.47	0.145	-0.644854	0.0967497
ED intervention	0.1633863	0.1372994	1.19	0.238	-0.1099013	0.4366739
Predictor Variables of time to CT Head	Coefficients	Std. Err	t	p > |t|	[95% Conf. interval]	
Age	0.00617341	0.0028299	2.18	0.032	0.0005458	0.0118009
Trauma team activation	-0.6133904	0.1255942	-4.88	0.000	-0.8631482	-0.3636326

Table 4 Times to CT head excluding patients with any need for emergency department intubation (or re-intubation)

No.of pts (72)	FTA (n = 53)	NTTR (n = 19)	p value
Age, median (IQR)	26 (21–46.5)	65 (43–77)	<0.0001
Gender, male	42 (79%)	12 (63%)	0.2
ISS, median (IQR)	29 (23.5-41.5)	25 (16–29)	0.0032
MAIS Head, median (IQR)	16 (16-25)	16 (16-25)	0.7
No.pts preintubated	49 (92%)	3 (16%)	<0.0001
No.pts who underwent any type of procedure in ED	22 (42%)	3 (16%)	0.0526
TTCTH-exclude intubation			
Time from ED adm to CT, median (IQR)	27 (19–36.5)	55 (30–107)	0.0015

is that of the responding trauma surgeons themselves. In systems that require the immediate or urgent presence of attending trauma surgeons this "non-surgical" task may exacerbate what has been perceived to be a crisis in trauma surgery human resources [4,11-14].

Contemporary initiatives have focused on identifying patients requiring specific emergency department procedures or operative interventions to define which of the many potential triage criteria are valuable or not [5]. In addition to identifying the need for a procedure, we suggest that significantly decreasing the delay until a critically injured patient with a potentially treatable space-occupying lesion detected on CT scanning is another critical aspect of full trauma activation. This needs to be evaluated as a process outcome. Simply put, time is brain. The duration of brain herniation before surgical decompression influences outcomes for acute epidural hematomas [15,16], and as such, obtaining urgent CT scans is typically a requisite part of brain injury preoperative resuscitation. As we believe that expediting the resuscitative and diagnostic workup of the critically

Table 5 Times to CT head for patients with no emergency department interventions

No. of pts (47)	FTA (n = 31)	NTTR (n = 16)	p valve
Age, median (IQR)	26 (20–48)	67 (45.5-77)	0.0005
Gender, male	22 (71%)	11 (69%)	1
ISS, median (IQR)	29 (20–41)	25 (16–25.5)	0.02
MAIS Head, median (IQR)	16 (16-25)	20.5 (16–25)	0.7
No.pts preintubated	30 (97%)	3 (19%)	<0.0001
TTCTH-no interventions			
Time from ED adm to CT, median (IQR)	25 (17–32)	60.5 (30–123.5)	0.0013

Table 6 A summary of the times from arriving in the ED until CT head for different subgroups of patients

No. of Pts	FTA n = 58	NTTR n = 30	p value
Median min. (IQR)	26 (19.5-36.5)	49.5 (32–80.5)	<0.001
Intubated	n = 50	n = 5	sample too small
Pre-hospital			
Median min (IQR)	26 (18.5-36.5)	33 (25–74.5)	
Intubated or	n = 5	n = 11	sample too small
Re-intubated in ED	*1 pt reintubated	*2 pts reintubated	
Median min (IQR)	25 (20.5-32)	45 (42–62)	
Pts w/o ED Intubation	n = 53	n = 19	0.0015
Median min (IQR)	27 (19–36.5)	55 (30–107)	
Pts w/o ED Intervention	n = 31	n = 16	0.0013
Median min (IQR)	25 (17–32)	60.5 (30–123.5)	
Intubated Pre-hospital or in ED	n = 54	n = 14	0.0002
Median min (IQR)	26 (19-36.5)	45 (36–67.5)	

injured is important to their outcome, we have included intubated head injuries as an activation criterion for full trauma activation.

CT scanning is considered the reference standard for diagnosing most traumatic injuries in the acutely injured patient [17-23] and specifically for detecting post-traumatic intra-cranial lesions [24,25]. Despite the primacy of CT scanning as the preferred definitive imaging modality however, there is limited information regarding the time factors and efficiency of different trauma systems in triaging and optimizing the prompt attainment of this imaging modality in the critically injured [10]. In one of the few reviews of CT efficiency, Fung Kon Jin and colleagues [10] found that the median start time in a high-volume "stream-lined" level-1 American trauma center for a severely injured cohort (median ISS 18) was 82 minutes, with the median time from arrival until completion of the diagnostic trauma evaluation being nearly 2 hours (114 minutes). The relevance of this time may be increased by noting that the mean time to CT head for non-traumatic neurological emergencies in a tertiary care academic institution that prioritized CT scanning for potential stroke over all other emergency department patients except trauma was either 99 or 101 minutes, depending on whether there were competing trauma activations [26].

In terms of patients with severe TBI, efforts to expedite diagnostic imaging in general include the introduction of CT scanning directly into the trauma room. Such a scanner in Amsterdam has reduced the time until completion of CT diagnostic imaging to 79 minutes in a cohort in whom the majority had an ISS < 16 [27]; to 23 minutes in a German CT equipped resuscitation room caring for a population with a mean ISS of 24 [28]; and to 12 minutes in an Austrian cohort (mean ISS = 27) in whom scanning was started immediately after admission. In the Austrian cohort a systolic BP > 70 mmHg was considered sufficient for CT scanning without cardiac arrest [25].

Based on our review however, we believe another strategy is to continue to retain the category of severe TBI as a criterion for full trauma team activation that is likely applicable to similar institutions. At least in our institution this associates with specifically decreased time to obtain head CT scans in those with severe head injuries, and mandates the presence of a surgeon to facilitate invasive interventions. Several groups have confirmed that a GCS < 8 was associated with high mortality [6,8], and such patients were 100 times more likely to die, 23 times more likely to require ICU, and 1.5 times more likely to need an operation among trauma patient admissions [6]. Although we cannot significantly prove in-hospital mortality, the designation of a trauma as requiring "activation" was associated with a 1.8 minute decrease per "unit" of activation in TTCTH statistically. We perceive this to be associated with the dedicated presence of the trauma surgeon as the team leader and to a general "entitlement" of the patient to all other human and technical resources available in our hospital resulting in markedly short durations to CT. Noting that a reported delay in NTTRs was "CT unavailable" reinforces this presumption. However, this study was not designed to compare the efficacy between a non-surgeon and a surgeon led trauma team activation.

There are limitations of this review that are both generic to retrospective reviews in general and specific to our data. Firstly, this non-randomized methodology can only note the association between FTAs at our institution and expedited transfers to CT scan and cannot delineate which specific factors or procedures were responsible. Further, we do not have exact data on the responding time for the trauma surgeons for all FTAs. There were further distinct differences between the two groups of patients with a greater need for definitive airway interventions in the non-FTA group. However, even after looking specifically at the TTCTH after secure airway control or after the performance of required resuscitative interventions it was still distinctly quicker in the FTA group. Finally we were surprised to realize that the time imprints embedded directly onto radiological images were inaccurate which has obvious implications for quality assurance and medico-legal review. We now regularly check for accuracy in this regard.

Conclusions
Full trauma activations involving attending surgeons were quicker at transferring seriously head-injured patients to CT. Patients with FTA were younger, higher ISS, lower scene GCS, and more often intubated in the pre-hospital setting. Discerning the reasons for delays to CT should be used to refine protocols aimed at minimizing unnecessary delays and maximizing workforce efficiency.

Abbreviations
ACS COT: American College of Surgeons Committee on Trauma; BP: Blood pressure; CT: Computed tomography; ED: Emergency department; FAST: Focused assessment with sonography; FMC: Foothills Medical Centre; FTA: Full trauma activation; GCS: Glasgow coma scale; ICU: Intensive care unit; ISS: Injury severity score; IQR: Interquartile ranges; LOS: Length of stay; MAIS: Maximum abbreviated injury scale; NTTR: Non-trauma team response; PACS: Picture archiving and communication system; TBI: Traumatic brain injury; TTCTH: Time to CT head.

Competing interests
The authors declare that they have no competing interests.

Authors' contributions
Study concept and design: AK, AR; Acquisition of data: AR, CT, AK; analysis and interpretation of data: AR, CT, AK, ZX, CB, PT; drafting of the manuscript: AK; critical revision of the manuscript: AK, ZX, CB. All authors read and approved the final manuscript.

Acknowledgements
The authors thank Dr David Zygun, MD FRCPC, University of Alberta, Dr Kevin Stevenson University of Saskatchewan, Viesha A. Ciura University of Calgary, Kimberley Musselwhite, MN RN, Alberta Health Services, Christine Vis Alberta Health Services for their assistance for this study.

Author details
[1]Regional Trauma Services, Foothills Medical Centre, University of Calgary, 29 Street, Calgary, NW 1403, Alberta. [2]Departments of Surgery, Foothills Medical Centre, University of Calgary, Calgary, Alberta. [3]Critical Care Medicine, Foothills Medical Centre, University of Calgary, Calgary, Alberta. [4]Radiology, Foothills Medical Centre, University of Calgary, Calgary, Alberta. [5]Emergency Medicine, Foothills Medical Centre, University of Calgary, Calgary, Alberta.

References
1. Committee on Trauma of the American College of Surgeons: *Resources for optimal care of the injured.* Chicago, IL: Committee on Trauma of the American College of Surgeons; 2006.
2. Davis T, Dinh M, Roncal S, Byrne C, Petchell J, Leonard E, *et al*: Prospective evaluation of a two-tiered trauma activation protocol in an Australian major trauma referral hospital. *Injury* 2010, 41(5):470–474.
3. Kouzminova N, Shatney C, Palm E, McCullough M, Sherck J: The efficacy of a two-tiered trauma activation system at a level I trauma center. *J Trauma* 2009, 67(4):829–833.
4. Norwood SH, McAuley CE, Berne JD, Vallina VL, Creath RG, McLarty J: A prehospital glasgow coma scale score < or = 14 accurately predicts the need for full trauma team activation and patient hospitalization after motor vehicle collisions. *J Trauma* 2002, 53(3):503–507.
5. Lehmann RK, Arthurs ZM, Cuadrado DG, Casey LE, Beekley AC, Martin MJ: Trauma team activation: simplified criteria safely reduces overtriage. *Am J Surg* 2007, 193(5):630–634. discussion 4–5.
6. Tinkoff GH, O'Connor RE: Validation of new trauma triage rules for trauma attending response to the emergency department. *J Trauma* 2002, 52(6):1153–1158. discussion 8–9.
7. Cook CH, Muscarella P, Praba AC, Melvin WS, Martin LC: Reducing overtriage without compromising outcomes in trauma patients. *Arch Surg* 2001, 136(7):752–756.

8. Cherry RA, King TS, Carney DE, Bryant P, Cooney RN: **Trauma team activation and the impact on mortality.** *J Trauma* 2007, **63**(2):326–330.

9. Region AHSC: *Trauma Services Annual Reports.* Calgary: Calgary Regional Trauma Services; 2010. [cited 2010 Feb 26 2010]; Available from: http://www.calgaryhealthregion.ca/programs/trauma/reports.htm.

10. Fung Kon Jin PH, van Geene AR, Linnau KF, Jurkovich GJ, Goslings JC, Ponsen KJ: **Time factors associated with CT scan usage in trauma patients.** *Eur J Radiol* 2009, **72**(1):134–138.

11. Grossman MD, Portner M, Hoey BA, Stehly CD, Schwab CW, Stotzfus J: **Emergency traumatologists as partners in trauma care: the future is now.** *J Am Coll Surg* 2009, **208**:503–509.

12. Shackford S: **How then shall we change?** *J Trauma* 2006, **60**(1):1–7.

13. Esposito TJ, Leon L, Jurkovich GJ: **The shape of things to come: results from a national survey of trauma surgeons on issues concerning their future.** *J Trauma* 2006, **60**(1):8–16.

14. Committee to Develop the Reogranized Specialty of Trauma SCC, and Emergency surgery: **Acute care surgery: trauma, critical care, and emergency surgery.** *J Trauma* 2005, **58**:614–616.

15. Bullock MR, Chesnut R, Ghajar J, Gordon D, Hartl R, Newell DW, *et al*: **Surgical management of acute epidural hematomas.** *Neurosurgery* 2006, **58**(3 Suppl):S7–S15. discussion Si-iv.

16. Haselsberger K, Pucher R, Auer LM: **Prognosis after acute subdural or epidural haemorrhage.** *Acta Neurochir (Wien)* 1988, **90**(3–4):111–116.

17. Committee on Trauma of the American College of Surgeons: *Advanced Trauma Life Support Course for Doctors.* 9th edition. Chicago: American College of Surgeons; 2012.

18. Trupka A, Waydhas C, Hallfeldt KKJ, Nast-Kolb D, Pfeifer KJ, Schweiberer L: **Value of thoracic computed tomography in the first assessment of se-verely injured patients with blunt chest trauma: results of a prospective study.** *J Trauma* 1997, **43**:405–412.

19. Willmann JK, Roos JE, Platz A, Pfammatter T, Hilfiker PR, Marincek B, *et al*: **Multidetector CT: detection of active hemorrhage in patients with blunt abdominal trauma.** *AJR Am J Roentgenol* 2002, **179**(2):437–444.

20. Self ML, Blake AM, Whitley M, Nadalo L, Dunn E: **The benefit of routine thoracic, abdominal, and pelvic computed tomography to evaluate trauma patients with closed head injuries.** *Am J Surg* 2003, **186**(6):609–613. discussion 13-4.

21. Salim A, Sangthong B, Martin M, Brown C, Plurad D, Demetriades D: **Whole body imaging in blunt multisystem trauma patients without obvious signs of injury: results of a prospective study.** *Arch Surg* 2006, **141**(5):468–473. discussion 73-5.

22. Tillou A, Gupta M, Baraff LJ, Schriger DL, Hoffman JR, Hiatt JR, *et al*: **Is the use of pan-computed tomography for blunt trauma justified? A prospective evaluation.** *J Trauma* 2009, **67**(4):779–787.

23. Rieger M, Czermak B, El Attal R, Sumann G, Jaschke W, Freund M: **Initial clinical experience with a 64-MDCT whole-body scanner in an emergency department: better time management and diagnostic quality?** *J Trauma* 2009, **66**(3):648–657.

24. Bullock MR, Chesnut R, Ghajar J, Gordon D, Hartl R, Newell DW, *et al*: **Surgical management of acute subdural hematomas.** *Neurosurgery* 2006, **58**(3 Suppl):S16–S24. discussion Si-iv.

25. Weninger P, Mauritz W, Fridrich P, Spitaler R, Figl M, Kern B, *et al*: **Emergency room management of patients with blunt major trauma: evaluation of the multislice computed tomography protocol exemplified by an urban trauma center.** *J Trauma* 2007, **62**(3):584–591.

26. Chen EH, Mills AM, Lee BY, Robey JL, Zogby KE, Shofer FS, *et al*: **The impact of a concurrent trauma alert evaluation on time to head computed tomography in patients with suspected stroke.** *Acad Emerg Med* 2006, **13**(3):349–352.

27. Fung Kon Jin PH, Goslings JC, Ponsen KJ, van Kuijk C, Hoogerwerf N, Luitse JS: **Assessment of a new trauma workflow concept implementing a sliding CT scanner in the trauma room: the effect on workup times.** *J Trauma* 2008, **64**(5):1320–1326.

28. Wurmb TE, Fruhwald P, Hopfner W, Keil T, Kredel M, Brederlau J, *et al*: **Whole-body multislice computed tomography as the first line diagnostic tool in patients with multiple injuries: the focus on time.** *J Trauma* 2009, **66**(3):658–665.

5

Children and adolescents deaths from trauma-related causes in a Brazilian City

Andrea Melo Alexandre Fraga[1*], Joaquim Murray Bustorff-Silva[2], Thais Marconi Fernandez[3], Gustavo Pereira Fraga[4], Marcelo Conrado Reis[1], Emilio Carlos Elias Baracat[5] and Raul Coimbra[6]

Abstract

Introduction: Injury is the first cause of death worldwide in the population aged 1 to 44. In developed countries, the most common trauma-related injuries resulting in death during childhood are traffic accidents, followed by drowning.

Methods: This retrospective study based on autopsy examinations describes the epidemiology profile of deaths by trauma-related causes in individuals younger than 18 years from 2001 to 2008 in the city of Campinas. The aim is to identify epidemiology changes throughout the years in order to develop strategies of prevention.

Results: There were 2,170 deaths from all causes in children < 18 years old, 530 of which were due to trauma-related causes, with a male predominance of 3.4:1. The age distribution revealed that 76% of deaths occurred in the 10-17 age group. The most predominant trauma cause was firearm injury (47%). Other frequent causes were transport-related injuries (138 cases-26%; pedestrians were struck in 57.2% of these cases) and drowning (55 cases-10.4%). Asphyxia/suffocation was the cause of death in 72% of cases in children < 1 year old; drowning (30.8%) was predominant in the 1-4 age group; transport-related deaths were frequent in the 5-9 age group (56%) and the 10-14 age group (40.4%). Gun-related deaths were predominant (68%) in the 14-17 age group. 51% of deaths occurred at the scene.

Conclusions: There was a predominance of deaths in children and adolescents males, between 15-17 years old, mainly from gun-related homicides, and the frequency has decreased since 2004 after the disarmament statute and the combating of violence.

Keywords: Wounds, Gunshot, Multiple trauma, Drowning, Brain injuries

Introduction

External causes of injuries are the leading cause of death among children and adolescents worldwide and each year more than 950,000 children under the age of 18 die of an injury [1]. Considering the high incidence and diversity of injury, solving this problem is one of the greatest challenges in the field of public health [1-3].

Brazil is the sixth most populous country in the world with approximately 195 million inhabitants, predominantly young. Blessed with abundant natural recourses, Brazil has the most powerful economy in Latin America and has acquired a strong position worldwide. Brazil is slowly improving several social indicators, but socioeconomic and regional disparities are still large [4]. In 2010, approximately 140,000 people died of external causes, and homicides and traffic related deaths accounted for two thirds of all deaths due to trauma-related causes [5]. In 2007, the homicide rate was 26.8 per 100,000 people and the violence has been associated with alcohol and illicit drug use [4].

The number of published studies in international literature from Brazil related to pediatric and adolescents injuries is small [4,6-8]. Fatal injury rates by age group per 100,000 inhabitants in 2003 were 17.7 in Brazilian children less than 5 years old, 10.7 in the 5-9 age group, 14.8 in the 10-14 age group, and 74.7 in the 15-19 age group. In developed countries, injuries due to motor vehicle accidents are the most common [2,9-11]. This high

* Correspondence: andreafrag@gmail.com
[1]Pediatric Emergency Division, Hospital de Clinicas, University of Campinas, Campinas, SP, Brazil
Full list of author information is available at the end of the article

incidence of transport-related deaths is observed in some developing countries such as China, India and Qatar [12-14].

Campinas is a city in the state of São Paulo with about one million inhabitants and each year there are 80 to 200 deaths from trauma-related causes among children. Although located in the most developed state in Brazil, compared with other countries this incidence is very high [8]. There is a need to develop an understanding of traumatic fatalities in children and adolescents to improve injury prevention strategies.

Developing an appropriate approach towards injury prevention in children depends on the knowledge of the epidemiology of traumatic deaths. The aim of this study is to analyze all fatal injuries from trauma-related causes among children and adolescents under 18 years old of age, occurring between 2001 and 2008 in Campinas, in order to identify age groups at risk, mechanism changes during this time period, and develop strategies to decrease the burden through injury prevention activities.

Materials and methods

Data from the Mortality Information System operated by Brazil's Ministry of Health reports 5,620 deaths from trauma-related causes in the city of Campinas in the period from January 1st, 2001 to December 31st, 2008 [5]. This represents 67 deaths from trauma-related causes per 100,000 inhabitants per year. Regarding the population under 18 years of age, there were 2,170 deaths independent of trauma-related causes. The present study selected 530 medico-legal examinations of individuals < 18 years of age who died from trauma-related causes.

In Brazil, by law, medico-legal autopsies are performed in all cases of sudden, suspicious or external cause related deaths. In Campinas there is only one medical examiner's office (Medical Legal Institute—IML) that performs autopsies on corpses from different cities. This study included only examinations confirmed as trauma-related and exclusively from the city of Campinas. The data for the causes of death were confirmed by the death certificate registry. The medical examiner is a forensic physician with expertise in investigating injury related deaths.

The study was retrospective and descriptive. Data were collected in a database using Excel for Windows (Microsoft™ Redmond, WA). The ages of children were categorized into five groups: less than 1 year, 1-4 years, 5-9 years, 10-14 years and 15-17 years, in order to correlate with causes and intents of death.

The deaths were grouped by cause: drowning, transport-related (car passengers, pedestrians hit by an automobile or train, bicycles, or motorcycles), asphyxia/suffocation, hanging/strangulation, poisoning, burning,

stab wound, firearm, fall, assault/blunt trauma, and others. The deaths were also grouped by intent: homicide, self-inflicted (suicide), and unintentional.

To compare trends of mortality, deaths were grouped into two periods, 2001-2004 and 2005-2008. Locations of death were described as: at the scene, pre-hospital care, and at the hospital. The times of death were classified as: immediate (at the scene), less than 24 hours, or more than 24 hours after the injury.

We analyzed the relationships between age group, cause of injury, intent, location, and time of death. The Chi-square test was used as a non-parametric statistical test and the Cochran-Armitage test of trend was carried out to determine the relationship between mechanisms of trauma deaths throughout the years. The level of $p < 0.05$ was considered as the cut-off value for significance.

Institutional Review Board approval from the IML and the University of Campinas was obtained.

Results

Overall, 530 deaths were analyzed. There was a decrease in the number of deaths and proportion of mortality by trauma-related causes in the period 2005-2008 compared to the period 2001-2004 ($p < 0.001$) (Figure 1).

There were 411 males (77.5%) and 119 females (22.5%). The proportion of males to females was 3.4:1 ($p < 0.001$). 76% of deaths were in children between 10-17 years old (Figure 2).

Gun-related injury was the most prevalent cause (249 deaths-47%), followed by transport-related injuries (138 deaths-26%) and drowning (55 deaths-10.4%). In the period from 2005 to 2008 the decrease of deaths was a consequence of a marked reduction in gun-related injuries (Figure 3). Using the Cochran-Armitage trend test there was a linear tendency of a decrease in deaths by firearms ($p < 0.0001$) and an increase in transport-related deaths ($p < 0.0001$) throughout the years.

Asphyxia/suffocation was the cause of injury in 72% of deaths in group < 1 year; drowning (30.8%) and transport-related injuries (22.8%) were more predominant in the 1-4 age group; transport-related deaths were frequent in the 5-9 age group (56%) and 10-14 age group (40.4%) whilst firearm injuries had the highest frequency in the group 14-17 age group (68%)-Table 1.

Pedestrian strike was the cause of injury in 57.2% of transport-related deaths. Two children (9 and 16 years old) were hit by a train. Motorcycle crashes are a public health problem in Brazil and 13 adolescents died this way (Figure 4).

Regarding times of death, 51% occurred at the scene, 4.7% during pre-hospital care, 25.6% occurred at the hospital within the first 24 hours after admission, and the remaining 18.7% of deaths occurred after 24 hours after admission to the hospital. Gun-related injuries

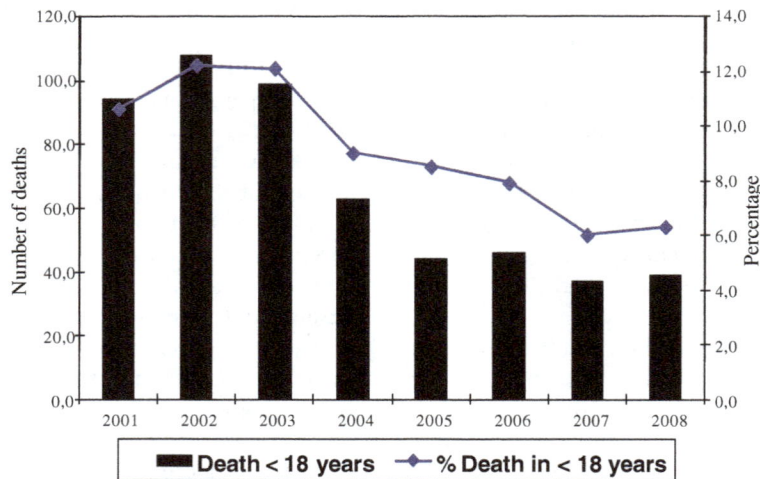

Figure 1 Deaths from external cause and proportion of all deaths among children < 18 years from 2001 to 2008.

carried a 49% mortality rate at the scene, followed by transport-related deaths (19%) and drowning (14%).

When we analyzed the deaths according to the intent, homicides occurred in 50.6% of cases and were more frequent in the 10-17 age group. Unintentional injuries occurred in 48.5% of deaths and traffic-related injuries were the most common. Self-inflicted injuries were identified in only 5 cases (0.9%).

Discussion

Studies related to mortality are useful in order to develop preventive strategies. In the present study deaths from trauma-related causes were predominantly amongst males. Studies conducted in various countries (the USA, Qatar, South Africa, Brazil, Sweden, China and India) showed the same pattern of results [6,9,11-15]. The reasons for this dominance, according to some authors, are greater exposures of males to risk factors such as alcohol abuse, drugs, increased interest in, and easier access to, firearms and vehicles such as cars or motorcycles, in addition to a greater integration into the labor market via legal or illegal activities. Another male-related feature is their greater impulsive and inquisitive nature, and their activities are more greatly related to intense emotions and adventure [12,16,17].

Several studies have shown that the majority of deaths from external causes in children under 18 years of age occurred between the ages of 10 and 17 years, as also reported in the present series. However, the causes of injury differ depending on the socioeconomic level of each country or region [8-14,16,18]. Another study conducted in African countries in 2009 differs from the above mentioned studies. The authors identified the group of greater mortality as the 1-4 year age group, and lack of adequate care was directed linked to those deaths [15].

In our series, the most prevalent causes of injury were gun-related injuries, traffic-related events and drowning. Adjusting for the total population growth, it was clear that gun-related injuries have decreased over time, while traffic-related events showed a slight increase in the period 2005-2008.

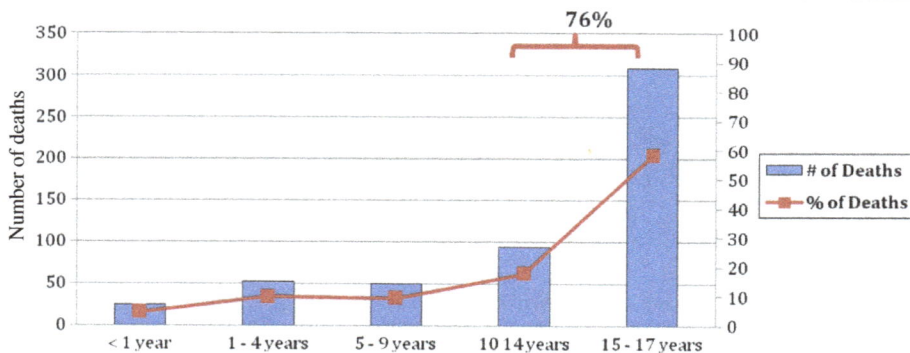

Figure 2 Deaths by age group.

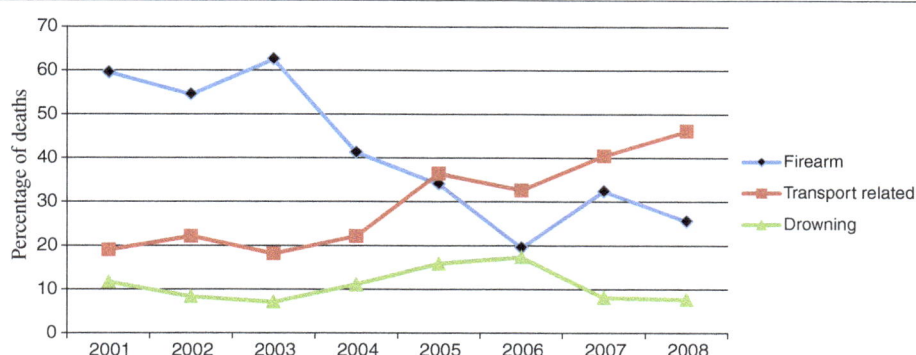

Figure 3 Deaths and most frequent causes of injuries between 2001 and 2008.

Currently, violence is a major public concern in all societies, especially in underdeveloped or developing countries. Gun-related injuries in this study were more prevalent in the 15-17 age group. These results were consistent with studies carried in other regions of Brazil [6,8]. One explanation for this fact is related to how urbanization has been developed in this country. There has been a high rate of internal migration, mostly young people in search of new employment opportunities in the large urban centers. However, most of these young people have not been absorbed by the labor market, thereby increasing marginalization on the periphery of large cities. This concentration of population associated with lack of employment and personal frustration causes

these young individuals to be exposed to different forms of violence [6,8].

In a recent U.S. study, conducted in 2008 by some of the present authors, in San Diego, California, it was shown that gunshot wounds were the third leading cause of death in children under 18 years of age [11]. In another Brazilian study, it was shown that the rate of violence-related death rates has increased almost five-fold during the period from 1979 to 1995 [6]. On the other hand, in some regions such as Qatar, South India, China and Canada, deaths from firearm-related injuries are uncommon [10,13,14,17].

Related to trauma-related injuries, the World Health Organization (WHO) considers traffic accidents as a major public health problem worldwide and that effective preventative measures are not taken, the trend is an overall increase of deaths with traffic accidents being the secondary cause [19]. This study shows that traffic accidents are a cause of death in all age groups, but the emphasis is on the > 10 year old age group. Literature data show that in most studies the main cause of deaths from trauma-related injuries in children under 18 years is related to traffic accidents [9,10,12-15].

Several studies have attempted to elucidate the risk factors related to deaths from traffic accidents [19-22]. There are human factors, such as driving under the influence of alcohol, stress and fatigue, and excessive speed and inexperience of young drivers. Factors related to the road system include poor road signs, bad road conditions such as poor surface maintenance and a lack of kerbs. Factors related to vehicles include inadequate tire, brake and engine maintenance and a lack of efficient airbags.

Specifically in relation to traffic accidents, this study demonstrated that up to the age of 14 years, there were more cases of injuries to pedestrians, struck by vehicles, than to vehicle occupants. According to studies on African countries, the increased mobility of children in this age group, the fact that they are care-free and walk in

Table 1 Deaths according to mechanism of injury and age groups

Mechanism	Total	<1 year	1-4	5-9	10-14	15-17
	530	25	52	50	94	309
–asphyxia / suffocation	25	18	5	1	-	1
–blunt trauma	14	1	3	1	1	8
–stabb	6	-	-	-	1	5
–drowning	55	1	16	6	14	18
–intoxication	3	1	-	-	-	2
–fall	21	2	5	4	5	5
–burn related	10	-	6	3	-	1
–firearm	249	-	2	4	33	210
–hanging / strangulation	8	1	-	2	2	3
–road traffic related	138	1	15	28	38	56
passenger	44	-	5	9	9	21
pedestrian	77	1	10	18	27	21
train	2	-	-	1	-	1
bicycle	2	-	-	-	1	1
motorcycle	13	-	-	-	1	12
–others	1	-	-	1	-	-

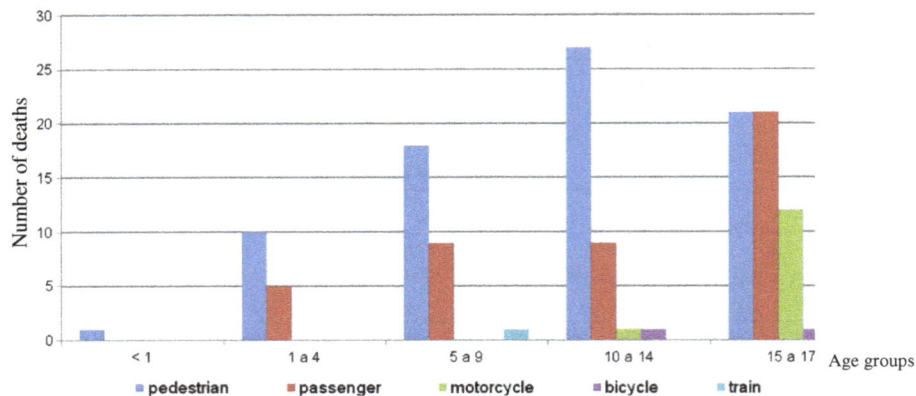

Figure 4 Transport-related deaths by age group.

groups, together with a lack of guidance, all justify a greater number of pedestrian accidents in this age group. The present study shows that in the 15-17 year age group, the frequency of deaths of pedestrians and vehicle occupants were similar. Studies show that in countries like Mexico and Colombia, accidents involving pedestrians are also more frequent [19,21]. This high frequency of accidents involving pedestrians can be related to the high influx of rural migrants to cities because they are not accustomed to the often chaotic traffic of the cities.

The present study revealed that 20% of deaths related to transport accidents were associated with motorcycles. In Brazil, the proportion of deaths related to motorcycle traffic rose from 4.1% in 1996 to 28.4% in 2007 [4]. Carrasco et al. [22] observed that the Campinas' motorcycle fleet is growing four times faster than its population. In 2009, Campinas had 126% more motorcycles than in 2001, and between 2001 and 2009, 479 people died as consequence of motorcycle crashes in the city of Campinas. This type of problem was also observed in parts of Asia and India [12]. Despite the obvious advantages of cost (purchase price, fuel costs per mile and maintenance), many studies have shown that the high risk of fatality and injury is much higher in motorcycle accidents than in other categories of motor vehicles. The vulnerability of motorcyclists is higher and fatality in an accident is 14 times more likely compared to car occupants [22,23]. Despite the laws regulating the use of helmets, safety equipment and the practice of traffic safety most of these rules are blatantly ignored in Brazil by motorcycle drivers.

The cause of death described as drowning is also described as an important cause of death in literature [11,15]. In this series there was a large number of drowning incidents among 1-4 year olds, and another peak among 10-17 year olds. The deaths in the younger age group may be due to negligence or absence of preventive measures such as grids or screens around pools. In a study from India

evaluating deaths in children under 5 years, drowning was the first cause. In the 10-17 age group, these deaths are more common in boys, usually engaged in work activities or recreation near ponds or rivers [15]. Another study conducted in China indicates that the majority of these accidents occur in rural areas [13].

Approximately 50% of deaths in this study occurred at accident scenes, and most of them were due to gunshot wounds. These data are consistent with a study conducted in another region in the state of São Paulo and in several American cities such as Los Angeles, San Francisco and Vermont [24,25]. In another American series, in Colorado, we found that most deaths occurring in less than 24 hours were due to traffic accidents [26].

Regarding intent, this study showed that the primary cause of death was homicide (50.6%), followed by accident (48.5%) and much lower, suicide (0.9%). These data are extremely alarming when considering the growing violence in our society and the social and economic repercussions that this may cause. The same pattern of intent was described in a study conducted in Recife, in the state of Pernambuco, and in another U.S. study conducted in Denver [6,27]. Other studies in Canada, Nepal, South Africa and China show accidents as the leading cause of death in children and adolescents [10,13,28,29]. It is interesting to note that a study in India, relating to the period of 1994 to 2005, showed that there were no cases of homicide in adolescents under 19 years of age [12].

In relation to suicide, this is an emerging problem in developed countries. In the U.S.A., it is the second most common cause of death in children in the 10-14 year age group and in a study conducted in Sweden in 2002, it was the first cause of death among 5-25 year olds [9,12].

Undisputed is the association between violence and alcohol misuse, illicit drug use and availability of firearms [4]. Other factors also related to homicide in younger children were described by Fujiwara et al. [30] in a study conducted in 2009, which used data from the National Violent Injury Statistics System in the U.S.A. The study indicated that the main victims of homicide aged less than 2 years were boys, whose parents had depression and financial problems [30].

The first measure in reducing deaths from trauma-related causes is prevention. These measures are specific to the host, the cause of death and the environmental and social factors surrounding the problem. Much of what has already achieved success in relation to prevention has been linked to active prevention associated with a mix of laws, educational programs and focuses on multidisciplinary and well-distributed teams, as well as the strengthening and organization of the state. In Brazil there are different initiatives bringing together the efforts of Federal, State and Municipal Governments and civil society aimed at addressing violence in general, and specifically among young people [4]. In 2003, the National Congress passed a law known as the Disarmament Statute, ruling on the registration, possession, and commercialization of firearms. In 2004 the government created the National Public Security Force to address urban violence and reinforce the state's presence in regions with high-crime rates [4]. These actions help to explain why gun-related homicides have been trending downward since 2004.

Several studies focused on the prevention of accidents have shown a decrease in the number of deaths, through actions such as the use of smoke detectors, containment systems specifically for children in transport (car seats), use of helmets, protective netting on windows, hedges or fences around swimming pools, and specific laws related to speed limits, zero tolerance to drinking and driving, among other measures [31-34].

This study has the limitation that the deaths occurring in Campinas cannot express the true situation in Brazil, a country with various social disparities. Another limitation is that this epidemiological study considered only deaths, the majority occurring at the scene, and this is not enough to guide prevention programs, since the pediatric trauma population admitted to the hospital is different, mainly according to the cause of trauma. Baracat et al. [35] studying 3,214 children (less than 14 years old) in trauma-related accidents admitted to our university hospital in 1997/1998 observed: males predominated (62.1%); injuries were more common in the 9-13 year age group (33.4%) and 2-5 year age group (27.2%); fall was the cause in 74% of cases, and 89.7% of admissions were of low complexity.

Conclusions

We conclude that among children and adolescents, there is a predominance of deaths arising from trauma-related

injuries amongst males aged 14-17 years, mainly from gunshots and with homicide as the main intention. The gun-related deaths have decreased since 2004. These findings are useful in guiding further development and implementation of intervention measures and prevention strategies in this municipality in order to reduce deaths from trauma-related injuries in children and adolescents.

Competing interests
The authors declare that they have no competing interests.

Authors' contributions
AMF and JB-S participated in the conception, design and intellectual content, literature review, collection, analysis and interpretation of data. TMF and GPF contributed to the medical records, literature review and manuscript writing. MCR and ECB contributed to the statistical analysis and manuscript writing. RC contributed to the conception, design, intellectual content, and manuscript writing. All authors read and approved the final manuscript.

Author details
[1]Pediatric Emergency Division, Hospital de Clinicas, University of Campinas, Campinas, SP, Brazil. [2]Division of Pediatric Surgery, Department of Surgery, School of Medical Sciences, University of Campinas (Unicamp), Campinas, SP, Brazil. [3]School of Medical Sciences, University of Campinas (Unicamp), Rua Alexander Fleming, 181, Cidade Universitária "Prof. Zeferino Vaz", Barão Geraldo, Campinas, SP, Brazil. [4]Division of Trauma Surgery, School of Medical Sciences, University of Campinas (Unicamp), Campinas, SP, Brazil. [5]Pediatric Emergency Division, Department of Pediatrician, School of Medical Sciences, University of Campinas (Unicamp), Campinas, SP, Brazil. [6]The Monroe E. Trout Professor of Surgery, Department of Surgery, Division of Trauma, Surgical Critical Care, and Burns, University of California San Diego, 200 West Arbor Dr, #8896, San Diego, CA 92103-8896, USA.

References
1. Peden M, Oyegbite K, Ozanne-Smith J, Hyder AA, Branche C, Fazlur-Rahman AKM, Rivara F, Bartolomeos K: *World report on child injury prevention.* Geneva: World Health Organization; 2008.
2. Nagaraja J, Menkedick J, Phelan KJ, Ashley P, Zhang X, Lanphear BP: **Deaths from residential injuries in US children and adolescents, 1985-1997.** *Pediatrics* 2005, **116**:454–461.
3. Committee on Child Abuse and Neglect; Committee on Injury, Violence, and Poison Prevention; Council on Community Pediatrics, American Academy of Pediatrics: **Policy statement–child fatality review.** *Pediatrics* 2010, **126**(3):592–596.
4. Reichenheim ME, De Souza ER, Moraes CL, De Mello Jorge MH, da Silva CM, De Souza Minayo MC: **Violence and injuries in Brazil: the effect, progress made, and challenges ahead.** *Lancet* 2011, **377**(9781):1962–1975.
5. Ministério da Saúde: *Sistema de Informação sobre Mortalidade.* Available from URL: http://www.datasus.gov.br/DATASUS Accessed August 30th, 2013.
6. Barros MD, Ximenes R, de Lima ML: **Child and adolescent mortality due to external causes: trends from 1979 to 1995.** *Rev Saude Publica* 2001, **35**:142–149.
7. Gawryszewski VP, Rodrigues EM: **The burden of injury in Brazil, 2003.** *Sao Paulo Med J* 2006, **124**:208–213.
8. Gawryszeski VP: **Injury mortality report for São Paulo State, 2003.** *Sao Paulo Med J* 2007, **125**:139–143.
9. Hjern A, Bremberg S: **Social aetiology of violent deaths in Swedish children and youth.** *J Epidemiol Community Health* 2002, **56**(9):688–692.
10. Pan SY, Ugnat AM, Semenciw R, Desmeules M, Mao Y, Macleod M: **Trends in childhood injury mortality in Canada, 1979-2002.** *Inj Prev* 2006, **12**(3):155–160.
11. Fraga AM, Fraga GP, Stanley C, Costantini TW, Coimbra R: **Children at danger: injury fatalities among children in San Diego County.** *Eur J Epidemiol* 2010, **25**(3):211–217.

12. Kanchan T, Menezes RG: **Mortalities among children and adolescents in Manipal, Southern India.** *J Trauma* 2008, **64**(6):1600–1607.

13. Jiang G, Choi BC, Wang D, Zhang H, Zheng W, Wu T, Chang G: **Leading causes of death from injury and poisoning by age, sex and urban/rural areas in Tianjin, China 1999-2006.** *Injury* 2011, **42**(5):501–506.

14. Bener A, Hussain SJ, Ghaffar A, Abou-Taleb H, El-Sayed HF: **Trends in childhood trauma mortality in the fast economically developing State of Qatar.** *World J Pediatr* 2011, **7**(1):41–44.

15. Ruiz-Casares M: **Unintentional childhood injuries in sub-Saharan Africa: an overview of risk and protective factors.** *J Health Care Poor Underserved* 2009, **20**(4 Suppl):51–67.

16. Brehaut JC, Miller A, Raina P: **Childhood behavior disorders and injuries among children and youth: a population based study.** *Pediatrics* 2003, **111**:262–269.

17. Jagnoor J, Bassani DG, Keay L, Ivers RQ, Thakur JS, Gururaj G, Jha P: **Million death study collaborators: unintentional injury deaths among children younger than 5 years of age in India: a nationally representative study.** *Inj Prev* 2011, **17**(3):151–155.

18. Agran PF, Winn D, Anderson C, Trent R, Walton-Haynes L: **Rates of pediatric and adolescent injuries by year of age.** *Pediatrics* 2001, **108**(3):E45.

19. Hijar M, Chu LD, Kraus JF: **Cross-national comparison of injury mortality: Los Angeles County, California and Mexico City, Mexico.** *Int J Epidemiol* 2000, **29**(4):715–721.

20. Galduróz JC, Caetano R: **Epidemiology of alcohol use in Brazil.** *Rev Bras Psiquiatr* 2004, **26**(Suppl 1):S3–S6.

21. Posada J, Ben-Michael E, Herman A, Kahan E, Richter E: **Death and injury from motor vehicle crashes in Colombia.** *Rev Panam Salud Publica* 2000, **7**(2):88–91.

22. Carrasco CE, Godinho M, De Azevedo Barros MB, Rizoli S, Fraga GP: **Fatal motorcycle crashes: a serious public health problem in Brazil.** *World J Emerg Surg* 2012, **7**(Suppl 1):S5.

23. Lin MR, Chang SH, Huang W, Hwang HF, Pai L: **Factors associated with severity of motorcycle injuries among young adult riders.** *Ann Emerg Med* 2003, **41**(6):783–791.

24. Masella CA, Pinho VF, Costa Passos AD, Spencer Netto FA, Rizoli S, Scarpelini S: **Temporal distribution of trauma deaths: quality of trauma care in a developing country.** *J Trauma* 2008, **65**(3):653–658.

25. Demetriades D, Murray J, Charalambides K, Alo K, Velmahos G, Rhee P, Chan L: **Trauma fatalities: time and location of hospital deaths.** *J Am Col Surg* 2004, **198**(1):20–26.

26. Cothren CC, Moore EE, Hedegaard HB, Meng K: **Epidemiology of urban trauma deaths: a comprehensive reassessment 10 years later.** *World J Surg* 2007, **31**(7):1507–1511.

27. Roaten JB, Partrick DA, Nydam TL, Bensard DD, Hendrickson RJ, Sirotnak AP, Karrer FM: **Nonaccidental trauma is a major cause of morbidity and mortality among patients at a regional level 1 pediatric trauma center.** *J Pediatr Surg* 2006, **41**(12):2013–2015.

28. Sharma G, Shrestha PK, Wasti H, Kadel T, Ghimire P, Dhungana S: **A review of violent and traumatic deaths in Kathmandu, Nepal.** *Int J Inj Contr Saf Promot* 2006, **13**(3):197–199.

29. Meel BL: **Mortality of children in the Transkei region of South Africa.** *Am J Forensic Med Pathol* 2003, **24**(2):141–147.

30. Fujiwara T, Barber C, Schaechter J, Hemenway D: **Characteristics of infant homicides: findings from a U.S. multisite reporting system.** *Pediatrics* 2009, **124**(2):e210–e217.

31. Scholer SJ, Hickson GB, Ray WA: **Sociodemographic factors identify US infants at high risk of injury mortality.** *Pediatrics* 1999, **103**(6 Pt 1):1183–1188.

32. Hoppe-Roberts JM, Lloyd LM, Chyka PA: **Poisoning mortality in the United States: comparison of national mortality statistics and poison control center reports.** *Ann Emerg Med* 2000, **35**(5):440–448.

33. Rimsza ME, Schackner RA, Bowen KA, Marshall W: **Can child deaths be prevented? The Arizona child fatality review program experience.** *Pediatrics* 2002, **110**(1 Pt 1):e11.

34. Gielen AC, McDonald EM, Wilson ME, Hwang WT, Serwint JR, Andrews JS, Wang MC: **Effects of improved access to safety counseling, products, and home visits on parents' safety practices: results of a randomized trial.** *Arch Pediatr Adolesc Med* 2002, **156**(1):33–40.

35. Baracat EC, Paraschin K, Nogueira RJ, Reis MC, Fraga AM, Sperotto G: **Accidents with children in the region of Campinas, Brazil.** *J Pediatr (Rio J)* 2000, **76**(5):368–374.

6

The utility of recombinant factor VIIa as a last resort in trauma

Rishi Mamtani[1], Bartolomeu Nascimento[2], Sandro Rizoli[3], Ruxandra Pinto[4], Yulia Lin[5], Homer Tien[6*]

From World Trauma Congress 2012
Rio de Janeiro, Brazil. 22-25 August 2012

Abstract

Introduction: The use of recombinant factor VII (rFVIIa) as a last resort for the management of coagulopathy when there is severe metabolic acidosis during large bleedings in trauma might be deemed inappropriate. The objective of this study was to identify critical degrees of acidosis and associated factors at which rFVIIa might be considered of no utility.

Methods: All massively transfused ($\geq$ 8 units of red blood cells within 12 hours) trauma patients from Jan 2000 to Nov 2006. Demographic, baseline physiologic and rFVIIa dosage data were collected. Rate of red blood cell transfusion in the first 6 hours of hospitalization (RBC/hr) was calculated and used as a surrogate for bleeding. Last resort use of rFVIIa was defined by a pH$\leq$ 7.02 based on ROC analysis for survival. In-hospital mortality was analyzed in last resort and non-last resort groups. Univariate analysis was performed to assess for differences between groups and identify factors associates with no utility of rFVIIa.

Results: 71 patients who received rFVIIa were analyzed. The pH> 7.02 had 100% sensitivity for the identification of potential survivors. All 11 coagulopathic, severely acidotic (pH $\leq$ 7.02) patients with high rates of bleeding (4RBC/hr) died despite administration of rFVIIa. The financial cost of administering rFVIIa as a last resort to these 11 severely acidotic and coagulophatic cases was $75,162 (CA).

Conclusions: Our study found no utility of rFVIIa in treating severely acidotic, coagulopathic trauma patients with high rates of bleeding; and thus restrictions should be set on its usage in these circumstances.

Introduction

Recombinant Factor VIIa (rFVIIa; Novoseven®, NiaStase®) is a hemostatic agent licensed for the management of hemorrhagic events and averting bleeding during invasive interventions in hemophilia A and B patients with FVIII and FIX inhibitors; acquired hemophilia; congenital deficiency of factor VII; and for the treatment of Glanzmann's thrombasthenia [1-3]. It has also been used off-label and studied in the treatment of coagulopathy in trauma patients [4-7].

The use of rFVIIa for non-approved indications has been formally evaluated in clinical trials (including two randomized controlled trials in trauma) [8-10], and shown to be of no survival benefit [11]; and with clear evidence of harm, particularly in the elderly [12]. Despite the lack of supporting evidence, transfusion guidelines in either military or civilian settings currently suggest the use of rFVIIa as a last resort for the management of refractory coagulopathy in trauma [13-16]. However, when the drug is used in these settings of massive hemorrhage, its efficacy as a pro-hemostatic agent may vary under different physiologic conditions, particularly in acidosis [17,18]. In metabolic acidosis, when pH levels are under 7.2, the activity of rFVIIa is significantly stunted. In fact, an investigation conducted by Meng et al. indicated that the activity of rFVIIa decreased by over 90% at a pH level of 7.0 [17]. Furthermore, high expenditures are associated with off-label use of rFVIIa [19]. Therefore, the use of rFVIIa as a last

* Correspondence: Homer.Tien@sunnybrook.ca
[6]Trauma Services, Division of General Surgery, Sunnybrook Health Sciences Centre and Canadian Forces Health Services, 2075 Bayview Avenue, Room H1 86, Toronto, ON M4N 3M5, USA
Full list of author information is available at the end of the article

resort when there is severe metabolic acidosis during significant hemorrhage in trauma might be considered inappropriate.

We reviewed a cohort of massively transfused trauma patients to whom rFVIIa was administered to evaluate its utility as a last resort for the management of traumatic coagulopathy. The objective of this study was to identify critical degrees of acidosis and associated factors at which the use of rFVIIa might be considered of no utility.

Methods

This study was conducted at Tory Regional Trauma Centre of Sunnybrook Health Sciences Centre (SHSC), a large Canadian Level I adult trauma facility. The study protocol was reviewed and approved by the Hospital Research Ethics Board.

Study cohort

Patient information was obtained from the Blood Bank information system (HCLL, Mediware, N.Y.) at SHSC and the computerized Trauma Registry. The cohort was comprised of patients admitted from January 1, 2000 to November 30, 2006, with the following inclusion criteria: (1) having been massively transfused, defined as having received 8 or more units of red blood cells (RBCs) within the first 12 hours (h) of admission (analogous to established criterion in recent randomized control trials on rFVIIa in trauma) [8,9]; (2) having received rFVIIa; (3) having recorded pH values; (4) and having recorded times during which dosages of rFVIIa were administered (from admission to administration).

Last resort use of rFVIIa was defined based on Receiver Operating Characteristics (ROC) curve analysis for survival. The ROC curve was determined to define a specific pH cutoff at which the test could appropriately discriminate the two groups based on the highest sensitivity for identifying potential survivors. The group with low survival based on the pH cutoff was defined as the group receiving last resort use of rFVIIa.

Data collection

Demographic data were obtained from the Trauma Registry and included the following: age, gender, type of injury, Abbreviated Injury Scale (AIS) score, Injury Severity Score (ISS), and note of discharge or in-hospital mortality. Electronic patient records and manual chart abstraction were used to gather data on in-hospital mortality and admission laboratory values including: platelet counts, hemoglobin level, arterial pH, International Normalized Ratio (INR), and plasma fibrinogen levels. The Blood Bank Information System (HCLL, Mediware, N.Y.) was used to determine patients who received rFVIIa for coagulopathy treatment within the first 24h of admission. The same database was utilized to obtain the time that RBC units were provided, and this information was verified by the hospital chart. The rate of transfusion for the first 6h of hospitalization was determined for all patients in the cohort. In our previous experience, this variable, used as a surrogate marker of the severity of bleeding, has shown to strongly predict 24h in-hospital death [20,21]. The rate of transfusion is also indicative of severity of injury and the urgency of treatment.

The price quote of the supplies of rFVIIa was obtained from the manufacturer and a recently published cost-effectiveness analysis [19,22]. We conducted cost analysis pertaining to the drug's administration as a last resort. We reviewed the monetary prices of rFVIIa dosages in the acidotic patients who died despite receiving the drug.

Outcome measures

The main outcome measure was in-hospital mortality. Secondary outcomes were patient's physiological covariates (ISS, AIS for head injury, gender, age, fibrinogen, rate of RBC transfusion within 6h of hospitalization and INR). The impact of rFVIIa administration was assessed by comparing outcomes between last resort and non-last resort cases. Also, sensitivity, specificity, negative predictive value (NPV) and positive predictive value (PPV) were calculated in relation to pH (defined by the best sensitivity on ROC cut-off for survival) and in-hospital mortality. An additional outcome measure was direct monetary costs associated with the use of rFVIIa for cases deemed inappropriate.

Statistical analysis

The main variables present in this study were pH and in-hospital mortality. Other covariates included pertained to the patient's physiological state (ISS, AIS for head injury, gender, age, base deficit, lactate, fibrinogen, rate of RBC transfusion within 6h of hospitalization and INR).

Last resort use of rFVIIa was defined based on ROC analysis for survival as aforementioned. The ROC curve was determined to define a specific pH cutoff at which the test could appropriately discriminate the two groups based on survival. From this value, the sensitivity, specificity, PPV and NPV were derived.

Potential determinants of rFVIIa failure were analyzed through a subgroup analysis of baseline characteristics, including degree of shock and acidosis, age, ISS, coagulopathy, rFVIIa dose regimens, and rates of RBC transfusion.

Continuous variables were expressed in standard deviations, medians, means, or interquartile ranges (IQR); these were compared using T-test or Mann-Whitney U test. Categorical variables were presented as percentages, and compared using chi-square or Fisher's exact test. All analyses were performed using SAS 9.1 (SAS Institute

Inc., Cary, NC). Two-sided p values were used and statistical significance was set at p < 0.05.

Results

A total of 7,076 patients were seen by the Sunnybrook trauma team during the 6-year study period. Within this group, 328 (4.6%) patients were massively transfused. Of these, 72 (22%) patients received rFVIIa. One patient was excluded due to absent pH data. Upon further investigation, it was noted that this subject had a low numerical ISS score, blunt trauma with no head injury, and received only one dose of 200 µg/kg of rFVIIa, given after 6.9 h in the hospital. He remained stable throughout his hospital stay. Therefore, our study cohort consisted of 71 massively transfused patients who received rFVIIa and had known pH values, meeting our entry criteria. All 71 patients had complete data sets for all variables studied.

The area under the ROC curve analysis for pH and survival was approximately 0.70 for the pH value 7.02, which had the highest sensitivity to identify survivors. The sensitivity of pH > 7.02 to identify survival was 100% and specificity of pH ≤ 7.02 for in-hospital mortality was 100%. The PPV was 56.7% and the NPV was 100%. The use of this best cut-off for pH based on the ROC curve for our subgroup analysis is supported by previous research suggesting that the efficacy of rFVIIa decreases by 90% when the body pH decreases from 7.4 to 7.0 [17]. Therefore, we divided our cohort into 2 groups based on admission pH (patients with pH ≤ 7.02 were analyzed in the last resort group while patients with pH > 7.02 in the non-last resort group). Clinical characteristics and demographics of the entire study cohort and subgroups based on pH are summarized in Table 1. Overall, there were no

significant differences between the two subgroups with respect to age, gender, type of injury, ISS, Head AIS, and dose of rFVIIa given. Baseline coagulation profiles showed significant differences in platelets (p < 0.01) and INR (p = 0.03), except for fibrinogen (p = 0.07). Additionally, the rate of bleeding using transfusion as a surrogate marker was significantly higher in the severely acidotic group (4 RBC units per hour ± 1.5 vs. 3 ± 1.7; p=0.03).

A comparison of mortality between the two groups is shown in Table 2. Of the 11 severely acidotic (pH ≤ 7.02) patients in the last resort group, all (100%) died. Of the 60 less acidotic (pH > 7.02) patients in the non-last resort group, 26 (43%) died.

The vast majority, 72% of rFVIIa-treated patients received only 1 dose, while 24% received 2 doses, and 4% received 3 doses after being admitted to the hospital. The first dose was administered after a median time interval of 4.5h (2.7, 7.7). Repeated doses were administered after an average time interval of 2.3h. This indicated that as the patient's condition deteriorated, more doses of rFVIIa were administered in an expedited fashion. The median initial dose was 85.7µg/kg (61.6, 102.8). This was also the overall median dosage, as most patients only received 1 dose.

Of note, a transfusion medicine specialist at SHSC approved the use of rFVIIa as a final alternative when all potential interventions failed. In the years 2000 and 2001, low doses of 17.1µg/kg of rFVIIa were administered after patients received more than 20 units of RBCs. However, following a supportive randomized control trial on rFVIIa in trauma [8], fewer units of RBCs were noted to be transfused prior to rFVIIa administration and more doses of rFVIIa were given from 2002 onwards.

Table 1 Demographics & Baseline Characteristics

Variable	Last resort (n=11)	Non-last resort (n=60)	P Value
Age (years)	27 (22, 39)	35 (24, 48)	0.14
Male (%)	82	63	0.3
Penetrating (%)	45	28	0.2
ISS	47 (±16)	43(±15)	0.4
Head AIS	0 (0, 2)	2 (0, 5)	0.1
Platelets	76 (±57)	184 (±95)	<0.01
Fibrinogen	0.64 (±0.3)	0.9 (±0.5)	0.07
INR	2.1 (1.8,2.7)	1.4(1.2, 1.6)	0.03
Hemoglobin	83 (±17)	100 (±28)	0.02
pH	6.87 (±0.11)	7.26 (±0.11)	<0.01
Rate of Bleeding (RBC/hr)	4 (±1.5)	3 (±1.7)	0.03
Time to rFVIIa (hr)	3.7 (±2.2)	6.2 (4.5)	0.04
rFVIIa Dose (ug/Kg)	89 (±43)	116 (±79)	0.14
> 1 rFVIIa doses (%)	9	33	0.05

Values are presented as mean (±SD) or median (IQR - Interquartile Range) when appropriate. ISS, injury severity score; AIS, abbreviated injury scale; INR, international normalized ratio; RBC/hr, units of red blood cells per hour in the first 6 hrs of admission; Statistical significance was set at p<0.05

Table 2 pH & In-hospital Mortality

	Alive	Dead	Hospital Mortality
pH > 7.02 (n=60)	34	26	43%
pH ≤ 7.02 (n=11)	0	11	100%
Sensitivity 100% (34/34)	**Specificity** 30% (11/37)	**(PPV)** 57% (34/60)	**(NPV)** 100% (11/11)

PPV, positive predictive value; NPV, negative predictive value

The total cost of administrating sufficient doses of rFVIIa to the 11 patients as a last resort was approximately $75,162 (CA). This monetary cost was measured solely based on the amounts of doses of rFVIIa given and excluded other expenditures associated with the administration of the drug. In the United States of America, a low dose (1,200 µg or 17.1µg/kg on a 70 kg average adult) of rFVIIa is the smallest available unit dose that costs approximately the same as 8 units of plasma [23]. The price of one unit of plasma is approximately $120 (USD), including expenditures related to administering them [23].

Discussion

Over the last decade, rFVIIa has been explored as a potential treatment for many coagulopathic states other than congenital conditions and hemophilias [7,11,24]. Theoretically, rFVIIa seems to be an appealing option following trauma because of its systemic intravenous administration and swift mechanism of action, acting at the injury site by binding to exposed tissue factor, and expediting the generation of thrombin on activated platelets to propel the coagulation cascade forward. However, in the context of massive hemorrhage, there are potential limiting factors such as acidosis and refractory shock.

From this study, a pH of 7.02 had the best sensitivity on the ROC curve for discriminating survivors and non-survivors. A pH > 7.02 was 100% sensitive at identifying potential survivors, reassuring the clinician that no probable survivors could have been missed if this pH cut-off was adopted. Thus, a pH of 7.02 may be used as a potential guideline or measure at which the administration of rFVIIa should not be considered for patients who are severely acidotic. The pH level of these patients appeared to be a key determining factor in the success of rFVIIa. As noted, there was a remarkable 100% mortality noted in coagulopathic and severely acidotic patients (pH ≤ 7.02) who had high bleeding rates, despite the use of rFVIIa. This is corroborated by recent research suggesting that the efficacy of rFVIIa decreases by 90% when the body pH decreases from 7.4 to 7.0 [17]. However, in a recent animal model of lactic acidosis, the effectiveness of rFVIIa in correcting abnormal

INR values at a mean pH of 7.14 was unaffected [18]. This suggests that other factors may influence its efficacy in clinical settings.

In keeping with our findings, data from the Australia and New Zealand Haemostasis Registry on 10 years of the use of rFVIIa in Australia and New Zealand which reports on the outcomes of 2181 trauma cases, the single most important predictor of the effect of rFVIIa on bleeding and 28-day mortality was pH [25]. In their multivariate analysis, for every 0.1 decline in pH, there were associated increases in non-responders to rFVIIa use and mortality rates [25]. Their unadjusted analysis on the relationship between 28-day mortality and pH showed that patients with pH < 6.90 had a mortality rate of 98% while the group with 7.30<pH<7.39 had a mortality of 23% [25]. Although the pH of 6.90 did not coincide with our threshold of 7.02, the pattern is apparent that mortality percentage drastically increases with decreases in pH. Logistic regression analysis was conducted and values for the odds ratio were obtained for the effect on bleeding and pH, as well as 28-day mortality and pH. For both, an inverse correlation was seen, in that when pH decreased, the odds ratio for mortality increased [25]. Furthermore, outside of the trauma literature, a study by Karkouti et al. found that the administration of rFVIIa should be expedited in order to increase its efficacy in cardiac surgery [24].

An additional factor that must be considered is the impact of other variables, such as rate of bleeding and baseline physiologic factors on rFVIIa, particularly temperature. Hypothermia is a well-known complication seen in the natural progression of traumatic injury, blood loss, hypovolemia, and shock [26]. While our study identifies correlations of pH with the effectiveness of rFVIIa, a recently conducted study by Meng et al., suggests that a decrease in temperature from 37°C to 33°C also results in a reduction of rFVIIa's activity by 20% [17]. The Australia and New Zealand Haemostasis Registry also presented graphical data pertaining to the effect of decreases in temperature and response of bleeding to rFVIIa administration in trauma patients. In fact, for ≤ 33.5°C, 70.7% of trauma patients had an unchanged bleeding response; and for normal physiologic temperature range (36.6-37.5°C), 38% had an unchanged bleeding response after receiving rFVIIa [25]. The registry also found that as pH is decreased, the activity of rFVIIa is reduced [25]. Finally, a study by Knudson et al analyzed subgroup of patients who received rFVIIa and lived at least 24 hr versus those who received rFVIIa and died. In this study, predictors of death included a low pH, a low platelet count, a more severe base deficit, and a higher transfusion rate [27]. In our present study, higher transfusion rates were also associated with failure of rFVIIa and increased mortality. These findings indicate that the efficacy of rFVIIa in coagulopathic, acidotic patients with high rates of bleeding is compromised with pH and temperature reductions.

As the patient's condition deteriorates over time due to failure of standard therapies, the pH drastically decreases and the activity of rFVIIa is virtually nonexistent, which makes it a challenge to consider the use of rFVIIa as a last resort. Thus, current recommendations on its use as an alternative to manage coagulopathy in trauma when other interventions fail should be taken with caution.

The high monetary cost of rFVIIa administration, with no strong evidence of survival benefit [7,11] and increased risks of thrombotic complications [12], also calls for a review of guidelines recommending the use of this medication for traumatic coagulopathy. The cost-effectiveness of using rFVIIa as a last resort therapy for critical bleeding requiring massive transfusion was recently evaluated [19]. The incremental costs of rFVIIa increased with severity of illness and transfusion requirement, and were unacceptably high (> US$100,000 per life-year) for most patients [19]. Overall, thought must be given to the expense of rFVIIa, and its utility as a last resort.

Alternatively, a more affordable and effective management strategy for traumatic coagulopathy is available. A recently conducted large randomized control trial (CRASH-2) involving 20,000 patients found that tranexamic acid reduced the risk of death in hemorrhaging trauma patients and should be recommended in bleeding trauma situations [28]. International cost-analyses supporting the use of tranexamic acid as opposed to administering rFVIIa found that the cost of giving tranexamic acid compared to not giving it was $18,025 in Tanzania, $20,760 in India and $48,002 in the UK [29]. The case being made for increased administration of tranexamic acid is bolstered by the lack of increased thromboembolic events observed in the CRASH-2 trial. In Total Knee Arthroplasty (TKA), a reduction in the number of blood transfusions has also been observed with no increase in symptomatic thromboembolic phenomena [30]. Tranexamic acid may not only be helpful from a biological perspective, but also in a monetary manner, in reducing resources in obtaining and providing blood products [30,31].

Limitations
The main limitations of this study are its retrospective nature, small size of the severely acidotic (pH ≤ 7.02) subgroup, and the changes over time with respect to the use of rFVIIa. Towards the start of the study period, this drug was dosed as low as 17.1μg/kg, and was considered as a final alternative therapy. However, further to research advances at the time, a shift towards increased doses and earlier use was noted by the year 2002, which continued to evolve until the end of the study period. This may also have had some impact upon observed results. The pH data reflects the patient's condition on arrival, which might not represent changes in degrees of acidosis immediately before the administration of the drug. However, the drug was administered only 3.7h after admission for the severely acidotic group and 6.2h for the less acidotic patients when other standard therapies had failed; thus a worsening pH level is intuitively expected in these clinical situations. The area under the ROC curve was tabulated to be 0.70, indicating potential for a more accurate cutoff for determining at which pH range the administration of rFVIIa should be more reserved. Finally, we did not have information on all co-morbidities that may have contributed to mortality.

Conclusions
Our study found no utility of rFVIIa in treating coagulopathic trauma patients with pH ≤ 7.02 and high rates of bleeding (4 units of RBC/h); and thus restrictions should be set on its usage in these circumstances. Furthermore, the lack of evidence demonstrating any survival benefit of rFVIIa in trauma, in conjunction with the potential increased risk of thromboembolic complications and high monetary costs of its off-label use, renders its utility highly questionable in such situations.

Future research should be conducted in finding alternatives to rFVIIa in the management of trauma coagulopathy. We hope our findings will guide physicians when deciding on the inclusion of this drug as part of massive transfusion protocols in trauma.

Abbreviations used
RBC: Red Blood Cell; rFVIIa: Recombinant Factor 7a; AIS: Abbreviated Injury Score; ISS: Injury Severity Score; INR: International Normalized Ratio.

Acknowledgments
The authors thank Cyndy Rogers, Bill Sharkey, Ahmed Coovadia and Connie Colavecchia for their contribution in providing trauma registry and blood bank data.
This article has been published as part of *World Journal of Emergency Surgery* Volume 7 Supplement 1, 2012: Proceedings of the World Trauma Congress 2012. The full contents of the supplement are available online at http://www.wjes.org/supplements/7/S1.

Author details
[1]Sunnybrook Health Sciences Centre, 2075 Bayview Avenue, Room H113, Toronto, ON M4N 3M5, Canada. [2]Trauma Program, Department of Surgery, Sunnybrook Health Sciences Centre, 2075 Bayview Avenue, Room B5 12, Toronto, ON M4N 3M5, Canada. [3]Departments of Surgery and Critical Care Medicine, Sunnybrook Health Sciences Centre, University of Toronto, Canada. [4]Sunnybrook Health Sciences Centre, 2075 Bayview Avenue, Room K3W-25, Toronto, ON M4N 3M5, Canada. [5]Sunnybrook Health Sciences Centre, 2075 Bayview Avenue, Room B2 04, Toronto, ON M4N 3M5, Canada. [6]Trauma Services, Division of General Surgery, Sunnybrook Health Sciences Centre

and Canadian Forces Health Services, 2075 Bayview Avenue, Room H1 86, Toronto, ON M4N 3M5, USA.

Authors' contributions
RM participated in the writing of the manuscript and was responsible for following the final submission guidelines. BN contributed to the study design; data collection and analysis; writing of the manuscript; and manuscript review. SR participated in the study design; its writing; and review. RP provided statistical support and reviewed the manuscript. YL participated in the writing and review of the manuscript. HT participated in the study conception; its writing; and review.

Competing interests and disclaimer
BN is the recipient of the 2010 National Blood Foundation Grant for the conduct of research related to coagulopathy in trauma. SR has been a consultant for Novo-nordisk, the manufacturer of Recombinant FVIIa. YL is a site investigator for a registry on the off-label use of recombinant factor VIIa that is funded by an unrestricted educational grant from Novo Nordisk. The other authors have no conflict of interest to declare.

References

1. Hedner U: **Mechanism of action, development and clinical experience of recombinant FVIIa.** *J Biotechnol* 2006, **124**(4):747-57, Epub 2006 May 12. Review.
2. Parameswaran R, Shapiro AD, Gill JC, *et al*: **Dose effect and efficacy of rFVIIa in the treatment of haemophilia patients with inhibitors: analysis from the Hemophilia and Thrombosis Research Society Registry.** *Haemophilia* 2005, **11**(2):100-6.
3. Hedner U: **Recombinant factor VIIa: its background, development and clinical use.** *Curr Opin Hematol* 2007, **14**:225-9, doi: 10.1097/MOH. 0b013e3280dce57b.
4. Kenet G, Walden R, Eldad A, *et al*: **Treatment of traumatic bleeding with recombinant factor VIIa.** *Lancet* 1999, **354**(9193):1879.
5. Martinowitz U, Kenet G, Lubetski A, *et al*: **Possible role of recombinant activated factor VII (rFVIIa) in the control of hemorrhage associated with massive trauma.** *Can J Anaesth* 2002, **49**(10):S15-20.
6. Mohr AM, Holcomb JB, Dutton RP, *et al*: **Recombinant activated factor VIIa and hemostasis in critical care: a focus on trauma.** *Crit Care* 2005, **9**(Suppl 5):S37-42, Epub 2005 Oct 7.
7. Barletta JF, Ahrens CL, Tyburski JG, *et al*: **A review of recombinant factor VII for refractory bleeding in nonhemophilic trauma patients.** *J Trauma* 2005, **58**(3):646-51.
8. Boffard KD, Riou B, Warren B, *et al*: **NovoSeven Trauma Study Group. Recombinant factor VIIa as adjunctive therapy for bleeding control in severely injured trauma patients: two parallel randomized, placebo-controlled, double-blind clinical trials.** *J Trauma* 2005, **59**(1):8-15, discussion 15-8.
9. Hauser CJ, Boffard K, Dutton R, *et al*: **CONTROL Study Group. Results of the CONTROL trial: efficacy and safety of recombinant activated Factor VII in the management of refractory traumatic hemorrhage.** *J Trauma* 2010, **69**(3):489-500.
10. Dutton RP, Parr M, Tortella BJ, *et al*: **Recombinant Activated Factor VII Safety in Trauma Patients: Results from the CONTROL Trial.** *J Trauma* 2011, **71**(1):12-19.
11. Lin Y, Stanworth SJ, Birchall J, *et al*: **Recombinant factor VIIa for the prevention and treatment of bleeding in patients without haemophilia.** *Cochrane Database Syst Rev* 2011, , **2**: CD005011.
12. Levi M, Levy JH, Andersen HF, *et al*: **Safety of recombinant activated factor VII in randomized clinical trials.** *N Engl J Med* 2010, **363**(19):1791-800, Erratum in: N Engl J Med. 2011 Nov 17;365(20):1944.
13. Wade CE, Eastridge BJ, Jones JA, *et al*: **Use of recombinant factor VIIa in US military casualties for a five-year period.** *J Trauma* 2010, **69**(2):353-9.
14. Woodruff SI, Dougherty AL, Dye JL, *et al*: **Use of recombinant factor VIIA for control of combat-related haemorrhage.** *Emerg Med J* 2010, **27**(2):121-4.
15. Rossaint R, Bouillon B, Cerny V, *et al*: **Management of bleeding following major trauma: an updated European guideline.** *Crit Care* 2010, **14**(2):R52.
16. Vincent JL, Rossaint R, Riou B, *et al*: **Recommendations on the use of recombinant activated factor VII as an adjunctive treatment for massive bleeding-a European perspective.** *Crit Care* 2006, **10**(4):R120.
17. Meng ZH, Wolberg AS, Monroe DM 3rd, *et al*: **The effect of temperature and pH on the activity of factor VIIa: implications for the efficacy of high-dose factor VIIa in hypothermic and acidotic patients.** *J Trauma* 2003, **55**(5):886-91.
18. Lesperance RN, Lehmann RK, Harold DM, *et al*: **Recombinant Factor VII is Effective at Reversing Coagulopathy in a Lactic Acidosis Model.** *J Trauma* 2011, [Epub ahead of print].
19. Ho KM, Litton E: **Cost-effectiveness of using recombinant activated factor VII as an off-label rescue treatment for critical bleeding requiring massive transfusion.** *Transfusion* 2011, doi: 10.1111/j.1537-2995.2011.03505.x. [Epub ahead of print].
20. Nascimento B, Lin Y, Callum J, *et al*: **Recombinant factor VIIa is associated with an improved 24-hour survival without an improvement in inpatient survival in massively transfused civilian trauma patients.** *Clinics (Sao Paulo)* 2011, **66**(1):101-6.
21. Rizoli SB, Nascimento B Jr, Osman F, *et al*: **Recombinant activated coagulation factor VII and bleeding trauma patients.** *J Trauma* 2006, **61**(6):1419-25.
22. David : **Recombinant Activated Human Factor VII (NovoSeven).** [http://www.canadianmedicine4all.com/recombinant-activated-human-factor-vii-novoseven.html].
23. Stein DM, Dutton RP, Hess JR, *et al*: **Low-dose recombinant factor VIIa for trauma patients with coagulopathy.** *Injury* 2008, **39**(9):1054-61.
24. Karkouti K, Beattie WS, Arellano R, *et al*: **Comprehensive Canadian Review of the Off-Label Use of Recombinant Activated Factor VII in Cardiac Surgery.** *Circulation* 2008, **118**(4):331-8, Epub 2008 Jul 7.
25. James I, John M: **Australia and New Zealand Haemostasis Registry.** Monsah University, Australia; 2010.
26. Hess JR, Brohi K, Dutton RP, *et al*: **The Coagulopathy of Trauma: A Review of Mechanisms.** *J Trauma* 2008, **65**(4):748-54, Review.
27. Knudson MM, Cohen MJ, Reidy R, *et al*: **Trauma, Transfusions, and Use of Recombinant Factor VIIa: A Multicenter Case Registry Report of 380 patients from the Western Trauma Association.** *J Am Coll Surg* 2011, **212**(1):87-95, Epub 2010 Nov 5.
28. CRASH-2 Trial Collaborators: **Effects of tranexamic acid on death, vascular occlusive events, and blood transfusion in trauma patients with significant haemorrhage (CRASH-2) a randomized, placebo-controlled trial.** *Lancet* 2010, **376**(9734):23-32, Epub 2010 Jun 14.
29. Guerriero C, Cairns J, Perel P, *et al*: **Cost-effectiveness analysis of administering tranexamic acid to bleeding trauma patients using evidence from the CRASH-2 trial.** *PLoS One* 2011, **6**(5):e18987.
30. Charoencholvanich K, Siriwattanasakul P: **Tranexamic Acid Reduces Blood Loss and Blood Transfusion after TKA: A Prospective Randomized Controlled Trial.** *Clin Orthop Relat Res* 2011, Epub ahead of print.
31. Sepah YJ, Umer M, Ahmad T, *et al*: **Use of Tranexamic acid is a cost effective method in preventing blood loss during and after total knee replacement.** *J Orthop Surg Res* 2011, **6**(1):22.

7

Right diaphragmatic injury and lacerated liver during a penetrating abdominal trauma

Antonino Agrusa[*], Giorgio Romano, Daniela Chianetta, Giovanni De Vita, Giuseppe Frazzetta, Giuseppe Di Buono, Vincenzo Sorce and Gaspare Gulotta

Abstract

Introduction: Diaphragmatic injuries are rare consequences of thoracoabdominal trauma and they often occur in association with multiorgan injuries. The diaphragm is a difficult anatomical structure to study with common imaging instruments due to its physiological movement. Thus, diaphragmatic injuries can often be misunderstood and diagnosed only during surgical procedures. Diagnostic delay results in a high rate of mortality.

Methods: We report the management of a clinical case of a 45-old man who came to our observation with a stab wound in the right upper abdomen. The type or length of the knife used as it was extracted from the victim after the fight. CT imaging demonstrated a right hemothorax without pulmonary lesions and parenchymal laceration of the liver with active bleeding. It is observed hemoperitoneum and subdiaphragmatic air in the abdomen, as a bowel perforation. A complete blood count check revealed a decrease in hemoglobin (7 mg/dl), and therefore it was decided to perform surgery in midline laparotomy.

Conclusion: In countries with a low incidence of inter-personal violence, stab wound diaphragmatic injury is particularly rare, in particular involving the right hemidiaphragm. Diaphragmatic injury may be underestimated due to the presence of concomitant lesions of other organs, to a state of shock and respiratory failure, and to the difficulty of identifying diaphragmatic injuries in the absence of high sensitivity and specific diagnostic instruments. Diagnostic delay causes high mortality with these traumas with insidious symptoms. A diaphragmatic injury should be suspected in the presence of a clinical picture which includes hemothorax, hemoperitoneum, anemia and the presence of subdiaphragmatic air in the abdomen.

Keyword: Diaphragmatic injury, Penetrating abdominal trauma, Diaphragmatic repair, Liver laceration, Stab wound

Background

Diaphragmatic injuries are a diagnostic and therapeutic challenge for the surgeon. They are often un recognized, and diagnostic delay causes high mortality from these injuries [1]. In countries with a low incidence of inter-personal violence, it is quite a rare trauma, with only 4-5% of patients undergoing laparotomy for trauma presenting a diaphragmatic injury [2]. These are mainly caused by blunt trauma of the chest and abdomen (75%) and, more rarely, by penetrating ones (25%) [3]. Clinical presentation varies from a state of hemodynamic instability secondary to bleeding of the diaphragm and organs involved in the trauma [4] to a condition of intestinal obstruction and respiratory failure that can occur months, or even years, after the trauma, due to diaphragmatic hernia [5]. Diagnosis is made difficult both by the frequent presence of concomitant multi-organ injuries that deviate the surgeon's attention from the diaphragm, and by the lack of adequate diagnostic imaging studies regarding the diaphragmatic muscle. In hemodynamically stable patients with penetrating wound of the abdomen, in which there is a strong suspicion of diaphragmatic injury, with a given negative diagnostic imaging, laparoscopy is considered a valuable

* Correspondence: antonino.agrusa@unipa.it
Department of General Surgery, Urgency and Organ Transplantation, University of Palermo, Via L. Giuffrè, Palermo 5 90127, Italy

diagnostic and therapeutic tool in the presence of experienced surgeons. In hemodynamically unstable patients a midline laparotomy is the recommended approach as it allows exploration of the entire abdominal cavity [6].

Methods

We report the clinical case of a 45 year-old man who came to our observation with a stab wound in the right upper abdomen, without cyanosis or dyspnea. Blood pressure was 130/80 mmHg and hemoglobin 12.5 mg/dl. On clinical examination, the patient had a lacerated, bleeding stab wound in the right upper quadrant through which part of the omentum, without other macroscopically visible injuries, could be seen. The type or length of the knife used as it was extracted from the victim after the fight. A focused assessment with sonography for trauma (FAST) test was carried out which showed subdiaphragmatic and perihepatic blood. Due to abundant tympanites and lack of cooperation on the part of the patient, nothing more could be seen. It was decided to have to patient undergo a CT scan of the abdomen to determine if there were any lesions to the abdominal organs.

From the scan, the presence of a right hemothorax without pulmonary lesions was seen, with moderate hemoperitoneum from an active bleeding parenchymal liver laceration and subdiaphragmatic air in the abdomen as a bowel perforation (Figure 1). Initially, the suspect of a bowel perforation suggested a laparoscopic approach, but the patient's hemodynamic condition rapidly changed. In the operating room, the patient presented pale with tachycardia; blood pressure decreased to 90/60 mm Hg and cardiac frequency increased to 115 bpm. A complete blood count check revealed a decrease in hemoglobin (7 mg/dl), and therefore it was decided to perform surgery in midline laparotomy [6,7]. After laparotomy, a significant amount of blood was evacuated to identify the site of bleeding. Liver inspection showed an 8 cm long, 1 cm deep laceration with active bleeding in segments IV-V (Grade II lesion classification AAST). A careful inspection of the abdominal cavity also showed a 12 cm length right diaphragmatic lesion with

signs of active bleeding that accounted for the presence of free air seen in the CT images. No other intestinal lesions were found. Temporary packing was used to treat the liver bleeding. After evacuating the right hemothorax, we proceeded with repair of the diaphragmatic lesion with nonabsorbable sutures, and by placing a thoracic Bouleau drainage. The suture was completed applying a medicated sponge containing thrombin and human fibrinogen in order to control hemostasis and facilitate the building of the tissues and healing process [8]. After stopping the bleeding from the liver and bile leakage it was decided to adopt a conservative approach applying hemostatic matrix on liver injury (Figure 2). Surgery was concluded with the placement of abdominal drains, in the right subphrenic space. One transfusion was carried out during surgery. In post-operative time, blood pressure was 120/80 mmHg, hemoglobin 9 mg/dl. Chest tube was removed 4 days post surgery, after an x-ray which confirmed resolution of hemopneumothorax.

Discussion

The diaphragm is the principle muscle of respiration. With the contraction of striated muscle fibers it carries more than 70% of the work creating a negative intrathoracic pressure which is necessary for the proper performance of respiratory mechanics, as well as encouraging proper venous return to the heart. The integrity of the diaphragm separates the chest cavity from abdominal positive pressure, which ensures proper maintenance of the different pressure regimes of the two chambers, and prevents the migration of the abdominal organs into the chest. A laceration of the diaphragm produces an alteration of these physiological mechanisms with possible migration of the abdominal viscera into the thorax and the disappearance of the thoraco-abdominal pressure gradient which causes alteration of respiratory mechanics, compression of the vena cava with reduced venous return to the heart, and consequential respiratory failure and cardiovascular collapse [9]. Diaphragmatic rupture is a potentially lethal clinical condition for the patient and a delayed or missed diagnosis causes high mortality with this type of trauma [1].

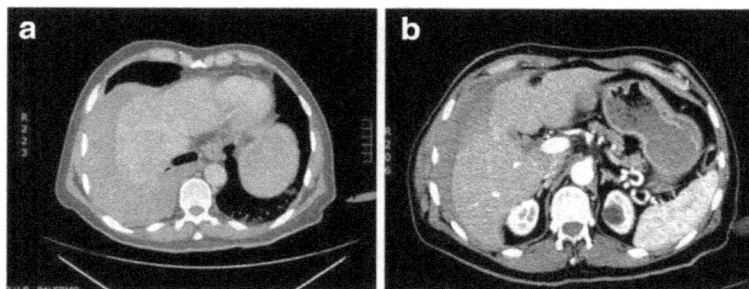

Figure 1 Computed tomography results of the patient. a) presence of a right hemothorax without pulmonary lesions; **b)** discrete hemoperitoneum by an active bleeding parenchymal liver laceration and "free air" in the abdomen.

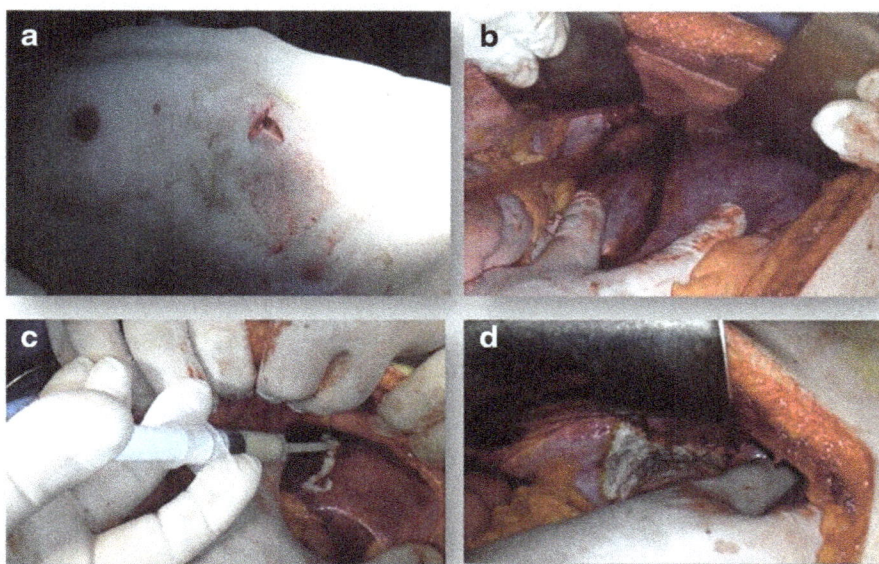

Figure 2 Characteristics of the stab wound and intra-operative findings. a) bleeding stab wound in the right upper quadrant; **b)** liver laceration and right diaphragmatic injury; **c)** application of hemostatic matrix (Floseal®) on liver lesion; **d)** repair of diaphragmatic lesion with non-absorbables sutures and positioning of medicated sponge containing thrombin and human fibrinogen (Tachosil®).

In literature, the first description of diaphragmatic trauma dates back to the sixteenth century when in 1853 Bowditch described a diaphragmatic injury, in a dead victim of a gunshot penetrating trauma, during the autopsy [5]. The first repair with favorable outcomes of a penetrating diaphragmatic injury was described by Riolfi in 1886, while in 1900 Walker published the first repair of traumatic diaphragmatic gunshot lesion with favorable outcomes [10].

It is difficult to accurately estimate the real incidence of diaphragmatic injuries due to delayed or missed diagnosis and pre-hospital deaths [1]. Approximately 5% of patients with abdominal trauma at the time of thoracotomy or laparotomy have a diaphragmatic injury [2]. They are mainly caused by blunt trauma of the chest and abdomen (75%) and more rarely by stabbing (25%) [3]. Diaphragmatic injuries mainly affect the male sex (M/F ratio 3:1) generally occur following closed thoracoabdominal trauma and more rarely penetrating trauma [11]. Mortality rate ranges from 1% to 28%; this high percentage depends upon frequency of associated injuries but also on the delay between diagnosis and the traumatic event [3]. Diaphragmatic injuries frequently occur during automobile accidents; frontal impact causes an increase of intra-abdominal pressure resulting in a lesion in the radial wall posterolateral to the diaphragm [3]. Side impacts also may be associated with lesions of the liver or spleen in 96% of cases [11]. Diaphragmatic injuries during penetrating trauma of the abdomen are extremely rare, making up 25%, of which 20% from gunshot and 5% from weapon [3]. In the course of

penetrating trauma to the abdomen small sized diaphragmatic lesions are often created, which may initially remain undetected and determinate the onset of a diaphragmatic hernia. Right hemidiaphragm trauma is less frequent than left trauma (with a ratio of 1:3) and also is diagnosed with greater delay. This is due to the protective function of the liver which lies on the right abdominal surface preventing herniation of the abdominal viscera into the thorax [9]. Furthermore, many studies performed on cadavers show that during closed trauma the pressure required to determine a lesion of the left hemidiaphragm is less than that required for the right side. [12]. Any discontinuity of the diaphragm leads to alterations of mechanical respiration and circulatory collapse until cardio circulatory system [13]. In severe multiple trauma with patient in a state of shock, respiratory failure and/or coma, diaphragmatic injuries can be misunderstood, as often the attention of the medical team is on damage to other organs which often occur in the course of this type of trauma. In acute phases, diaphragmatic rupture usually occurs with thoracoabdominal pain, hypotension, hemodynamic instability, dyspnea, and cyanosis. Hemodynamic instability and shock are often the result of associated injuries and bleeding of the diaphragmatic muscle injury [14]. When the diaphragmatic lesion is small, it may go unrecognized for several hours, weeks or even months and manifest late and progressively as a diaphragmatic hernia with the appearance of typical symptoms of intestinal obstruction, tachycardia, dyspnea [15]. Small injury of the right hemidiaphragm may even remain undetected due to the protective function offered by the liver, which prevents bowel herniation into the thorax cavity. There is rarely herniation of the liver [16]. Preoperative diagnosis of diaphragmatic injury still represents a diagnostic challenge for the radiologist. The high mortality of this trauma is also linked to the difficulty of studying this anatomical site in emergency conditions [1]. In a chest x-ray, a diaphragmatic injury should be suspected when the hemidiaphragm is not correctly placed. The specific signs of a diaphragmatic lesion on chest x-rays are represented by the presence of air-fluid levels in the chest and the salience of a hemidiaphragm compared to the contralateral side. Chest x-ray has a diagnostic accuracy of less than 40% and can only detect indirect signs described, the absence of which does not rule out a diaphragmatic lesion [17]. Diagnostic accuracy is four times greater for lesions of the left hemidiaphragm (42%) compared to the right (17%) [8]. Chest x-ray has been replaced by computed tomography (CT) which has a diagnostic sensitivity of 50% for right hemidiaphragm lesions and of 70% for the left side ones. It allows the physician to see any discontinuity of the diaphragmatic profile and the presence of loops or omentum in the thoracic cavity, as well as the presence of hemoperitoneum and hemothorax [17]. Historically, CT showed poor visualization of the diaphragm due to motion of the muscle itself, but the advent of multiphasic spiral CT has led to a sensitivity of 80% and a specificity of 90% [18]. CT is a valuable diagnostic tool, readily available in trauma centers and executable in hemodynamically stable patients with multiple trauma. In hemodynamically unstable patients, ultrasound (US), and in particular FAST in real time can demonstrate the absence or reduced motility of the diaphragm suggestive of lesions of the muscle itself, with an accuracy of 30%. In addition, the US can identify the presence of indirect signs such as hemothorax and hemoperitoneum [19]. Magnetic resonance imaging (MRI) has a sensitivity and specificity of 95% in identifying a diaphragmatic lesion, it is not always available in emergency rooms, but extremely helpful in the diagnosis of post-traumatic diaphragmatic hernias [20].

Thus, in the absence of a bowel herniation through the lesion, it is very difficult to diagnose a diaphragmatic lesion with the conventional images that are readily available in emergency conditions [21]. This observation is even more valid when penetrating injuries affect the right upper quadrant of the abdomen. In these cases, the liver, due to its particular anatomical position, stands between the lesion and the viscera preventing diaphragmatic herniation of the latter into the chest through the opening in the diaphragm, accounting for the delay in diagnosis of this type of diaphragmatic injury [22]. In this case, there are indirect signs such as effusion into the thorax and abdomen, principally if there is a lacerated liver (98% of cases) and the presence of subdiaphragmatic air in the abdomen. In hemodynamically stable patients with penetrating injury of the abdomen in which there is a strong clinical suspicion of diaphragmatic hernia, laparoscopy is indicated as, in addition to having a diagnostic role [6,23] inidentifying the presence of associated lesions, when possible, it also allows repair of the torn diaphragm with a non-absorbable suture sutures [6]. In hemodynamically unstable patients a midline laparotomy is the recommended approach as it allows exploration of the entire abdominal cavity. The diaphragmatic lesion is repaired with non-absorbable suture after placement of chest tube.

In countries with a low incidence of inter-personal violence, stab wound diaphragmatic injury is particularly rare, in particular involving the right hemidiaphragm. Diaphragmatic injury may be underestimated due to the presence of concomitant lesions of other organs, to a state of shock and respiratory failure, and to the difficulty of identifying diaphragmatic injuries in the absence of high sensitivity and specific diagnostic instruments. Diagnostic delay causes high mortality with these traumas with insidious symptoms. A diaphragmatic injury should be suspected in the presence of a clinical picture which includes hemothorax, hemoperitoneum, anemia and the presence of subdiaphragmatic air in the abdomen.

Consent

Written informed consent was obtained from the patient for publication of this case report and accompanying images. A copy of the written consent is available for review by the Editor-in-Chief of this journal on request.

Competing interests
The authors declare that they have no competing interests.

Authors' contributions
AA, RG and CD study design and writing; DVG, FG, DBG and SV data analysis and writing; GG study the design. All authors read and approved the final manuscript.

Authors' information
Agrusa Antonino and other co-authors have no study sponsor.

References
1. Duzgun AP, Ozmen MM, Saylam B, Coskun F: **Factors influencing mortality in traumatic ruptures of diaphragm.** *Ulus Travma Acil Cerrahi Derg* 2008, 14(2):132–138.
2. Lewis JD, Starnes SL, Pandalai PK, Huffman LC, Bulcao CF, Pritts TA, Reed MF: **Traumatic diaphragmatic injury: experience from a level I trauma center.** *Surgery* 2009, 146(4):578–584.
3. Clarke DL, Greatorex B, Oosthizen GV, Muckart DJ: **The spectrum of diaphragmatic injury in a busy metropolitan surgical service.** *Injury* 2009, 40:932–937.
4. Bosanquet D, Farboud A, Lunckraz H: **A review of diaphragmatic hernia.** *Resp Med CME* 2009, 2:1–6.
5. Bowdich HI: **Diaphragmatic hernia.** *Buffalo Mad J* 1853, 9:65–94.
6. O'Malley E, Boyle E, O' Callaghan A, Coffey JC, Walsh SR: **Role of laparoscopy in penetrating abdominal trauma: a systematic review.** *World J Surg* 2013, 37(1):113–22.

7. Mattews BD, Bui H, Harold KL, Kervher KW, Adrales G, Park A, Sing RF, Heniford BT: **Laparoscopic repair of traumatic diaphragmatic injuries.** *Surg Endsc* 2003, **17:**254–258.

8. Toro A, Mannino M, Reale G, Di Carlo I: **TachoSil in abdominal surgery: a review.** *J Blood Med* 2011, **2:**31–36.

9. RamonVilallonga V, Pastor L, Alvarez R, Charco M, Armengol S, Navarro A: **Right-side diaphragmatic rupture alter blunt trauma.** *An Unusual entity WJES* 2011, 6–3.

10. Hedblom CA: **Diapragmatic hernia.** *JAMA* 1925, **85:**947–953.

11. Morgan BS, Atcyn-Jones TW, Garner GP: **Traumatic diaphragmatic injury.** *J R Army Med Corps* 2010, **156**(3):139–144.

12. Boulanger BR, Mizman DP, Rosati C, Rodriguez A: **A comparison of right and left blunt traumatic diaphragmatic rupture.** *J Trauma* 1993, **35:**255–260.

13. Sacco R, Quitadamo S, Rotolo N, Di Nuzzo D, Mucilli F: **Traumatic diaphragmatic rupture: personal experience.** *Acta Bio Medica* 2003, **74:**71–73.

14. Okada M, Adachi H, Kamesaki M, Mikami M, Ookura Y, Yamakawa J, Hamabe Y: **Traumatic diaphragmatic injury: experience from a tertiary emergency medical center.** *Gen Thorac Cardiovasc Surg* 2012, **60:**649–654.

15. Goi G, Callegaro D, Villa R, Moroni E, Bondurri A, Danelli P: **Large-bowel obstruction as a result of occult diaphragmatic hernia 11 years after injuries.** *Ann Ital Chir* 2012, **83**(5):425–428.

16. Kuppusamy A, Ramanathan G, Gurusamy J, Ramamoorthy B, Parasakthi K: **Delayed diagnosis of traumatic diaphragmatic rupture with herniation of the liver: a case report.** *Turk J Trauma Emerg Surg* 2012, **18**(2):175–177.

17. Matsevych OY: **Blunt diaphragmatic rupture: four year's experience.** *Hernia* 2008, **12:**73–78.

18. Stein DM, York GB, Boswell S, Shanmuganathan K, Haan M, Scalea TM: **Accuracy of computed tomography scan in the detection of penetrating diaphragm injury.** *J Trauma* 2007, **63**(3):538–543.

19. Boussuges A, Gole Y, Blanc P: **Diaphragmatic motion studied by M-mode ultrasonography: method, reproducibility and normal values.** *Chest* 2009, **135**(2):391–400.

20. Sanmuganathan K, Mirvis SE, White CS, Pomerantz SM: **MR imagining evaluation of hemidiaphragms in acute blunt trauma: experience with 16 patients.** *AJR* 1996, **167:**397–402.

21. Leppaniemi A, Haapiainen R: **Occult diaphragmatic injuries causated by stab wouds.** *J Trauma* 2003, **55:**646–650.

22. Desser TS, Edwards B, Hunt S, Rosenberg J, Purtill MA, Jeffrey JB: **The dangling diaphragm sign: sensitivity an comparison with existing CT signs of blunt traumatic diaphragmatic rupture.** *Emerg Radiol* 2010, **17:**37–44.

23. Agrusa A, Romano G, Di Buono G, Dafnomili A, Gulotta G: **Laparoscopic approach in abdominal emergiences: a 5-year experience at single centre.** *G Chir* 2012, **33:**400–403.

8

Penetrating arterial trauma to the limbs: outcome of a modified protocol

Antonio Krüger[1]*, Carla Florido[1], Amelie Braunisch[1], Eric Walther[1], Tugba Han Yilmaz[3] and Dietrich Doll[2,4,5]

Abstract

Background: Penetrating arterial injuries to the limbs are common injuries in high volume trauma centers. Their overall surgical results reported in the literature are satisfactory - apart of those of the popliteal artery that still may lead to a significant incidence in amputations. With the present study we assessed our outcome with penetrating arterial injuries to the limb as to see if the direct involvement of vascular surgeons in the management of popliteal artery injuries leads to an improved (lowered) amputation rate. Results were benchmarked with our published results from previous years.

Methods: All patients sustaining penetrating arterial injuries to the limbs admitted to the Chris Hani Baragwanath Academic Hospital during an 18- month period ending in September 2011 were included in this study. Axillary, brachial and femoral artery injuries were operated on by the trauma surgeons as in the past. All popliteal artery injuries were operated on by the vascular surgeons (new).

Results: There were a total of 113 patients with 116 injuries, as some patients had multiple vascular injuries: 10 axillary, 47 brachial, 34 femoral and 25 popliteal artery injuries. Outcome of axillary, brachial and femoral artery injury repair were excellent and not significantly different from our previous reported experience. Injury to the popliteal artery showed a diminished re-exploration rate from 34% down to 10% (p = 0,049) and a decrease of amputation rate from 16% to 11% which was statistically not significant (p = 0,8).

Conclusion: Penetrating arterial trauma to the axillary, brachial and femoral artery is followed by excellent results when operated by trauma surgeons. In the case of popliteal artery injury operated by the vascular surgeons, the results of this study do not show any statistically significant difference related to amputation rate from our previous reported studies when operated by trauma surgeons. Taking into consideration the diminished re-exploration rate and a tendency to a lower amputation rate, we feel that there is possible tendency of better outcome if operated by vascular surgeons. Multicenter studies with large number of enrolled patients will be required to prove the validity of this suggestion.

Keywords: Popliteal artery, Penetrating trauma, Treatment protocol, Outcome, Amputation rate, Vascular repair, Vascular surgeon

Introduction

Penetrating arterial injuries to the limbs generally show a good outcome if an experienced trauma team operates on them without undue delay. Several articles studying this subject were published from our institution within the last two decades [1-5]. In the last few years we proceeded to certain changes in our management protocol of this type of injury: popliteal artery injuries, formerly done by trauma surgeons, were now done by vascular surgeons. The purpose of this study was to assess the effect of these changes in our management protocols to patient outcome in terms of re-exploration rate as well as the rate of limb loss (amputation).

Patients and methods

Chris Hani Baragwanath Academic Hospital with approximately 3000 beds is Teaching Hospital of the University of Witwatersrand, as it is the largest hospital in the southern hemisphere. The trauma unit deals with

* Correspondence: akrueger@med.uni-marburg.de
[1]Department of Trauma-, Hand- and Reconstructive Surgery, Philipps-University, Baldingerstr. 1, Marburg, Germany
Full list of author information is available at the end of the article

neck, cardiothoracic, abdominal and vascular trauma as well as with polytrauma patients. It is run by general surgeons with a subspecialty in trauma. The hospital services care for approximately 3, 5 million people living in SOWETO (South West Township), Johannesburg, South Africa.

In this study we included all patients with penetrating trauma of the major arteries of the extremities who were admitted to hospital over 18 months (from the 1st of March 2010 to 1st of September 2011. Arterial injuries distal to the bifurcation of the brachial or the trifurcation of the popliteal artery were not included in the study.

Patient variables extracted included gender, age, injury mechanism, admission vital signs, Glasgow Coma Scale (GCS), preoperative investigations, initial management and outcomes. Data were entered into a computerised spreadsheet (Microsoft Excel 2007) and analyzed using SPSS for Windows©, version 18.0. Graphic presentation was done by Microsoft Excel 2007 and Graph Pad Prism©. Discrete variables are presented as proportions (percentages), unless stated otherwise and were analysed by Fischer's exact test. Statistical significance was accepted if $p < 0, 05$.

The majority of the patients sustained gunshot injuries through commercially available handheld low velocity weapons (pistols). Patients with high-velocity weapons contact, as the AK-47 been the most common high velocity weapon used in our society, were rarely seen arriving in the hospitals. Amongst the 61 patients out of the 113 patients who sustained gunshot injuries, it was generally difficult if not impossible to determine the caliber of weapon used and from what distance it was fired.

The trauma surgeon on call is present on the hospital premises at a 24 hour rotation. He is responsible for the management of all patients, from their arrival via the resuscitation room treatment (if needed) to the operating theatre. He is also responsible for the care of patients admitted to ICU or to the trauma ward. All arterial injuries irrespective of the anatomical site are dealt with by the trauma surgeons. The only exception is the popliteal artery injuries which according to our new management protocol are operated by the vascular surgeons.

All patients were admitted and resuscitated in the trauma resuscitation area applying the world wide standardized Advanced Trauma Life Support (ATLS ®) principles. On admission to the trauma resuscitation area all patients – only if haemodynamically stable - received a full body X- Ray examination with a Lodox ® (Low Dose X-Ray) scanner, so that the presence of bullet fragments or fractures could be visualized.

Our protocols stress the importance of emergency room hemorrhage control; direct digital pressure being the most effective method, which was maintained until definitive operative control was established. Balloon tamponade has been a useful adjunctive measure, where one ore more Foley catheters are inserted into the tract of the missile or stab and the balloon inflated with fluid until hemorrhage is controlled. Large skin wounds are rapidly closed around the catheter(s) with skin sutures to prevent dislodgement during balloon inflation and to assist in creating a tamponade.

Physical examination was the cornerstone of the diagnosis and relied mostly on the presence of "hard" or "soft" signs of arterial injury (Tables 1 & 2). "Hard" signs are indicative of ischemia or ongoing hemorrhage and include absent distal pulses, extensive external bleeding, expanding or pulsatile hematoma, palpable thrill, continuous murmur, or other signs of distal ischemia (pain, pallor, coolness). The presence of "hard" signs mandated immediate surgical exploration. "Soft" signs of arterial injury included a history of severe bleeding at the trauma scene, nonexpanding hematoma, diminished but palpable pulses, and peripheral neural deficit. Doppler pressure measurements were undertaken in our department as an adjunct to stratify risk in patients with arterial trauma. In the absence of "hard" signs, a Doppler pressure deficit of greater than 10 per cent, compared with the contralateral limb, was considered a "soft" sign of arterial injury. As recommended by Frykberg et al. and confirmed in our previous published experience,

Table 1 Hard clinical signs in n = 113 patients with arterial vascular injuries

Clinical signs*	Femoral		Popliteal		Axillary		Brachial		Total	
	all pts: n = 34		all pts: n = 25		all pts: n = 10		all pts: n = 47		all pts: n = 113	
	pts [n]	pts [%]	pts [n]	pts [%]	pts [n]	pts [%]	pts [n]	pts [%]	pts [n]	pts [%]
Cold ischemic extr.	8	24%	18	72%	2	20%	11	23%	39	35%
Absent pulses	14	41%	14	56%	7	70%	19	40%	54	48%
Bruit or thrill	1	3%	0	0%	0	0%	0	0%	1	1%
Exp. or pulsating H	3	9%	2	8%	0	0%	2	4%	7	6%
Pulsatile bleeding	6	18%	5	20%	3	30%	12	26%	26	23%

Seven of the patients underwent immediate amputation. *Please note that multiple signs are possible. Pts = patients; extr. = extremity; Exp. or pulsating H. = patients with expanding or pulsating hematoma.

Table 2 Soft clinical signs in n = 113 patients with arterial vascular injuries

Clinical signs*	Femoral		Popliteal		Axillary		Brachial		Total	
	all pts: n = 34		all pts: n = 25		all pts: n = 10		all pts: n = 47		all pts: n = 113	
	pts [n]	pts [%]	pts [n]	pts [%]	pts [n]	pts [%]	pts [n]	pts [%]	pts [n]	pts [%]
Nonexpanding H.	7	21%	1	4%	2	2%	3	6%	13	12%
Paraesth./Paresis	6	18%	6	24%	6	60%	17	36%	35	31%
Decreased pulses	5	15%	3	12%	1	10%	11	23%	20	18%

Seven of the patients underwent immediate amputation. *Please note that multiple signs are possible. Pts = patients; Nonexpanding H. = patients with nonexpanding hematoma; Paraesth./Paresis = paraesthesia and / or paresis of the extremity in the awake patient.

proximity of injury to major vessels was not considered a "soft" sign [6].

According to our previous recommendations the most reliable tool for detection of arterial injury was the arteriography. This slowly changed over the years with the use of multi-slice CT scanners. According to our new protocol we are performing only CT- arteriography if this is indicated by the clinical presentation. Patients with "soft" signs of vascular injury underwent CT- arteriography with a 64 or 128 detector row CT scanner if hemodynamically stable. CT- arteriography was also performed on physiologically stable patients if there was uncertainty regarding the site of injury, e.g., multiple gunshot wounds or shotgun wounds. If the patient requiring arteriography was physiologically too unstable to be transferred to the CT scanner (approximately 50 meters from our trauma resuscitation area), then arteriography was carried out in the trauma resuscitation area with the use of the Lodox - Scanner (Figure 1) or preoperatively in theatre with a C- Arm.

All patients were given a dose of Cefazolin 1 g. intravenously perioperatively, and the dose was administered every 12 hours for a total of 48 hours. In patients with associated abdominal injury the antibiotic regime consisted of Amoxicillin-Clavulanic acid 1,2 g. intravenously.

After operative exploration of the injured artery we proceeded with the debridement of the site of the injury.

The distal part of the vessel routinely underwent thrombectomy with a Fogarty catheter to ensure sufficient backflow. Primary repair or primary anastomosis was practiced if it was not leading to any narrowing to the injury site or to undue anastomotic tension. If narrowing or tension were pending, a graft was inserted. Although an autologous saphenous vein graft from the contralateral site was our first choice, PTFE (Polytetrafluoroethylene) graft was used if the saphenous vein was unavailable, of the vein was of insufficient diameter or if the time needed to harvest the vein would be detrimental to the patient's outcome. Whenever graft was used, great care was taken to cover it with viable muscle or other well perfused soft tissues available. In most cases venous injuries were dealt with by ligation. In cases of injury of large diameter veins which could be repaired by simple suturing, ligation could be avoided. We never attempted to repair any venous injuries by complex techniques, such as fashioning of a spiral graft. In all cases venous repair preceded the arterial one.

In cases of skeletal injury accompanied by significant bone instability or length shortening, distal revascularisation was initially achieved by the use of a temporary arterial shunt. In these cases, skeletal fixation followed immediately, as did removal of the temporary shunt and replacement of it by a vein or PTFE graft. Temporary shunting (Figure 2) also was used in cases of physiologically instability of the

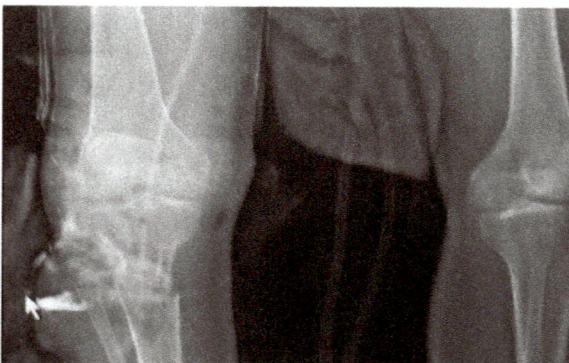

Figure 1 Transection of the right popliteal artery at the level of the trifurcation after gunshot injury (Lodox picture). Bullet fragment can be seen right to white arrow.

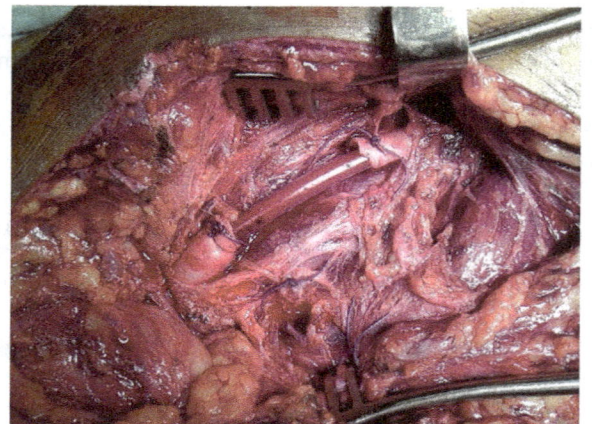

Figure 2 Temporary shunting of the femoral artery.

patient which enforced postponement of definitive management of the injured (damage control situations; pending or obvious DIC).

Early fasciotomy was performed in the presence of distal swelling, severe distal muscular- skeletal injury, delayed restoration of blood flow (more than 4 to 6 hours after accident/injury) and venous ligation. There was a tendency to perform fasciotomy in any doubtful cases or in the presence of an anticipated reperfusion injury [7]. Compartment syndrome was clinically diagnosed and at no stage intra-compartmental pressures were measured.

Nerve injury was repaired at the time of the arterial repair only if the patient was haemodynamically stable and the repair of the nerve was considered technically easy [8].

Methodologywise, in three patients with bilateral femoral arterial injury (with side different treatment and outcome), each side was treated, analyzed and counted as a single injury.

Results

There were a total of 113 patients who underwent operation for 116 penetrating arterial injury to the limbs. There were 103 male and 10 female patients. The mean age was 25 years (range 13–66 years). Of these 113 patients, 61 had received gunshot wounds and 30 received stab knife wounds. 20 injuries were inflicted by other sharp instruments and in two patients injury was related to dog bites. There were 10 axillary artery, 47 brachial artery, 34 femoral artery (15 common, 14 superficial and 5 profunda femoral artery) and 25 popliteal artery injuries. Three patients had simultaneous profunda femoral and superficial femoral artery injury.

Fifty-nine out of the 113 (52%) patients who underwent operation presented with additional trauma to other anatomical areas including bones / fracture dislocations and nerve lesions.

Tables 3 and 4 illustrate the operative findings and the type of arterial repair done depending on the site of the injury.

Sixteen of these 59 patients (27%) with additional injuries were hypotensive with a systolic BP < 90 mm Hg on admission. In contrast to them, only 10 patients of the 54 patients without concomitant injuries (19%) presented with systolic hypotension.

Limb-saving surgery

113 patients were receiving an operation, and 92 (81%) of them had a successful primary reconstruction. This were all patients with axillary artery injury, 40 out of 46 (87%) patients with brachial artery injury, 24 out of 30 (80%) patients with femoral and 18 out of 20 (90%) patients with popliteal artery injury. There were 12 (11%) patients who developed complications related to the initial interposition graft (bleeding, thrombosis); all of them were re-explored. All re-explorations were performed by the trauma surgeon in charge.

Brachial artery results

Of the 47 patients with brachial artery injury, one already presented with severe ischemia of the forearm and he underwent primary amputation for already overt muscle necrosis. Of the 46 patients who underwent brachial artery repair or graft, 6 (13%) patients had to be re-explored. These were the 2 patients with saphenous vein interposition graft who developed thrombosis and 2 patients with basilic vein interposition graft who developed postoperative bleeding. The use of basilic vein graft was a diversion to our protocol. A new saphenous vein graft was used in all four cases with satisfactory result. Another patient with saphenous interposition graft had to be taken back to theatre for postoperative bleeding from the anastomosis site that was controlled with stitches. Another patient developed thrombosis in a feeding tube which was used as a temporary emergency shunt. All 46 patients operated with brachial artery injury were discharged with a good radial pulse (Table 5).

Femoral artery results

One grossly avital limb which was amputated straight away was not calculated as treated or treatment failure (early amputation). There were overall 6 out of 34 (18%) cases with femoral artery injury that had to be re-explored, 3 of them were associated with initially delayed presentation (approximately 12 hours post injury) and with

Table 3 Intraoperative findings in n = 113 patients with arterial vascular injuries

| Intrap. findings* | Femoral | | Popliteal | | Axillary | | Brachail | | Total | |
| | all pts: n = 34 | | all pts: n = 25 | | all pts: n = 10 | | all pts: n = 47 | | all pts: n = 113 | |
Artery	pts [n]	pts [%]	pts [n]	pts [%]	pts [n]	pts [%]	pts [n]	pts [%]	pts [n]	pts [%]
Thrombosed	3	9%	1	4%	3	30%	3	6%	10	9%
Fully transsected	17	50%	19	76%	5	50%	28	60%	69	61%
incompletely transs.	11	32%	5	20%	4	40%	11	23%	31	27%
Dissected	2	6%	0	0%	0	0%	4	9%	6	5%
AV fistula	2	6%	0	0%	0	0%	1	2%	26	23%

*Please note that multiple signs are possible. Pts = patients; AV fistula = traumatic arterio-venous fistula discovered.

Table 4 Intraoperative vascular procedures done in n = 113 patients with arterial vascular injuries

Vasc. Procedure	Femoral all pts: n = 34		Popliteal all pts: n = 25		Axillary all pts: n = 10		Brachial all pts: n = 47		Total all pts: n = 113	
	pts [n]	pts [%]	pts [n]	pts [%]	pts [n]	pts [%]	pts [n]	pts [%]	pts [n]	pts [%]
Lateral arteriorraphy	2	6%	0	0%	0	0%	1	2%	3	3%
Primary end-to-end	3	9%	2	8%	2	20%	15	32%	22	19%
Vein interpositiona	12	35%	17	68%	5	50%	28	60%	62	55%
PTFE interposition	12	35%	0	0%	2	20	0	0%	114	12%
Shunt/Stent	1	3%	1	4%	1	10%	2	4%	5	4%

Pts = patients; PTFE = Poly-tetra-fluoro-ethylen interposition graft.

pulseless cold limb. They were all referred from one smaller district hospital to our hospital. These three had all unsuccessful re-exploration that led to amputation. One of these patients died after repeated amputations. Of the other three patients one had successful re-exploration and two others underwent amputation. Therefore 5 of 33 femoral artery injuries underwent amputation after unsuccessful primary reconstruction, an overall amputation rate of 15%. If we exclude the 3 patients who were transferred to us from the other hospital with an approximately 12 hours post injury delay and signs of severe ischemia, there were only 2 amputations out of 30 cases of adequately treated limb injuries of the femoral arterial axis (7%; Table 5).

Popliteal artery results

4 of the 25 patients with popliteal artery injury (16%) underwent immediate amputation as muscles were found to be not viable during 4-compartment-fasciotomy. A fifth patient also underwent amputation as he was physiologically unstable and it was not possible to use an arterial shunt, with the injury being very close to the trifurcation, so the popliteal artery needed to be ligated proximally. This patient developed severe ischemia of the leg that was amputated at a second stage. Two patients with saphenous vein grafts developed

complications regarding thrombosis or insufficient reperfusion of the limb. They were explored unsuccessfully and finally underwent limb amputation. Therefore, of the 20 patients with popliteal artery injury that underwent arterial grafting, 2 underwent amputation, with an amputation rate of 10% (Table 5).

Additional injuries

Seven patients had an exploratory laparotomy because of concomitant abdominal injury. Abdominal surgery preceded the vascular repair in 4 times, whereas limb surgery was done in 3 patients. Abdominal surgery preceded limb surgery in cases of life threatening abdominal hemorrhage. There was concomitant bone injury in 32 out of 113 (28%) patients, two out of 10 (20%) in the axillary group, eight out of 47 (17%) were in the brachial group, six out of 34 (18%) were in the femoral group and 16 out of 25 (64%) in the popliteal group. Fourteen of those patients required external fixation, 1 in the axillary, 3 in the brachial, 3 in the femoral and 7 in the popliteal group.

There were 33 out of 113 (29%) patients documented with additional nerve injury - one out of 10 (10%) with axillary, 29 out of 47 (62%) with brachial and three out of 25 (12%) with popliteal artery injury.

Table 5 Results and outcome of surgical therapy

Outcome		Femoral all inj: n = 34		Popliteal all pts: n = 25		Axillary all pts: n = 10		Brachial all pts: n = 47		Total all pts: n = 113	
		pts [n]	pts [%]	pts [n]	pts [%]	pts [n]	pts [%]	pts [n]	pts [%]	pts [n]	pts [%]
Immediate amputation		1	3%	4	16%	0	0%	1	2%	6	5%
DCS amputation		0	0%	1	4%	0	0%	0	0%	1	1%
Revisions	total	6	18%	2	8%	0	0%	6	13%	14	12%
	successful	1	3%	0	0%	0	0%	6	13%	7	6%
	amputation	5	15%	2	8%	0	0%	0	0%	7	6%
Long ischemia & amputatio		3	9%	12%	0	0		0	0%	3	3%
Deaths		3	9%	0	0%	1	10%	1	2%	5	4%
Successful repair		29	85%	18	72%	10	100%	46	98%	103	91%

DCS amputation = vascular repair was aborted because of trauma load leading to damage control procedures. All deaths were due to trauma severity and consecutive DIC. Death does not exclude a good vascular result, while amputation does. Patent vascular repair with good flow before death - without pending amputation - were judged a good result. Pts = patients.

There was a 31% overall venous trauma rate with 35 concomitant vein injuries.

Compartment syndrome was clinically diagnosed and at no stage intra-compartmental pressures were measured. As fascial compartment measures are known to be notoriously unreliable, fasciotomy was done on the base of clinical judgment alone. Four out of 47 (9%) patients with brachial artery injury, 9 out of 31(29%) patients with femoral artery injuries and 6 out of 25 (24%) patients with popliteal artery injuries already presented compartment syndrome at the time of admission. Early full- thickness fasciotomies were performed in 2 out of 10 (20%) patients with axillary, 20 out of 47 (43%) with brachial, 8 out of 31 (26%) patients with femoral and 17 out of 25 (68%) with popliteal artery injuries.

There was an average of 22% incidence of postoperative wound infection, with no significant late morbidity. This was unrelated to the anatomical site of the injury.

Mortality

There were five postoperative deaths, of whom were 2 deaths following femoral artery injury. Another patient with gunshot injuries to the abdomen and femoral artery underwent damage control laparotomy and shunting of the artery (Figure 2). He had to be re-taken to theatre 16 hours later for relook laparotomy. There was no specific bleeding source found, which was due to DIC. The arterial shunt was left in place and the patient demised the next day in ICU from disseminated intravascular coagulopathy. One patients with injury to the brachial artery went into cardiac arrest intraoperatively. He was successfully resuscitated and operated; unfortunately he demised postoperatively. There was one patient with stab wounds to the axillary artery, neck, chest, abdomen and lower extremities who developed DIC and demised postoperatively in ICU at the day of admission.

Thus concomitant trauma to neighbouring organ regions outweighed the vascular trauma in terms of mortality by far.

Discussion and conclusion

Over the last 20 years there has been a gradual reduction in the incidence of penetrating trauma presenting in our hospital, with a corresponding reduction of penetrating arterial injuries. In 1994 the incidence of penetrating trauma presenting at the Chris Hani Baragwanath Academic Hospital was 95% compared to 5% of blunt trauma. In 2008 the incidence of penetrating trauma was 47% compared to 53% of blunt trauma. As penetrating trauma is directly related to crime, it would seem that crime in Soweto has diminished over the years.

The reason for this is three fold: Firstly, the establishment of democracy led to the disappearance of political violence. Secondly, there are more employment opportunities for the previously disadvantaged population groups. Thirdly, the population now considers police as their protector and not as an oppressior of the Apartheid regime, this leading to increased population - police cooperation.

Another change that has developed over the years is that there are more patients referred from the district hospitals that are covered by our hospital. This results in a significant number of patients with delayed presentation, leading to a considerable number of primary amputation or thrombotic postoperative complications in this group of patients.

Diagnosticwise, the use of CT arteriography (CTA) has completely replaced the conventional "invasive" arteriography in our hospital and has greatly facilitated the investigations of arterial trauma. In our experience it has been satisfactory in all cases and it there was never any need to perform conventional arteriography. Hitherto, especially if there is clinical presence of hard symptoms of vascular injury, the positive predictive value is close to 100% [9]. Mindbogglingly, infrapopliteal vasospasms have not been found in surgical explorations with pathological CTA.

The mortality within our patient group is 5/113 patients, with 3 deaths attributed to DIC and coagulopathy. It may be pointed out that associated penetrating trauma to nerves, veins, and other body regions are still not uncommon in South Africa. We noticed a relatively small incidence on nerve injury in popliteal injuries in our collective (12%), which is said to ultimately to determine the functional outcome of the limb [10,11]. If we compare our patients' trauma with penetrating injuries from other studies, 2/3 of all penetrating vascular injuries here are gunshot-related, where others studies are dominated by stab injuries [12,13]. Thus the force and destruction to the neurovascular bundle, bones, soft tissues and remote body regions should have been expected to be substantially higher in our study [14]. Indeed, 32 of our 113 patients arrived with combined vascular and bony injuries, among them the highest incidence at 60% of all patients in the popliteal group. Thus the high amputation rate in the popliteal group of 7/25 (4 primary amputations, one amputation related to hemodynamic instability of the patient and 2 late amputations) is not surprising.

The mean time between injury and operation in our previous reported experience as well as in our present are comparable. It was thus interesting to compare our previous experience outcome on each different anatomical site of injury with the actual results and with the literature. As pointed out, isolated vascular injury may come with an amputation rate as low as 3% [15], but penetrating trauma, increased transport times (longer warm ischemia time) and coagulopathy may push the amputation rate up to 33% and higher [16], as do combined arterio-venous trauma, fractures [17,18], hypotension and torso injuries increase mortality [19].

Comparing brachial, popliteal and femoral mortality, the latter will be the highest (3/34), as the proximal femoral vessel has the highest flow, no collaterals, may not easy be assessable for bleeding with tourniquet and may come as multiple vascular injury, as was present in three of our femoral patients.

Focussing on the arterial injury of the upper limb, we see that the overall outcome in the past and the present studies is very satisfactory particularly in the present study: all operated patients with axillary and brachial injuries had successful outcome. The same applies for the patients with femoral artery injury if we do not take into consideration the 3 patients who were referred from other hospital to us with a more than 12 hours delay between injury and surgery. In all the studies (previous and present) reported from our institute, the injuries were operated by trauma surgeons.

In contrast to that, if we compare our patients outcome for gunshot popliteal artery injury, we see that there is a difference between our present and our past reported experience. Previously the amputation rate of the combined experience of this type of injury was 11 out of 68 (16%), not considering the primary amputations [20]. At our present study again taking into consideration only the gunshot injuries to the popliteal artery (21 out of 25 patients of our study), there were 2 out of 18 patients (11%) who underwent amputation. Again we did not include patients with primary amputation due to muscle necrosis on arrival in this calculation. All the penetrating popliteal artery injuries not caused by gunshot wound had a positive outcome. So the amputation rate of the present study compared with the old ones is 11% to 16% (p-value = 0, 8). It is also interesting to see that the number of re explorations in the past experience is 23 out of 68 patients (34%) compared to the present experience that is 2 out of 18 patients (11%), which just touches the statistical level of significance with p = 0,049.

Knowing that the overall injury to operation time interval between the 2 groups has been comparable, we have the impression that our present results are better than those of the past. The patients in the older study were operated by the trauma surgeons. In the recent study - because of the change of management protocol - the injury in this specific popliteal site was operated by the vascular surgeons. This is the only parameter that would logically lead to a difference in outcome.

Patients presenting with penetrating arterial injuries are in their great majority young men and, to a lesser extent, woman. As a consequence their arteries are of good quality. Particularly with arteries of the upper limb and the femoral artery, there is a significant network of collaterals that overall contribute to satisfactory outcome, by providing critical distal blood supply and many times keeping muscle viability for a considerable length of time. These factors can lead us to the conclusion that the operations in young people at these sites are not only technically easier due to the good quality of the arteries but are also probably forgiving minor technical imperfections. This is not the case with the popliteal artery, particularly the distal one that is not supported by an extensive collateral network. A further "aggravating" factor at this site is the difficulty in access and position of the graft. Taking into consideration the above characteristics of the popliteal artery and our significantly improved results after the change of our protocol management, we are tempted to assume that this change is due to the fact that patients were operated by vascular surgeons. At the end of the day they are more experienced in dealing with difficult vascular operative situations.

Four patients with popliteal artery injuries in the authors' recent experience underwent immediate amputation. Perhaps this fact alone accounted for the small improvement in outcomes. By increasing the rate of early amputations, this might reduce the number of graft failures and late amputations as the result of a more favourable selection bias. This fact could also have accounted for the better results rather than "better technique" employed by the vascular surgeons.

The remaining question arising from our results is: should all patients with arterial trauma to the limbs be operated by vascular surgeons? Our opinion is that they should not, taking into consideration our results with the axillary, brachial and femoral artery injuries. This is supported by the international literature as well that reports excellent results with this type of injury.

We are therefore convinced that patients with penetrating trauma to the axillary, brachial and femoral arteries are getting excellent service when operated by trauma surgeons of a Level I Trauma centre. On the other hand we feel that popliteal arteries, particularly the distal ones, should be operated by vascular surgeons through the trauma service.

In conclusion penetrating trauma to the arteries of the limbs is an injury that should be dealt with as an absolute emergency. In the presence of "soft" signs of arterial injury, the use of new generation spiral CT- scanners leads to excellent diagnostic results, compared to those of arteriography. The outcome with axillary, brachial and femoral artery injuries - when operated by experienced trauma surgeons - are satisfactory. When it comes to popliteal artery injury there is a statistically significant reduced rate of popliteal artery re-exploration if vascular surgeons do the primary repair. Thus we believe it is related to better surgical technique, due to the involvement of the vascular surgeons. There is a higher percentage – although not statistically significant rate - of limb salvage with vascular surgeons and popliteal repair. We are wondering if a study with a larger number of patients will lead to a statistically significant reduction of amputation rate. We therefore feel that this issue should further be explored through a multi-center study so that we come to a solid and universally acceptable conclusion, related to our suggestion that popliteal artery injury should rather be operated by vascular and not trauma surgeons.

Competing interests
The authors declared that they have no competing interests.

Authors' contributions
Conception and design: DD, CF. Acquisition of data: CF, AB, EW. Statistical analysis: CF. Analysis and interpretation of data: CF, DD, AK. Drafting the article: DD, CF, AK. Critically revising the article: all authors. All authors read and approved the final manuscript.

Disclosure
The authors report no conflict of interest concerning the materials or methods used in this study or the findings specified in this paper.

Author details
[1]Department of Trauma-, Hand- and Reconstructive Surgery, Philipps-University, Baldingerstr. 1, Marburg, Germany. [2]Department of Visceral, Thoracic and Vascular Surgery, Philipps-University of Marburg, Marburg, Germany. [3]Department of Surgery, Izmir, Turkey, Baskent University, Ankara, Turkey. [4]Department of Trauma, Chris Hani Baragwanath Academic Hospital, Johannesburg, Soweto, South Africa. [5]Department of Surgery, St.-Marien-Hospital Vechta, Teaching Hospital of the MHH Hannover University, Vechta, Germany.

References
1. Degiannis E, Bowley DM, Bode F, Lynn WR, Glapa M, Baxter S, Shapey J, Smith MD, Doll D: Ballistic arterial trauma to the lower extremity: recent South African experience. Am Surg 2007, 73:1136–1139.
2. Degiannis E, Levy RD, Sofianos C, Florizoone MG, Saadia R: Arterial gunshot injuries of the extremities: a South African experience. J Trauma 1995, 39:570–575.
3. Degiannis E, Levy RD, Potokar T, Saadia R: Penetrating injuries of the axillary artery. Aust N Z J Surg 1995, 65:327–330.
4. Bowley DM, Degiannis E, Goosen J, Boffard KD: Penetrating vascular trauma in Johannesburg, South Africa. Surg Clin North Am 2002, 82:221–235.
5. Degiannis E, Smith MD: (2005) Vascular injuries. In Ballistic Trauma. 2nd edition. Edited by Mahoney PF, Ryan JM, Brooks AJ, Schwab CW. London: Springer; 2005.
6. Frykberg ER: Arteriography of the injured extremity: are we in proximity to an answer? J Trauma 1992, 32:551–552.
7. Barros D'Sa AA, Harkin DW, Blair PH, Hood JM, McIlrath E: The Belfast approach to managing complex lower limb vascular injuries. Eur J Vasc Endovasc Surg 2006, 32:246–256.
8. Shergill G, Bonney G, Munshi P, Birch R: The radial and posterior interosseous nerves. Results fo 260 repairs. J Bone Joint Surg Br 2001, 83:646–649.
9. Frykberg ER, Dennis JW, Bishop K, Laneve L, Alexander RH: The reliability of physical examination in the evaluation of penetrating extremity trauma for vascular injury: results at one year. J Trauma 1991, 31:502–511.
10. Wali MA: Upper limb vascular trauma in the Asir region of Saudi Arabia. Ann Thorac Cardiovasc Surg 2002, 8:298–301.
11. Graham JM, Mattox KL, Feliciano DV, DeBakey ME: Vascular injuries of the axilla. Ann Surg 1982, 195:232–238.
12. Ergunes K, Yilik L, Ozsoyler I, Kestelli M, Ozbek C, Gurbuz A: Traumatic brachial artery injuries. Tex Heart Inst J 2006, 33:31–34.
13. Ekim H, Tuncer M: Management of traumatic brachial artery injuries: a report on 49 patients. Ann Saudi Med 2009, 29:105–109.
14. Zellweger R, Hess F, Nicol A, Omoshoro-Jones J, Kahn D, Navsaria P: An analysis of 124 surgically managed brachial artery injuries. Am J Surg 2004, 188:240–245.
15. Rasouli MR, Moini M, Khaji A: Civilian traumatic vascular injuries of the upper extremity:report of the Iranian national trauma project. Ann Thorac Cardiovasc Surg 2009, 15:389–393.
16. Fox CJ, Perkins JG, Kragh JF Jr, Singh NN, Patel B, Ficke JR: Popliteal artery repair in massively transfused military trauma casualties: a pursuit to save life and limb. J Trauma 2010, 69(Suppl 1):S123–S134.
17. Cakir O, Subasi M, Erdem K, Eren N: Treatment of vascular injuries associated with limb fractures. Ann R Coll Surg Engl 2005, 87:348–352.
18. Feliciano DV, Herskowitz K, O'Gorman RB, Cruse PA, Brandt ML, Burch JM, Mattox KL: Management of vascular injuries in the lower extremities. J Trauma 1988, 28:319–328.
19. Asensio JA, Kuncir EJ, Garcia-Nunez LM, Petrone P: Femoral vessel injuries: analysis of factors predictive of outcomes. J Am Coll Surg 2006, 203:512–520.
20. Degiannis E, Velmahos GC, Florizoone MG, Levy RD, Ross J, Saadia R: Penetrating injuries of the popliteal artery: the Baragwanath experience. Ann R Coll Surg Engl 1994, 76:307–310.

9

Establishment and implementation of an effective rule for the interpretation of computed tomography scans by emergency physicians in blunt trauma

Yukihiro Ikegami*, Tsuyoshi Suzuki, Chiaki Nemoto, Yasuhiko Tsukada, Arifumi Hasegawa, Jiro Shimada and Choichiro Tase

Abstract

Introduction: Computed tomography (CT) can detect subtle organ injury and is applicable to many body regions. However, its interpretation requires significant skill. In our hospital, emergency physicians (EPs) must interpret emergency CT scans and formulate a plan for managing most trauma cases. CT misinterpretation should be avoided, but we were initially unable to completely accomplish this. In this study, we proposed and implemented a precautionary rule for our EPs to prevent misinterpretation of CT scans in blunt trauma cases.

Methods: We established a simple precautionary rule, which advises EPs to interpret CT scans with particular care when a complicated injury is suspected per the following criteria: 1) unstable physiological condition; 2) suspicion of injuries in multiple regions of the body (e.g., brain injury plus abdominal injury); 3) high energy injury mechanism; and 4) requirement for rapid movement to other rooms for invasive treatment. If a patient meets at least one of these criteria, the EP should exercise the precautions laid out in our newly established rule when interpreting the CT scan. Additionally, our rule specifies that the EP should request real-time interpretation by a radiologist in difficult cases. We compared the accuracy of EPs' interpretations and resulting patient outcomes in blunt trauma cases before (January 2011, June 2012) and after (July 2012, January 2013) introduction of the rule to evaluate its efficacy.

Results: Before the rule's introduction, emergency CT was performed 1606 times for 365 patients. We identified 44 cases (2.7%) of minor misinterpretation and 40 (2.5%) of major misinterpretation. After introduction, CT was performed 820 times for 177 patients. We identified 10 cases (1.2%) of minor misinterpretation and two (0.2%) of major misinterpretation. Real-time support by a radiologist was requested 104 times (12.7% of all cases) and was effective in preventing misinterpretation in every case. Our rule decreased both minor and major misinterpretations in a statistically significant manner. In particular, it conspicuously decreased major misinterpretations.

Conclusion: Our rule was easy to practice and effective in preventing EPs from missing major organ injuries. We would like to propose further large-scale multi-center trials to corroborate these results.

Keywords: Blunt trauma, Computed tomography, Rule, Misinterpretation

* Correspondence: yikegami@fmu.ac.jp
Department of Emergency and Critical Care Medicine, School of Medicine,
Fukushima Medical University, 1 Hikarigaoka, Fukushima 960-1295, Japan

Introduction

In recent years, the use of computed tomography (CT) has enabled rapid and accurate diagnoses in cases of primary trauma [1-5]. CT can be used to detect injuries that are otherwise invisible, but this requires a high level of skill in interpretation. Regular corroboration by a radiologist is therefore necessary to maintain an acceptable level of accurate diagnoses. However, some studies have reported real-time interpretation by a radiologist to be impossible because of a serious shortage of radiologists [6,7]. Additionally, in Japan, emergency physicians (EPs) must currently interpret CT results themselves to decide on a suitable treatment plan in many trauma cases.

Even a slight misdiagnosis may cause death in severe multiple trauma. Most EPs have abundant knowledge of trauma and a high level of skill in primary trauma care, but they cannot provide adequate treatment if they do not correctly identify injured organs. EPs are therefore required to have a high level of skill in interpreting CT results, while knowing that they should always exercise caution in doing so. In our opinion, it is most important to prevent misdiagnosis of traumatic injuries at the first stage of treatment to avoid potentially wrong or unnecessary treatment and any resulting consequences.

In this study, we proposed a precautionary rule to guide our EPs and prevent CT misinterpretation. Through this study, we hope to contribute to the establishment of a safe and effective emergency CT interpretation system for use in blunt trauma patients.

Materials and methods

Our emergency department (ED) is equipped with a multi-slice CT machine (from Toshiba Medical Systems Corporation) with 64 channels and is always in a state of standby for trauma patients. In blunt trauma, the EP in charge of the ED carries out a primary survey based on a standardized protocol, which actively employs whole body CT. EPs interpret the CT scan at the time of imaging and record their image diagnoses in an electronic clinical chart. From there, the hospital procedure to definitive diagnosis based on CT is as follows. A radiologist interprets the emergency CT obtained in the ED within several hours, and this image report is uploaded to the electronic clinical chart. Every morning, the EPs discuss the radiologist's report in a trauma conference and then arrive at a final CT diagnosis.

To reduce CT misinterpretation by EPs, we established a simple precautionary rule, which advises EPs to interpret CT scans with particular care when a complicated injury is suspected per the following criteria: 1) unstable physiological condition; 2) suspicion of injuries in multiple regions of the body (e.g., brain injury plus abdominal injury); 3) high energy mechanism of injury; and 4) requirement for rapid movement to other rooms for invasive treatment. If a patient meets at least one of these criteria, the EP should carefully interpret the CT scan. Namely, the EP should undertake the following actions: 1) employment of enhanced CT for chest, abdomen, and pelvis; 2) re-interpretation of the images more than twice after short intervals; 3) changing the window levels according to the organs interpreted; 4) evaluation using not only an axial view but also a sagittal or coronal view when necessary; 5) use of a three-dimensional view to evaluate bone injuries; and 6) repetition of the CT after time has passed.

Additionally, our rule specifies that the EP should request real-time interpretation by a radiologist in difficult cases per the following guidelines: 1) the patient's physiological condition deteriorates in spite of treatment; 2) laboratory data show the development of anemia or metabolic acidosis in spite of treatment; or 3) unclear points remain in spite of re-interpretation or repetition of the CT. We posted this rule in the CT control room and the ED conference room, and we held a briefing session for our EPs introducing this new rule. We implemented the practice that the EP in charge of the ED must follow the rule. Our precautionary rule is shown in Table 1.

This study comprised two periods. In the first period (before introduction of the rule), the records of CT interpretations in ED blunt trauma cases during January 2011 and June 2012 were reviewed, and the accuracy of the EPs' interpretations as well as resulting patient outcomes were investigated. In the second period (after introduction of the rule), the accuracy of the EPs' CT interpretations and the resulting patient outcomes were investigated for July 2012 and January 2013. Finally, we evaluated whether our rule was effective by comparing the accuracy of the EPs' interpretations and patient outcomes both before and after implementation of the rule.

In both periods, the interpretation accuracy was evaluated by comparing the initial interpretation recorded by the EP and the definitive diagnosis. Each evaluation was independently performed by a senior EP (authorized by the Japanese Association for Acute Medicine) who did not directly participate in the study. When one patient underwent a simultaneous CT scan of several body regions, the results were classified by region and analyzed separately. The evaluation of image diagnoses was performed by dividing the body into the following regions: head, face, neck, chest, abdomen, and pelvis. Checkpoints in each region were evaluated in accordance with the Abbreviated Injury Scale (AIS) (Table 2). In this study, we defined standards for the level of misinterpretation (minor versus major) and the level of gravity (effect on the patient) to evaluate how the level of misinterpretation influenced the clinical course of the patient (namely, we thought that a major misinterpretation, in which an anatomic abnormality was missed, was more likely to lead to a fatal prognosis). Those

Table 1 Precautionary rule for CT interpretation by emergency physicians in blunt trauma

Caution	#1	Unstable physiological condition
		1> GCS < 10 points
		2> Systolic pressure < 90 mmHg
	#2	Suspected injury to multiple regions of the body
		1> severe pain in more than 2 of the 6 regions (head, face, neck, chest, abdomen, pelvis)
		2> bleeding, wounds, deformities, or contusions in more than 2 of the 6 regions
	#3	Injury due to high energy mechanism
		1> traffic accident:
		pedestrian, bicycle vs. vehicle, motorcycle crash, highway crash
		victim thrown from vehicle, death of fellow passenger
		case involving a difficult rescue, sideslip of the vehicle, etc.
		2> fall (3 m)
		3> crushed under heavy object
		4> other high energy mechanisms
	#4	Case that requires invasive emergency treatment necessitating movement to other rooms
		1> case that requires an emergency operation
		2> case that requires emergency angiography (embolization)
		3> other invasive treatment required
Action		**If patient's condition agrees to one of above criteria at least, EP should take action as follows**
		1) EP should actively employ enhanced CT for chest, abdomen and pelvis if possible.
		2) EP should re-interpret emergency CT more than twice after a short interval.
		3) EP should change window level according to organs to interpret.
		4) EP should evaluate not only in an axial view but also in a sagittal view or coronal view if needed.
		5) EP should actively evaluate bone injuries using three-dimensional view.
		6) EP should repeat CT after time has passed if there are unclear points.
Additional advice		**If there problems as follows, EP should consider real-time consultation with a radiologist**
		1) Patient's physiological condition deteriorates in spite of treatments.
		2) Data of laboratory findings show development of anemia or metabolic acidosis in spite of treatments.
		3) Unclear points remain in spite of re-interpretation CT or repetition of CT.

We established a new precautionary rule for the interpretation of emergency CT scans in cases of blunt trauma.

definitions were designed in accordance with past reports (Table 2) [8-10].

For this study, we used unpaired t-tests for continuous data and chi-squared tests for categorical data, except when the number of expected cells was found to be less than five, in which case we used Fisher's exact test. IBM SPSS version 21 was employed and all tests were two-tailed, with differences reported as significant for $p < 0.05$. This study was approved by the ethics committee of Fukushima Medical University, and we tried to protect personal information as much as possible.

Results

In the first period, 365 patients (280 males and 85 females) were identified as blunt trauma patients. Emergency CT was used 1606 times on these patients (361 times for the head, 77 times for the face, 272 times for the neck, 306 times for the chest, 295 times for the abdomen, and 295 times for the pelvic area). The mean patient age was 50.1 ± 23.3 years (expressed as mean ± standard deviation [SD]), and the mean Injury Severity Score (ISS) was 11.9 ± 11.1 (mean ± SD). The cause of trauma was a traffic accident in 186 cases, a fall in 117 cases, and other mechanisms in 62 cases.

The accuracy and outcomes of the EPs' interpretations from the first period are shown in Table 3. Of the 1606 cases, 44 (2.7%) minor misinterpretations and 40 (2.5%) major misinterpretations were identified. There were no duplicated diagnostic mistakes within an individual case and no pattern of diagnostic mistakes from specific doctors.

Table 2 Checkpoints for the interpretation of each region and definitions

Checkpoint	Head	Skull fracture, Basal skull fracture, Brain contusion, Intracranial hemorrhage, Subarachnoid hemorrhage, Subdural hemorrhage, Epidural hemorrhage, Vascular injury
	Face	Bone injury (Ophthalmology wall, Maxilla, Mandible, Zygomatic, Nose), Eyeball injury, Optic nerve injury, Vascular injury (if enhanced)
	Neck	Bone injury (Cervical spine, Spinous process, Transverse process), Pharyngeal injury, Bronchial injury, Vascular injury (if enhanced)
	Chest	Bone injury (Rib, Clavicle, Scapula, Sternum), Thoracic spine injury, Pneumothorax, Hemothorax Pulmonary injury, Bronchial injury, Cardiac injury, Cardiac tamponade, Esophageal injury Diaphragmatic injury, Vascular injury (if enhanced)
	Abdomen	Bone injury (Lumber spine), Parenchymal organ injury (Liver, Gallbladder, Pancreas, Spleen, Kidney, Adrenal gland), Digestive tract injury, Free air, Mesenteric injury, Ureteral injury, Vascular injury (if enhanced)
	Pelvis	Bone injury (Lumber spine, Ilium, Sacrum, Pubis, Ischium, Acetabular cartilage, Femur), Bladder injury, Urinary tract injury, Genital organ injury, Vascular injury (if enhanced)
Definition of misinterpretation		
No misinterpretation		All checkpoints were accurately cleared.
Minor misinterpretation		Anatomical abnormalities were identified, but details were incomplete or incorrect. (e.g., rib fracture was identified but the injured number was misinterpreted; brain injury was pointed out, but the correct diagnosis such as subdural hemorrhage was not recorded.)
Major misinterpretation		Anatomical abnormality described on CT was apparently missed even if EP received support by radiologist.
Gravity level		The gravity level was determined upon review of the patient's clinical course.
	Level 1	Clinical course was not affected by the EP's interpretation.
	Level 2	Clinical course was affected by the EP's misinterpretation.
		1) More invasive treatment was required because of the delayed detection of organ injuries.
		2) Temporary functional disorders or persistent cosmetic problems
		3) The course of treatment was unavoidably changed.
		4) Hospital stay was prolonged.
	Level 3	Clinical prognosis was seriously affected by the EP's misinterpretation.
		1) Permanent, severe functional disorders or cosmetic problems (e.g., persistent disorder of consciousness, limb palsy, large scars)
		2) Death

Checkpoints for each region were established in accordance with the Abbreviated Injury Scale (AIS).

In this period, there were eight major misinterpretations out of 361 cases (2.2%) that underwent head CT (3 subarachnoid hemorrhages, 2 brain contusions, 2 skull fractures, and 1 epidural hemorrhage). One patient judged as a gravity level 2 had a traumatic subarachnoid hemorrhage, brain contusion, and skull fracture detected by the attending EP, but a conscious disorder developed owing to progression of a missed slight epidural hemorrhage. An emergency operation to remove the hemorrhage was successfully performed. Other patients recovered with conservative treatment. There were five major misinterpretations from the 77 cases (6.5%) of orbital plate fractures on face CT, but none of the patients required surgical treatment or experienced persistent functional disorders. There were three major misinterpretations from the 272 cases (1.1%) of spinous process fractures in the cervical spine, but surgical treatment was not required in any.

There were 19 major misinterpretations (6.2%) out of the 306 cases that underwent chest CT (7 costal fractures,

4 transverse process fractures in the thoracic spine, 1 sternum fracture, 1 scapula fracture, 3 pulmonary contusions, 2 cases of pneumothorax, and 1 intercostal artery injury). The patient with intercostal artery trauma did not survive and was categorized as gravity level 3. Three patients with costal fractures and one patient with pneumothorax were categorized as gravity level 2 because a chest drain was required. There were two major misinterpretations from the 295 cases (0.7%) that underwent abdominal CT (1 of liver trauma and 1 of kidney trauma). Neither required any surgical treatment. Anemia did not develop, and both recovered fully without intensive treatment. There were three misinterpretations out of the 295 cases that underwent pelvic CT (1 each for fractures of the pubis, ischium, and neck of the femur). The patient with the femoral neck fracture was operated on by orthopedic surgeons, but the other two patients did not require any surgical treatment. Anemia did not develop in either case, and both recovered fully without intensive treatment.

Table 3 Accuracy and outcomes of EPs' CT interpretations in the first period

Region	Number	Correct interpretation	Minor misinterpretation	Gravity level		Major misinterpretation	Gravity level	
Head	361	338 (93.6%)	15 (4.2%)	1	15		1	7
				2	0	8 (2.2%)	2	1
				3	0		3	0
Face	77	59 (76.6%)	13 (16.9%)	1	12		1	5
				2	1	5 (6.5%)	2	0
				3	0		3	0
Neck	272	267 (982%)	2 (0.7%)	1	2		1	3
				2	0	3 (1.0%)	2	0
				3	0		3	0
Chest	306	281 (91.8%)	6 (2.0%)	1	4		1	14
				2	1	19 (6.2%)	2	4
				3	0		3	1
Abdomen	295	288 (97.6%)	5 (1.7%)	1	5		1	2
				2	0	2 (0.7%)	2	0
				3	0		3	0
Pelvis	295	289 (98.0%)	3 (1.0%)	1	2		1	2
				2	1	3 (1.0%)	2	1
				3	0		3	0
Total	1606	1522 (94.8%)	44 (2.7%)	1	40		1	33
				2	3	40 (2.5%)	2	6
				3	0		3	1

Abbreviation: EPs emergency physicians.
Minor misinterpretations occurred in 44 out of 1606 cases (2.7%), and major misinterpretations occurred in 40 cases (2.5%). There were no duplicated diagnostic mistakes within an individual case.

In the second period, 177 patients presented with blunt trauma, of whom 129 were male and 48 female. In total, emergency CT was used 820 times (171 times for the head, 49 times for the face, 155 times for the neck, 151 times for the chest, 147 times for the abdominal area, and 147 times for the pelvic area). The mean patient age was 50.3 ± 23.4 years (mean ± SD), and the mean ISS was 11.7 ± 9.1 (mean ± SD). There was no statistically significant difference in mean age or ISS compared with the first period. The cause of trauma was a traffic accident in 99 cases, a fall in 44 cases, and other mechanisms in 34 cases.

The accuracy and outcomes of EPs' interpretation in the second period are shown in Table 4. Of the 820 cases, 10 (1.2%) minor misinterpretations and two (0.2%) major misinterpretations were identified. The improvements between the first and second period were statistically significant. Minor misinterpretations occurred in 2.7% of cases (95% confidence interval, 1.9% to 3.5%) in the first period versus 1.2% of cases (95% confidence interval, 0.5% to 2.0%) in the second period (Fisher's exact test, $p = 0.02$). For major misinterpretations, the difference was even greater; major misinterpretations occurred in 2.5% of cases (95% confidence interval, 1.7% to

3.3%) in the first period versus 0.2% of cases (95% confidence interval, −0.1% to 0.6%) in the second period (Fisher's exact test, $p < 0.01$). In the second period, the frequency of minor misinterpretations on face CT was significantly decreased compared with the first period, and there were no minor misinterpretations on pelvic CT in the second period. For head, face, neck, abdomen, and pelvis, there were no major misinterpretations in the second period. For chest CT, two slight costal fractures were missed, but they were categorized as gravity level 1 because they did not require any advanced treatment. In total, real-time radiological support was requested 104 times (12.7% of all cases). In all of these cases, it was difficult to accurately detect injured organs because of complicated trauma, and the additional support meant that effective treatment was carried out.

Discussion

In severe blunt trauma cases, the rapid and accurate detection of injured organs is critical in saving lives. Recently, CT has been reported to be an effective tool for the detection of blunt trauma [3]. In the past, active employment of CT was not recommended because it was thought to expose patients to the risks associated with

Table 4 Accuracy and outcomes of EPs' CT interpretations in the second period versus the first period

Region	Number	Correct interpretation	Minor misinterpretation	Gravity level		P value	Major misinterpretation	Gravity level		P value	Real-time support
Head	171	169 (98.8%)	2 (1.2%)	1	2	0.07	0	1	0		
				2	0			2	0	(−)	17
				3	0			3	0		
Face	49	47 (95.9%)	2 (4.1%)	1	2			1	0		
				2	0	0.03*	0	2	0	(−)	4
				3	0			3	0		
Neck	155	154 (99.3%)	1 (0.6%)	1	1		0	1	0		
				2	0	0.05		2	0	(−)	14
				3	0			3	0		
Chest	151	146 (96.7%)	3 (2.0%)	1	3			1	2		
				2	0	0.38	2(1.3%)	2	0	0.02*	23
				3	0			3	0		
Abdomen	147	145 (98.7%)	2 (1.3%)	1	2			1	0		
				2	0	0.47	0	2	0	(−)	23
				3	0			3	0		
Pelvis	147	147 (100%)	0	1	0			1	0		
				2	0	(−)	0	2	0	(−)	23
				3	0			3	0		
Total	**820**	**808 (98.5%)**	**10 (1.2%)**	**1**	**8**			**1**	**2**		
				2	**0**	**0.02***	**2 (0.2%)**	**2**	**0**	**<0.01***	**104 (12.7%)**
				3	**0**			**3**	**0**		

Fisher's exact test was performed to compare the number of misinterpretations between the first and second periods.
*Indicates a significant difference, with p < 0.05. Abbreviation: EPs emergency physicians.
In the second period, minor misinterpretations occurred in 10 out of 820 cases (1.2%), and major misinterpretations occurred in 2 out of 820 cases (0.2%). The new rule significantly decreased both minor and major misinterpretations (p < 0.05).

high levels of radiation [11]. However, CT can detect very subtle organ trauma, and it is applicable to many areas of the body. Nowadays, it does not require the risky long distance transport of severely injured patients because most emergency medical institutions are equipped with highly efficient CT machines. In fact, CT is becoming one of the most indispensable primary examination tools for the diagnosis of acute diseases in addition to its use in trauma cases [12-14].

However, the present interpretation system for CT has not kept up with the modality's technological development, and real-time interpretation by radiologists is not available in many institutions in Japan because of a nationwide shortage of radiologists. Many EPs, therefore, must make decisions regarding trauma treatment plans without radiological support. Hunter et al. reported that only wet reading was available in the majority of medical institutions surveyed and that emergency CT was usually supported only by radiology residents even in university hospitals [15]. Torreggiani et al. reported that real-time interpretation by radiologists was not available in many institutions and that, in some, radiologist interpretation

took more than 48 hours to prepare [16]. They also reported that EPs and radiologists felt very differently about whether the interpretation system was adequate. Many EPs complained of a deficiency in the current interpretation system. Such problems are likely to continue into the long term unless effective measures are taken. Our hope is that this study may provide an effective CT interpretation system for EPs to use in blunt trauma cases.

In this study, EPs misinterpreted 40 of 1606 cases (2.5%) in the first period. Seven of the 365 total patients (1.9%) were most likely placed at a disadvantage by a major misinterpretation; these patients were categorized as gravity level 2 or 3, and they required additional treatments (such as emergency surgery). Chung et al. studied the accuracy of 4768 interpretation reports of torso CT performed by a radiology resident [9]. In this study, serious misdiagnosis occurred in 2.0% of the cases, and changes in treatment were required in 0.3%. Petinaux et al. reported major discrepancies between the interpretations from EPs and radiologists in 3% of cases (for plain chest and abdominal X-rays) [17]. Most of the discrepancies were considered misdiagnoses, and changes in treatment were required in 0.05% of the cases. Gray comprehensively surveyed the occurrence of diagnostic mistakes in the ED [18] and found that 79.7% of mistakes were associated with bone trauma and that most misdiagnoses could likely be avoided by careful interpretation.

There were no large differences in the number and level of diagnostic mistakes between these studies and our study. However, even a small misinterpretation by the EP may lead to irrelevant treatment or a potentially fatal delay in appropriate treatment. This must be avoided wherever possible, but is difficult to achieve in actuality. One solution is to further train EPs to improve their interpretations of CT results. However, a high level of skill is required to interpret CT results, and we believe that it would be almost impossible to improve interpretation ability with unsystematic short-term training. Keijzers et al. evaluated the effect of imaging training in a randomized study and concluded that short-term training did not improve the skill of EPs in interpreting chest CT [19]. The systematic introduction of long-term training would be impossible in our hospital, because EPs are too busy working during the day.

Our study suggested that a simple precautionary rule could significantly decrease misinterpretations without requiring long-term EP training. In particular, the frequency of major misinterpretations decreased in a remarkable manner after implementation of the rule. Our procedure is simple and easy to put into practice, but it proved to be very effective in maximizing the safe interpretation of CT scans by EPs in blunt trauma. Essentially, the rule advised that EPs should interpret emergency CT scans with particular care when a complicated injury was suspected. We believe that the interpretational skill of our EPs is by no means low, but in unstable cases or cases that need invasive emergency treatments, there is a high risk that exact interpretation cannot be carried out. We believe that promoting cautious and meticulous interpretation in every case, but particularly in the cases mentioned above, is effective in preventing misdiagnosis. Our procedure is simple to implement, allowing interpretation to be finished in a short time.

Additionally, our rule specifies that the EP should request the support of real-time interpretation by a radiologist in difficult cases. The interpretations made by a radiologist are not always perfect, but we think that objective evaluation by a professional third party is effective in preventing misinterpretation. We have recently refined our cooperative arrangements, and a radiologist now voluntarily participates in the primary evaluation of major trauma cases. However, success depends on a relatively small group of dedicated radiologists, and it might not be possible to obtain similar cooperation in other medical institutions. Saketkhoo et al. reported that very few radiologists were dedicated to cooperation with the ED [20]. In this study, online interpretation with an electronic chart was used in all cases, which was effective in providing real-time radiology support because radiologists did not have to physically attend the ED. In our study, the incorporation of collaborative real-time support from a radiologist helped to maximize the efficacy of our method.

The problems caused by CT misinterpretation in the ED need to be avoided, and this study represents a first step in establishing an effective and safe CT interpretation system. However, our study has several limitations. First, the number of CT interpretations evaluated was slightly low because our study was conducted in a single medical institute. Second, the definition of the checkpoints may not have been ideal, as severe anatomical injuries were mixed with slight anatomical injuries. Third, the standard for requesting cooperation with a radiologist was not precisely defined. We think that further work is needed to ensure that our method is more widely applicable, and we plan to request cooperation from other critical care centers in Fukushima Prefecture to test it more widely in the future.

Conclusions

The introduction of a simple precautionary rule, together with collaboration with a radiologist, was effective in improving the accuracy of EPs' CT interpretations. In the future, we would like to continue these efforts to establish a comprehensive CT interpretation system for blunt trauma patients.

Abbreviations
AIS: Abbreviated injury scale; CT: Computed tomography; ED: Emergency department; EPs: Emergency physicians; ISS: Injury severity score; SD: Standard deviation.

Competing interests
The authors declare that they have no competing interests.

Authors' contributions
YI designed this study and obtained approval from the ethics committee and cooperation from the radiology department. CT supervised the conduction of the study. TS, CN, and YT managed the data, including quality control. JS and AH provided statistical advice regarding the study design and analyzed the data. YI drafted the manuscript, and all authors contributed substantially to its revision. YI takes responsibility for the study as a whole. Editorial assistance was provided by Edanz, a professional editing company. All authors read and approved the final manuscript.

References
1. Soto JA, Anderson SW: **Multidetector CT of blunt abdominal trauma.** *Radiology* 2012, **265**:678–693.
2. Merchant N, Scalea T, Stein D: **Can CT angiography replace conventional bi-planar angiography in the management of severe scapulothoracic dissociation injuries?** *Am Surg* 2012, **78**:875–882.
3. Flohr TG, Bruder H, Stierstorfer K, Petersilka M, Schmidt B, McCollough CH: **Image reconstruction and image quality evaluation for a dual source CT scanner.** *Med Phys* 2008, **35**:5882–5897.
4. Wing VW, Federle MP, Morris JA Jr, Jeffrey RB, Bluth R: **The clinical impact of CT for blunt abdominal trauma.** *AJR* 1985, **145**:1191–1194.

5.   Huber-Wagner S, Lefering R, Qvick LM, Körner M, Kay MV, Pfeifer KJ, Reiser M, Mutschler W, Kanz KG, Working Group on Polytrauma of the German Trauma Society: **Effect of whole-body CT during trauma resuscitation on survival: a retrospective, multicenter study.** *Lancet* 2009, **373**:1455–1461.

5.   O'Leary MR, Smith M, Olmsted WW, Curtis DJ: **Physician assessments of practice pattern in emergency department radiograph interpretation.** *Ann Emerg Med* 1988, **17**:1019–1023.

7.   James MR, Bracegirdle A, Yates DW: **X-ray reporting in accident and emergency departments-an area for improvements in efficiency.** *Arch Emerg Med* 1991, **8**:266–270.

8.   Tienq N, Grinberg D, Li SF: **Discrepancies in interpretation of ED body computed tomographic scans by radiology residents.** *Am J Emerg Med* 2007, **25**:45–48.

9.   Chung JH, Strigel RM, Chew AR, Albrecht E, Gunn ML: **Overnight resident interpretation of torso CT at a level 1 trauma center: an analysis and review of the literature.** *Acad Radiol* 2009, **16**:1155–1160.

10. Vorhies RW, Harrison PB, Smith RS, Helmer SD: **Senior surgical residents can accurately interpret trauma radiographs.** *Am Surg* 2002, **68**:221–226.

11. Tien HC, Tremblay LN, Rizoli SB, Gelberg J, Spencer F, Caldwell C, Brenneman FD: **Radiation exposure from diagnostic imaging in severely injured trauma patients.** *J Trauma* 2007, **62**:151–156.

12. Broder J, Warshauer DM: **Increasing utilization of computed tomography in the adult emergency department, 2005–2006.** *Emerg Radiol* 2006, **13**:25–30.

13. Lee J, Pawa KS, Kirschner J, Pawa S, Wiener DE, Newman DH, Shah K: **Computed tomography use in the adult emergency department of an academic urban hospital from 2001 to 2007.** *Ann Emerg Med* 2010, **56**:591–596.

14. Smith CB, Barrett TW, Berger CL, Berger CL, Zhou C, Thurman RJ, Wrenn KD: **Prediction of blunt traumatic injury in high-acuity patients: bedside examination vs. computed tomography.** *Am J Emerg Med* 2011, **29**:1–10.

15. Hunter TB, Krupinski EA, Hunt KR, Erly WK: **Emergency department coverage by academic department of radiology.** *Acad Radiol* 2000, **7**:165–170.

16. Torreggiani WC, Nicolaou S, Lyburn ID, Harris AC, Buckley AR: **Emergency radiology in Canada: a national survey.** *Can Assoc Radiol J* 2002, **53**:160–167.

17. Petinaux B, Bhat R, Boniface K, Aristizabal J: **Accuracy of radiographic readings in the emergency department.** *Am J Emerg Med* 2011, **29**:18–25.

18. Gray HR: **Diagnostic errors in an accident and emergency department.** *Emerg Med J* 2001, **18**:263–269.

19. Keijzers G, Sithirasenan V: **The effect of a chest imaging lecture on emergency department doctors' ability to interpret chest CT images: a randomized study.** *Europ J Emerg Med* 2012, **19**:40–45.

20. Saketkhoo DD, Bhargavan M, Sunshine JH, Forman HP: **Emergency department image interpretation services at private community hospitals.** *Radiology* 2004, **231**:190–197.

10

The scientific production in trauma of an emerging country

Gustavo Pereira Fraga[1*], Vitor Augusto de Andrade[2], Ricardo Schwingel[2], Jamil Pastori Neto[2], Sizenando Vieira Starling[3], Sandro Rizoli[4]

Abstract

Background: The study aims to examine whether the end of specialty in trauma surgery in 2003 influenced the scientific productivity of the area in Brazil.

Methods: We identified and classified the manuscripts and their authors, from databases such as *PubMed*, *Scielo* and *Plataforma Lattes* and sites like *Google*, in addition to the list of members of SBAIT, the sole society in Brazil to congregate surgeons involved in trauma care in the country. We applied statistical tests to compare the periods of 1997-2003 and 2004-2010. We also analyzed the following variables: impact factor of journals in which manuscripts were published, journals, regional origin of authors, time since graduation, and conducting post-doctorate abroad.

Results: We observed a significant increase in publication rates of the analyzed groups over the years. There was a predominance of quantitative studies from the Southeast (especially the state of São Paulo). More time elapsed after graduation and the realization of postdoctoral studies abroad influenced the individual scientific productivity.

Conclusion: The number of articles published by authors from the area of trauma has been growing over the past 14 years in Brazil. The end of the specialty in trauma surgery in the country did not influence the scientific productivity in the area.

Background

Brazil is an emerging economy and a member of the "BRIC" countries, which also includes Russia, India and China. Its research labor force and research and development investment are rapidly expanding opening many new possibilities in a diversifying research portfolio. With around 85,000 papers published over a 5 year period (2003-2007), Brazil is responsible for 1.83% of the world's papers published in journals indexed by Thomson Reuters, the agency that regularly indexes over 10,000 scientific journals worldwide [1,2].

Along with the recent economic and scientific growth of the country, the number of injuries has also grown to an astounding 130.000 deaths per year in Brazil with over 300.000 victims suffering some sequelae. Most victims of trauma in Brazil are between 5 and 14 years of age [2]. Not all is bad in Brazil that over the last decade, Brazil experienced major improvements in this scenario with the creation of stricter laws and changes in it's traffic code leading to notable reductions in interpersonal violence and automobile crashes, which were the leading causes of death [3-7].

Despite the overall growth in trauma, in 2003 the residency training in trauma surgery during a two years program was abolished in Brazil. This change in our opinion, lead to a reduction in the number of trained professionals and academic exposure to this surgical specialty that could reduce the impetus of doing more research on the treatment of trauma disease. Therefore we hypothesized that despite the overall scientific growth in Brazil, specifically in trauma, the termination of training in trauma surgery would reduce the country scientific production

* Correspondence: fragagp2008@gmail.com
[1]Division of Trauma Surgery, Department of Surgery, School of Medical Sciences, University of Campinas (Unicamp), Rua Alexander Fleming, 181 Cidade Universitária "Prof. Zeferino Vaz" - Barão Geraldo, Campinas - SP, Brazil
Full list of author information is available at the end of the article

in this area [8-10]. The objective of this study is to evaluate the scientific productivity in trauma, comparing the number of publications before and after the residency training in trauma was terminated in 2003 in Brazil.

Methods

For the purpose of this study, academic production was defined as the number of publications in "trauma". The University of Campinas (UNICAMP) Research Institutional Ethics Board approved the study and the Sociedade Brasileira de Atendimento Integrado ao Traumatizado (SBAIT) gave us consent to do the study and access to the list of all its members on December 2010.

SBAIT is the only society in Brazil to congregate surgeons dedicated to trauma care. The vast majority of the Brazilian general surgeons committed to trauma, with academic activities in trauma and holding a University appointment are members of SBAIT. It is not a governmental agency, membership is voluntary and its members are trained in general surgery and not in orthopedics or neurosurgery that congregate under the auspices of other Societies. The manuscripts published by the SBAIT members are the best sample of Brazil's scientific production in the area of trauma.

After obtaining the list of all SBAIT members in December 2010, we identified all manuscripts they authored after 2003 (2004 to 2010). To determine whether any significant changes occurred, we performed a similar search for the same number of years, but prior to 2003, thus from 1997 to 2003. The manuscripts were retrieved from PubMed (http://www.pubmed.com), Scielo (http://www.scielo.org), the open-access online web curriculum vitae Plataforma Lattes (http://www.lattes.cnpq.br) commonly used by Brazilian investigators and a general search at Google (http://www.google.com.br).

Data collection was performed in February 2011. The manuscripts were classified as trauma when the focus was clearly on this area, or otherwise as non-trauma. For the few manuscript where the focus was uncertain, the classification was decided by consensus. The manuscripts authored by more than one SBAIT member were counted only once. Considering our goal of investigating the scientific production in Brazil, the manuscripts authored by SBAIT members that were done overseas and published in non-Brazilian journals were excluded. To evaluate the quality of the manuscripts and identify the journals favored by the Brazilian investigators, we gathered the name of the Journal, year of publication and the Impact Factor (IF) as calculated by the *Thompson Web of Knowledge* (*Institute for Scientific Information* – ISI) [11].

The first analysis aimed at studying the variations in the number of published papers before and after 2003, the year residency in trauma surgery was abolished. To this end, we tabulated the number of all publications and of all publications in trauma as well as the name of the Journals and their yearly Impact Factor since 1997. We then performed a simple comparison of the number of publications before and after 2003 and the Impact Factor of the journals.

To characterize the SBAIT members most successful in publishing in trauma, the authors were separated according to: 1. the place (state) of residence at the time of the publication; 2. the number of publications; 3. year of graduation from medical School and 4. whether they had graduate studies overseas. The year of graduation and overseas training was obtained from the open publicaly available online web CV Plataforma Lattes (http://www. lattes.cnpq.br). Next we analyzed the association between years of graduation and number of publications, as well as whether overseas training resulted in sustained increase in scientific production. The papers published during the overseas training were not included in the present analysis.

The statistical analysis used mean/median, standard deviation and maximum/minimum values for the numeric variables. The Spearman correlation was used to analyze the variation in the total number of publications, year of publication and Impact Factor. Linear regression analysis was used to estimate the association of the total number of publications, while the Mann-Whitney test was used to compare publications between the two study periods (before and after 2003). Due to the sample size and lack of normal distribution, the Kruskal-Wallis test was used to analyze time from graduation from medical School. Pearson qui-square and the exact Fisher test were used for values below 5. Significance was determined to be of 5% ($p<.05$) and SAS for Windows was used (version 9.1.3. SAS Institute Inc, 2002-2003, Cary, NC, USA).

Results

In December 2010 SBAIT had a total of 320 members, which consists of the group of surgeons analyzed in the present study. Of these 320 surgeons, 104 (32.5%) published a total of 627 original papers in all areas of knowledge, of which 178 were in trauma. Considering only the work developed and published in Brazil, there were a total of 571 papers, of which 160 were in trauma. These 160 trauma papers were authored by a total of 52 surgeons, all SBAIT members.

We found a significant correlation between the year of publication and the overall number of publications ($r = 0.89890$, $p = 0.001$), the number of publications in trauma ($r = 0, 65560$, $p =0.0109$) as well as the number of papers in trauma published in journals with any impact factor ($r = 0.60824$, $p =0.0210$). This analysis reveals a continuing and significant increase in publication rates of the analyzed groups over the years (Figure 1). Graphs 1A (Straight regression: $Y = -7995.23 +01.04 X$, $P <0.001$),

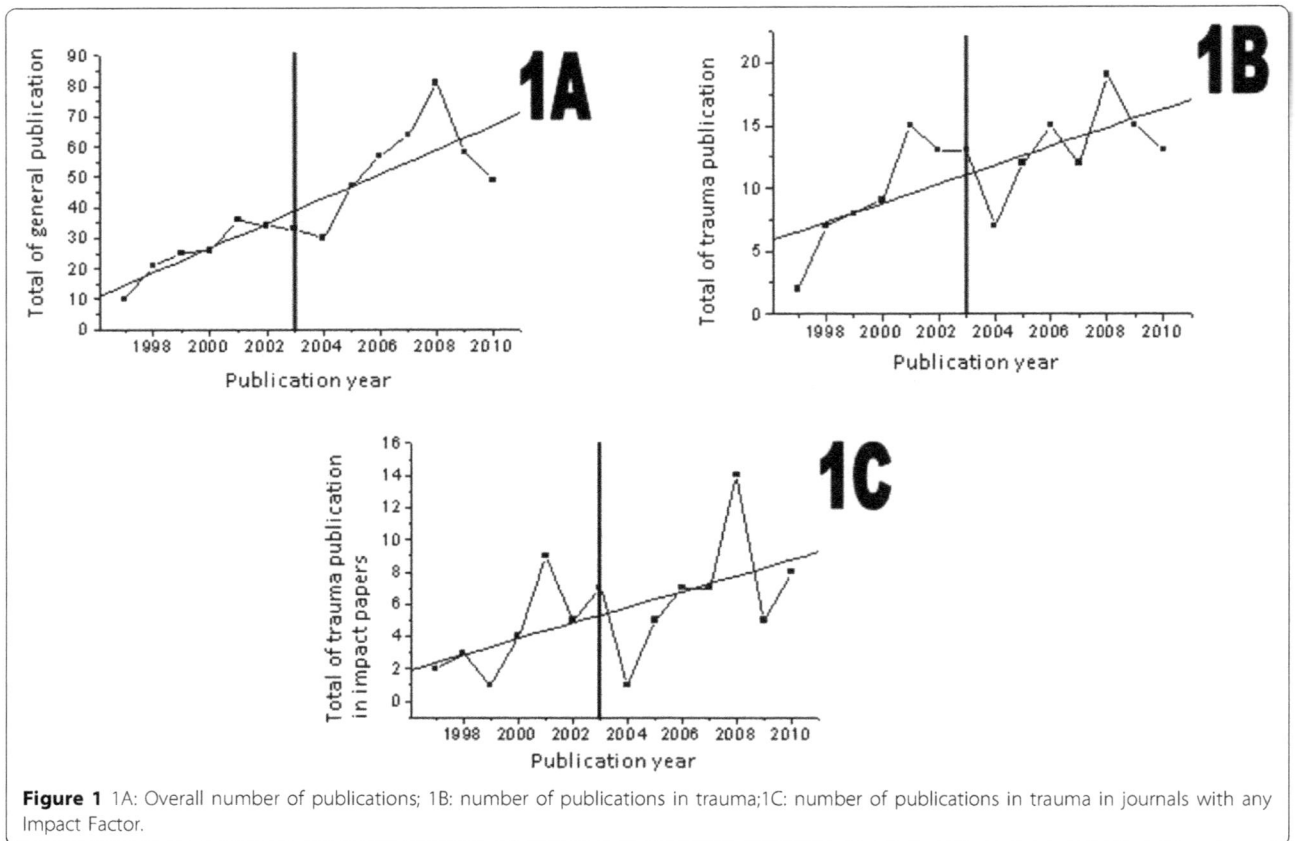

Figure 1 1A: Overall number of publications; 1B: number of publications in trauma;1C: number of publications in trauma in journals with any Impact Factor.

1B (Straight regression: Y=-1494.50 + 0.75 X, P = 0.004) and 1C (Straight regression: Y=-71.96 00:49 + X, P = 0.029) disclose the linear regression analysis and the association between the year of publication and total number of publications and the trend towards an increased number of publications.

The comparative analysis between the periods before (1997 to 2003) and after 2003 (2004 to 2010) showed a statistically significant difference only on the overall number of publications, which was higher after 2003 (p = 0.006). The total number of publications in trauma (p = 0.196) and trauma in journals with impact factor (p = 0.245) was not statistically different. No statistically significant difference was found on the year of publication and impact factor of journals published (p = 0.3683), the study of linear trend between years and the impact factor by linear regression (p = 0.510) and comparison of the impact factor among two periods (p = 0.477).

Table 1 show the list of top 10 journals in the world that have published Brazilian papers in trauma.

Table 2 shows the regional distribution of the SBAIT members with publications in trauma between 1997 and 2010.

The Southeastern region of Brazil had 160 surgeons that were members of SBAIT in December 2010. Of

these, 101 were from Sao Paulo state, 45 had published at least 1 paper and 30 had authored papers in trauma. Sao Paulo state had the highest number of publications in Brazil. Compared to the other states, Sao Paulo had significantly more SBAIT members with publications (p =0.002) and more publications per author in trauma (p = 0.003). When the two periods were compared, the number of publications from Sao Paulo continued to be

Table 1 List of top 10 journals that have published Brazilian papers in trauma.

Journal	Number of papers
Revista do Colégio Brasileiro de Cirurgiões	54
Journal of Trauma	16
Revista da Associação Medica Brasileira	15
Acta Cirúrgica Brasileira	12
Injury - International Journal of the Care of the Injured	7
Revista do Hospital das Clínicas	6
World Journal of Emergency Surgery	4
Revista de Saúde Pública	3
Jornal Vascular Brasileiro	3
Sao Paulo Medical Journal	3

Table 2 SBAIT member distributions by region and publication.

Region	Total of members	Published	Published on trauma
Southeast	160	66	35
Northeast	64	11	4
South	46	16	9
North	37	8	4
Midwest	13	3	0

significantly higher (p = 0.003). Of the 160 papers published, 52 were authored by surgeons from Sao Paulo. The same was observed with trauma publications authored by 30 (57.7%) surgeons from the State of Sao Paulo. About ¼ of the authors from Sao Paulo (12 or 23%) published more than five papers in this period. Figure 2 shows the distribution of the 52 authors by number of papers published in trauma.

The number of years from graduation from medical school of the 104 SBAIT members authoring papers in Brazil on all topics over the study period was of 22.4 years, varying from 1 to 49 years. Table 3 shows the number of years since graduation for the 104 authors. Statistical analysis revealed significant correlation between the elapsed time after graduation and the number of publications of each author in trauma, the authors show that with more time graduation held the largest number of published studies (p =0.0373).

Of the 320 SBAIT members in December 2010, 10 had post-doctoral training overseas: 6 in the United States, 1 in Canada, 1 in both the United States and Canada, 1 in France and 1 in Germany. There was a significant difference between the number of publications by these 10 surgeons and the 94 other ones on the number of publications in Brazil and overseas (p <0.001; p <0.001 respectively) (Table 4).

Discussion

This study is important because is the first to examine the scientific contribution of an emerging country in trauma. Overall the number of publications undertaken and supported by Brazilian continuously grew over the last 14 years (Figure 1A, 1BA, 1C). This increase, demonstrated in Figure 1A, paralleled the trend in scientific production in surgery over the last decade demonstrated by Heldwein et al [2]. Possible explanations for this increase may be inputed to increasing funding for research by the Brazilian government, particularly the Ministry of Health that over the last decade increased the opportunities for international exchange and dissemination of Internet use [2,12,13].

The number of publications devoted to trauma, analyzed as a whole and also in relation to the proportion published in journals with impact factor, followed the increased productivity of Brazilian researchers, showing that the production has grown not only in absolute numbers, but also in quality [2,14]. Thus, the end of residency in trauma surgery in Brazil did not seem to have affected the scientific development of the area nor the enthusiasm of the authors [8,9,15]. The sustained growth may be explained by the greater diffusion of courses such as the Advanced Trauma Life Support (ATLS) and scientific events throughout the country, which also grew enormously over the last decade (results not shown). We consider that the greater involvement of professionals in trauma is very welcome in our country, given the increasing numbers of motor vehicle collisions and domestic violence. According to the Information System (SIM), which collects national data, the period comprising the years 1998 and 2008, the total number of homicides rose from 41,950 to 50,113 (an increase of 17.8%, higher than the population growth of 17.2% over the same period, despite the disarmament policies developed mainly from 2004), and deaths from traffic crashes increased from 30,994 to 39,211 (an increase of 20.8%, also higher population growth, despite the enactment of the last Traffic Code in 1997 which led to a decrease in the quantity of violence, but in absolute terms, lasted only three years - 1997 to 2000) [4,6,7,16-19].

In this study, we chose not to analyze the quality of studies, which could be done by analyzing the number of times they were actually cited. We still performed an evaluation of the quality when we analyzed the impact factor of the journals that published the studies. We opted for the impact factor, since it provides a global assessment of the insertion of Brazilian investigators in the national and international setting of scientific publications. It is important to mention that no single parameters is ideal for determining the quality of publications since high-impact journals can still publish low impact studies [16,20].

Zhi Li et al. [20] analyzed the characteristics of publications in urgent and emergency care by Chinese authors. He reported that over a period of 10 years 932 studies were published and the number of publications grew

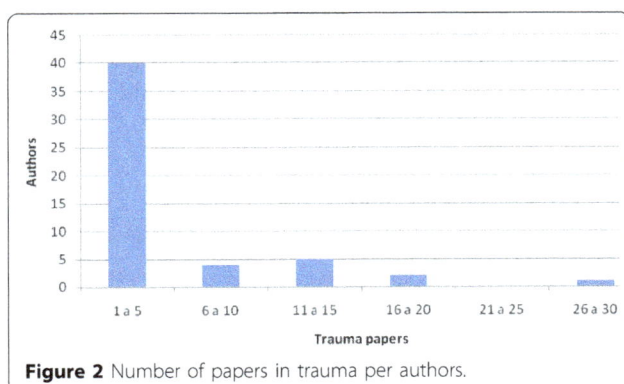

Figure 2 Number of papers in trauma per authors.

Table 3 Number of years from graduation from medical schools and number of publications.

Time of graduation	Number of authors	Average general publications	Average numbers of publications in trauma
< 5 years	5	2,2	0,6
6 – 10 years	11	2,2	0,3
11 – 15 years	6	1,3	0,7
16 – 20 years	23	10,9	3,6
21 – 25 years	18	3,6	1,4
26 – 30 years	19	8,6	2,0
31 – 35 years	14	7,8	1,6
> 35 years	8	23,8	8,9

over the years. The Journal of Trauma was used the most by the authors surveyed. When he analyzed the 18 major journals specialized in trauma, this author found that the United States (from 1999 to 2008) was the country with the highest number of publication in trauma with 9956 articles. It was followed by Germany, Britain, France and Japan, with 2668, 2460, 1301 and 998 publications each. Despite many major differences that which prevent a reasonable comparison, our study shows that Brazilian surgeons published less than the countries described above with 160 publications in 38 journals. However we must also consider that significant social, cultural, economical and scientific differences between Brazil and the other countries. Under this perspective, we think that the number of publications by Brazilian surgeons is encouraging particularly when one considers the continuous growth remains significant, especially considering the scientific context of the country.

The Journal of the Brazilian College of Surgeons (Revista do Colegio Brasileiro de Cirurgioes) was the journal with the largest number of publications by Brazilian surgeons including trauma papers. The JBCS is published bimonthly and was founded in 1930 by the Brazilian College of Surgeons. The non-Brazilian with the largest number of publications was the Journal of Trauma, founded in 1961 and specialized in trauma and emergency surgery (Table 1). In the Chinese study by Zhi Li et al. [20] the Journal of Trauma was also the one that published most Chinese papers.

The southeast region of Brazil has the highest population density in the country, housing 42% of the Brazilian population. The State of São Paulo alone is home to about 50% of all the southeast population and 55% of all the SBAIT members living in the southeast region. Sao Paulo has the largest Gross Domestic Product (GDP) of the country [21,22], the largest vehicle fleet and rate of urbanization, all social factors that are directly related to the leading causes of death from trauma: motor vehicle collisions and homicides [3]. The southeast has five of the largest universities in the country resulting in the State of Sao Paulo alone producing 38% of all Brazilian publications and in 2008, 1.83% of all publications in the world [1,2,13].

Our results demonstrate that after Sao Paulo Minas Gerais, Rio Grande do Sul and Parana are the ones with the largest number of publications in general surgery.

Despite the observed growth in research we observed, the number of publications being done in Brazil remain small [1,23]. The Coordination for the Improvement of Higher Education Personnel (CAPES) recently reported that more than 50% of all dissertations and doctoral thesis made in Brazil are not published, a fact that can make the country invisible to the scientific community [24,25].

Another interesting finding of the present study is that ¾ of the authors (76.9%) published up to five papers, 1/6 (17.3%) 6 to 20 papers and 1/20 (5.76%) published 26 to 30 papers. The group of surgeons that were SBAIT members in 2010 that published studies is small but considerable 16.3%. Seniority, measured in this study as years from graduation, correlated with scientific productivity: those with the highest number of publications were also the most seniors, especially those with more than 35 years since graduation. If 3 of the 8 investigators with more than 35 years since graduation were excluded from the analysis, the average number of publications would be much lower (7.2 for all publications and 1.4 for trauma) and the most productive group would consist of those between 16 and 20 years of graduation.

Table 4 SBAIT members with post-doctoral training overseas and number of publications.

Post doctorate at exterior	Number of years since graduation	Number of papers published during overseas post-doctoral training	Number of papers published in Brazil
No = 94	1 – 49 (Average: 22,2)	-	1 - 56 (Total: 520; Average: 5,6)
Yes = 10	17 - 33 (Average: 24,3)	0 - 6 (Total: 17; Average: 3,4)	3 - 86 (Total: 249; Average: 24,9)

Our study also shows the significant and positive influence of post-doctoral training overseas on scientific publications. Of the 104 authors, only 10 had post doctoral training overseas but their a average number of publications was 4.4 times higher than the others. These results are in agreement with the work of other authors [24,25]. Such training foster collaboration between institutions and investigators and reinforce the importance of promoting such training, promoting cooperation between institutions, evolution of organizations, and development of scientific production [24,25].

Conclusion

The number of papers published in Brazilian journals by Brazilian surgeons in surgery and trauma has experienced a linear growth over the past 14 years. We were unable to identify any evidence that the end of residency in trauma surgery in Brazil negatively influenced the scientific production in this area. The main characteristics of the Brazilian surgeons that write papers in trauma can be described as someone that lives in the southeast of Brazil, most likely in the State of São Paulo and graduated from medical school more than 16 years ago. The observed growth in the number of publications parallels the economic growth of the country and the investments made by the Brazilian government in research and development over recent years. New possibilities of research in this area of knowledge can be offered, with options for expansion of partnership and international cooperation for the development of science. Our study suggests that the scientific growth in this specific area of surgery (trauma) is more likely the result of an overall growth in research and development and less due to specific growth in trauma as can be attested by the fact that the end of the residency program in trauma surgery in 2003 had no apparent effect in the number of publications in trauma.

Acknowledgements

This article has been published as part of *World Journal of Emergency Surgery* Volume 7 Supplement 1, 2012: Proceedings of the World Trauma Congress 2012. The full contents of the supplement are available online at http://www.wjes.org/supplements/7/S1.

Author details

[1]Division of Trauma Surgery, Department of Surgery, School of Medical Sciences, University of Campinas (Unicamp), Rua Alexander Fleming, 181 Cidade Universitária "Prof. Zeferino Vaz" - Barão Geraldo, Campinas - SP, Brazil. [2]School of Medical Sciences, University of Campinas (Unicamp), Campinas - SP, Brazil. [3]Hospital João XXIII, Belo Horizonte - MG, Brazil. [4]Departments of Surgery and Critical Care Medicine, Sunnybrook Health Sciences Centre, University of Toronto, Canada.

Authors' contributions

GPF had overall responsibility for the study including conception, design and intellectual content, collection, analysis and interpretation of data. VAdA participated in the conception, design and intellectual content, collection, analysis and interpretation of data. RS participated in the conception, design and intellectual content, collection, analysis and interpretation of data. JPN participated in the conception, design and intellectual content, collection, analysis and interpretation of data. SVS participated in the intellectual content, revision of the manuscript, figures and tables. SR participated in the intellectual content, revision of the manuscript, figures and tables.

Competing interests

None.

References

1. Country Profiles: 2009: Top 20 Countries in ALL FIELDS, 1999- August 31, 2009. Avaible at: http://sciencewatch.com/dr/cou/pdf/09decALL.pdf..
2. Heldwein FL, Hartmann AA, Kalil AN, Neves BVD, Ratti GSB, Beber MC Jr, *et al*: Cited Brazilian papers in general surgery between 1970 and 2009. *Clinics* 2010, **65**(5):521-529.
3. Waiselfisz JJ: **Map of Violence 2011. The young people of Brazil**. *Brasília: Ministry of Justice* 2009.
4. Reichenheim ME, Souza ER, Moraes CL, Jorge MHPM, Silva CMFP, Minaya MCS: **Violence and injuries in Brazil: the effect, progress made, and challenges ahead**. *Lancet* 2011, **377**:1962-1975.
5. Paim J, Travassos C, Almeida C, Bahia L, Macinko J: **The Brazilian health system: history, advances, and challenges**. *Lancet* 2011, **377**:1778-1797.
6. Victora GC, Barreto ML, Leal MC, Monteiro CA, Schmidt MI, Paim J, *et al*: **Health conditions and health-policy innovations in Brazil: the way forward**. *Lancet* 2011, **377**:2042-2053.
7. Almeida-Filho A: **Higher education and health care in Brazil**. *Lancet* 2011, **377**:1898-1900.
8. Birolini D: **Trauma: social and medical challenge**. *J Am Coll Surg* 2008, **207**(1):1-6.
9. Green SM: **Trauma surgery: discipline in crisis**. *Ann Emerg Med* 2009, **53**:198-207.
10. The Committee to Development the Reorganized Specialty of Trauma, Surgical Critical Care, and Emergency Surgery: **Acute Care Surgery: Trauma, Critical care, and Emergency Surgery**. *J Trauma* 2005, **58**:614-616.
11. ISI Web of knowledge database. Available at: http://apps.isiknowledge.com.
12. Ministry of Health Department of Science and Technology, Ministry of Science, Technology and Strategic Inputs: **Decentralization in the context of promoting health research**. *Rev. Saúde Pública* 2011, **45**(3):626-630.
13. Marques F: **Advances and challenges**. *Fapesp* 2011, **185**:26-33.
14. Berwanger O, Riberio RA, Finkelsztejn A, Watanabe M, Suzumura EA, Duncan BB, *et al*: **The quality of reporting of trial abstracts is suboptimal: Survey of major general medical journals**. *Journal of Clinical Epidemiology* 2009, **62**:387-392.
15. Ciesla DJ, Moore EE, Moore JB, Johnson JL, Cothren CC, Burch JM: **The Academic Trauma Center Is a Model for the Future Trauma and Acute Care Surgeon**. *J.Trauma* 2005, **58**(4):657-662.
16. Schimidt MI, Duncan BB, Silva GA, Menezes AN, Monteiro AC, Barreto SM, *et al*: **Chronic non-communicable diseases in Brazil: burden and current challenges**. *Lancet* 2011, **377**:1949-1961.
17. Mello Jorge M, Koizumi M: **Traffic accidents in Brazil: an atlas of their distribution**. *São Paulo* ABRAMET; 2007.
18. Krug EG, Dahlberg LL, Mercy JA, Zwi AB, Lozano R: **World report on violence and health**. Geneva: World Health Organization; 2002.
19. WHO: **Age-standardized mortality rates by cause (per 100 000 population)**. Geneva: World Health Organization; 2008, Avaible at: http://www.who.int/whosis/indicators/compendium/2008/1mst/en/index.htm.
20. Li Z, Liao Z, Wu FX, Yang LQ, Sun YM, Yu WF: **Scientific publications in critical care medicine journals from Chinese authors: a 10-year survey of the literature**. *J Trauma* 2010, **69**(4):E20-3.
21. BRAZIL. Ministry of Planning, Budget and Management. Brazilian Institute of Geography and Statistics: **Population Count.**, Available at: http://www.censo2010.ibge.gov.br.
22. BRAZIL. Ministry of Planning, Budget and Management. Brazilian Institute of Geography and Statistics: **Population Count.**, Available at:http://www.ibge.gov.br/home/download/estatistica.shtm.
23. Andrade VA, Carpini S, Schwingel R, Calderan Fraga GP: **Publication of papers presented in a Brazilian Trauma Congress**. *Rev Col Bras Cir* 2011, **38**(3):172-176.

Fatal motorcycle crashes: a serious public health problem in Brazil

Carlos Eduardo Carrasco[1], Mauricio Godinho[2], Marilisa Berti de Azevedo Barros[3], Sandro Rizoli[4], Gustavo Pereira Fraga[2*]

Abstract

Introduction: The numbers of two-wheel vehicles are growing across the world. In comparison to other vehicles, motorcycles are cheaper and thus represent a significant part of the automobile market. Both the mobility and speed are attractive factors to those who want to use them for work or leisure. Crashes involving motorcyclists have become an important issue, especially fatal ones. Specific severe injuries are responsible for the deaths. Defining them is necessary in order to offer better prevention and a more suitable medical approach.

Methods: All fatal motorcycle crashes between January 2001 and December 2009 in Campinas, Brazil, were analyzed in this study. Official data have been collected from police incident reports, hospitals' registers and autopsies. Both incidents and casualties were analyzed according to relevant variables. The Injury Severity Score (ISS) was calculated, describing the most potentially fatal injuries.

Results: There were 479 deaths; 90.8% were male; the mean age was 27.8 (range 0-73); 86.4% were conductors of the vehicles; blood alcohol was positive in 42.3%; 49.7% died at a hospital; 32.6% died at the scene; 26.1% of the accidents occurred at night, 69.1% were urban and 30.9% occurred on highways. The main causes of injury were collisions (63%) and falls (14%). The mean ISS was 38.5 (range 9-75). With regard to injuries, head trauma (67%) and thoracic trauma (40%) were the most common, followed by abdominal trauma (35%). Traumatic brain injury (67%) and hypovolemic shock (38%) were the most frequent causes of death.

Conclusions: Alcohol was a significant factor in relation to the accidents. Head trauma was the most frequent and severe injury. Half of the victims died before receiving adequate medical attention, suggesting that prevention programs and laws should be implemented and applied in order to save future lives.

Introduction

The number of motorcycles is increasing worldwide, particularly in developing countries. A World Health Organization (WHO) study on the Americas concluded that in countries like Brazil, Mexico, Canada and the United States [1], motorcycle crashes are responsible for 20-30% of all deaths due to trauma.

In Singapore, motorcycle crashes are responsible for 54% of all deaths caused by any motor vehicle accidents [2]. In Italy in 1997 [3], 20% of all deaths due to traffic accidents involved motorcycles while in the United States the number of deaths due to motorcycle crash increased 103% between 1997 and 2006 [4], numbering 2,300 deaths in 1994 and 4,000 in 2004 [5]. In the United Kingdom in 1998 [6] motorcycle crashes were responsible for 15% of all deaths or serious injuries by traffic accidents.

The number motorcycles has increased especially in large urban areas possibly due to increasing fuel costs, intense traffic and low purchase price for motorcycles [1,7-10]. Despite being considered dangerous, motorcycles are an attractive and cheap option for leisure and/or work, particularly in urban areas.

* Correspondence: fragagp2008@gmail.com
[2]Division of Trauma Surgery, Department of Surgery, Faculty of Medical Sciences, University of Campinas (FCM/UNICAMP), Campinas, SP, Brazil
Full list of author information is available at the end of the article

In Brazil, motorcycles are widely used to transport correspondence in high traffic urban areas by a special class of workers known as *"motoboys"*, as well as taxis (*"moto-taxis"*). Despite a few studies demonstrating the enormous impact in mortality of motorcycle crashes, this issue has been mostly neglected by scholars, the public and registries, and the extent deaths due to motorcycle accidents occur in Brazil remains unknown [11-13].

Despite the laws regulating the use of helmets, safety equipment and the practice of traffic safety most of these rules are blatantly ignored in Brazil by motorcycle drivers, which is unfortunately also observed in many other places in the world particularly developing countries [14]. It is essential to understand better the injuries, the causes leading to the accident and other important data in order to prevent and reduce all injuries, particularly the fatal ones.

The purpose of this study is to investigate the epidemiological aspects of the deaths in motorcycle crashes, to define the most frequent and severe injuries observed in these accidents and analyze the Injury Severity Score (ISS) [16] of the casualties. Secondary goals are to warn on the urgent actions in injury prevention and regulation required in order to reduce the number of deaths and serious injuries in the future.

Material and methods

All motorcycle crashes within the borders of Campinas, in the period from 2001 to 2009, were included in this study. Data analyzed included whether the driver and/or passenger were involved, whether the victims died or survive and excluded occupants from other vehicles that might also been involved in the same crash. Accidents occurring on highways or within city streets were included.

Campinas has over 1 million inhabitants and is the 3rd most populous city in the state of São Paulo and 14th in Brazil. Over the last few years the population has grown by 1.2% per year while the motorcycles fleet grew by 4.9% per year [14]. Thus Campinas motorcycle fleet is growing 4 times faster than its population. In 2009, Campinas had 126% more motorcycles than in 2001 and 69% of the motorcycle crashes had at least one severely injured or dead victim [14]. Between 2000 and 2008, Marín-León *et al.* [15] observed that motorcycles in Campinas were responsible for the highest pedestrian fatality rate (4 deaths/1,000 accidents).

Sources

After Institutional Review Board (IRB) approval, data were obtained through an official city institution in Campinas (*EMDEC – Empresa Municipal de Desenvolvimento de Campinas*) which controls and manages the traffic within the borders of the city. Casualties, injury severities and autopsy reports were individually analyzed at the Institute of Legal Medicine, whose records also contain medical reports and police bulletins.

Collecting data

A specific form was developed to suitably collect all the information required: age, gender, place of accident, cause of accident, moments of accident and death, injury(ies), medical procedures carried out and blood alcohol (victims were considered intoxicated when the blood alcohol analyses were positive).

Trauma indices

Both the Abbreviated Injury Scale (AIS) and Injury Severity Score (ISS) were calculated for all those included in this study.

Statistical analyses

Continuous variables were expressed by their means. Categorical data were expressed as frequencies and percentages. Comparisons between groups were made using the Chi square test or the Fisher exact test for categorical variables as appropriate.

Results

Victims

Between 200 and 2009 479 people died as consequence of a motorcycle crash in the city of Campinas in Brazil. Most, 90.8% were male and 86.4% were the driver of the motorcycle. The mean age was 27.8 (range: 0-73); blood alcohol was positive in 42.24% of the victims (mean rate: 0.627 g/L), 49.7% died in a hospital, 32.6% at the scene and 17.7% on route to a hospital or the time of death was unknown.

Accidents

69.1% of the events occurred within the urban area and 30.9% on the highways. The most common accidents were collisions (63%) and falls (14%). The collisions involved cars in 37% of the occasions and trucks or buses in 32%. There were several different objects and vehicles that motorcycles collided with. Cars and large vehicles such as buses or trucks have emerged as the main protagonists (Figure 1). Street lamps, trees, walls, containers, animals and pedestrians were less common, but showed that even fixed objects can represent a serious danger to motorcyclists, especially when drivers are under the influence of alcohol. The most common time for accidents to occur was at night (between 6pm and midnight), when 26.1% of the collisions occurred.

Injuries

Traumatic brain injury (TBI) was found as the most common injury (67%), followed by thoracic trauma and

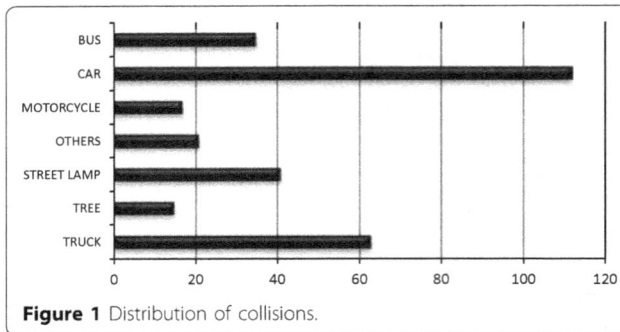

Figure 1 Distribution of collisions.

abdominal trauma (Figure 2). The results included injuries which occurred separately or together with other injuries. Hypovolemic shock was the cause of death in 38% of the cases, frequently associated with TBI.

Trauma indices

Mean ISS was 38.51 (range: 9-75) and 11.89% of the victims had ISS = 75, the maximum value of the index (Figure 3). 80.4% scored ISS > 24 (very severe injuries).

AIS shows that head and neck traumas are the most potentially fatal and severe injuries, followed by thorax, abdomen and pelvic organ injuries (Figure 4).

ISS was higher for victims of highway crashes (median ISS: 41.0) than urban areas (Median ISS: 33.0) (p < 0.001). For the casualties who had ISS between 9 and 24 (n=94), the causes of death are illustrated in Figure 5.

Time of death and its relations

1) Alcohol: most victims with positive blood alcohol died at the scene (p < 0.001); those with negative blood alcohol had similar time-of-death results when comparing the numbers of deaths at the scene or at a hospital (Figure 6).

2) ISS: Median ISS gradually decreases when considering the number of deaths at the scene (ISS=43), on route to a hospital (ISS=35) or at a hospital (ISS=30) respectively (p < 0.001).

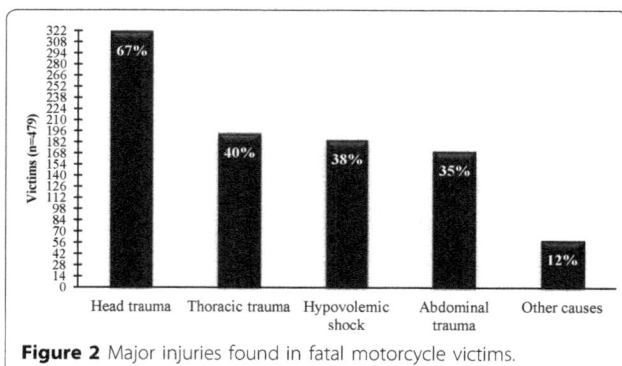

Figure 2 Major injuries found in fatal motorcycle victims.

Surgical procedures

For those arriving alive at a hospital (238), 106 (44.53%) underwent surgery. Thoracic drainage was performed on 34 patients (32.1%), followed by a laparotomy on 29.2% and craniotomy on 23.6%. Orthopedic procedures, tracheotomies and other procedures were performed on just a few cases.

Discussion

Most deaths observed in motorcycle crashes occur in young men and alcohol had a prominent role. Tests for blood alcohol levels are positive in many more motorcyclists than registered since these tests cannot be performed when there is either massive body destruction or urgent medical treatment. Literature has recognized that alcohol is the major contributing risk factor to fatal crashes [10,17]. Brazil has very strict laws on the question of driving under the influence of alcohol and this appears to be an influence in the reduction of accidents and deaths, as also demonstrated in other parts of the world [17].

Almost half of the patients reached a hospital alive, but the other half didn't survive before pre-hospital teams had arrived at the scene of the accident, or before advanced trauma treatment could be put into practice. In accordance with local cultural habits regarding the consumption of alcohol, accidents frequently occur on Saturday nights.

Most accidents occurred in urban areas, but the most severe and potentially fatal injuries occurred on highways, where higher speeds are reached, which in turn exacerbates the severity of accidents.

When motorcycle accidents occur, injuries are often found in multiple body parts, being much more common than only in isolated ones. Even in relatively simple accidents, it is usual for wounds to the head and extremities to be found simultaneously. Associated with other injuries or not, head trauma was the most common injury found, despite the use of helmets being obligatory in Brazil, and this trend can be witnessed worldwide and is documented in associated literature [17-19]. This suggests that the trauma dynamics are so aggressive that even the use of appropriate equipment is not enough to avoid brain damage. Helmets, actually, change the forces applied on the head, but even so, those forces are extremely high, causing skin and muscle injuries when directly applied, or brain injuries when indirectly applied [18].

As the most frequent occurrence is blunt trauma, injuries to the intra-thoracic and intra-abdominal organs are common and cause serious bleeding, resulting in hypovolemic shock.

Trauma indices continue to be a very useful tool in evaluating trauma patients. In this study, for every ten

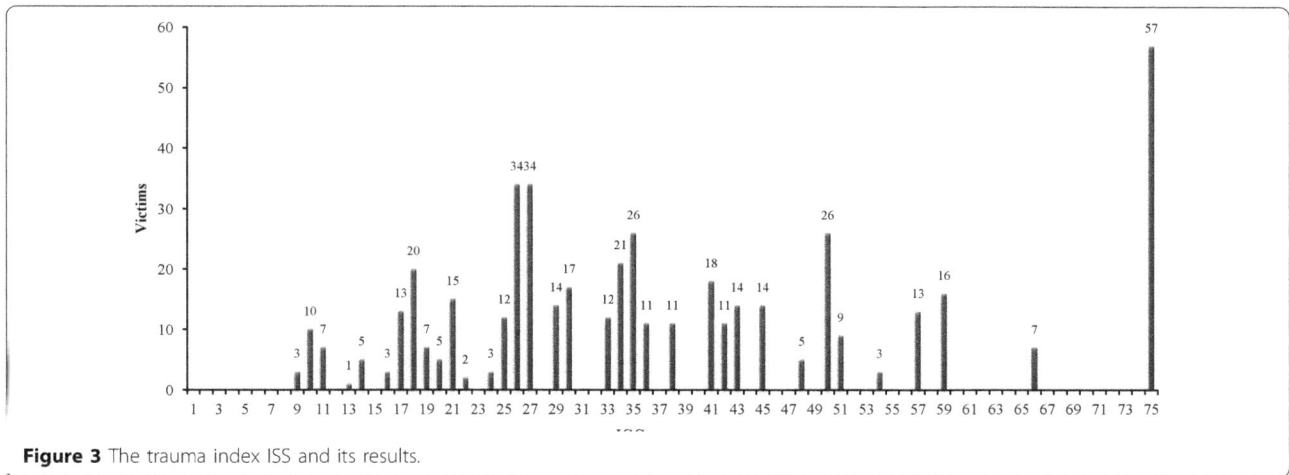

Figure 3 The trauma index ISS and its results.

victims, approximately eight suffered very severe injuries (ISS > 24), and fifty-seven casualties (11.9%) received maximum score (ISS = 75). This value is reached when potentially life-threatening injuries are found. Such results make clear that accidents involving motorcyclists usually result in serious damage to health or death. Something that must also be considered, however, is that almost 20% of the casualties had ISS < 24. In other words, those injuries considered minor or even moderate can result in death, depending on the causes of injury and the individuals' health.

Regarding the six AIS body segments, motorcyclists receive the most severe injuries to the head and neck, followed by the thorax and abdomen. It's notable that heart and liver injuries usually lead to severe or very severe stratification.

It may be further mentioned that ISS deviates according to the moment of death. As may be expected, deaths at the scene are likely to be more "severe" and deaths at a hospital not so. In general, ISS decreases as the victims near advanced trauma life support since it offers better diagnosis and treatment.

For those who reached hospital, survivability was improved via clinical support and/or surgical procedures. However, only 44.5% survived until surgery. According to injury frequency, surgical procedures were carried out on the thorax, abdomen and head. Other injuries, for example in extremities, are not usually life-threatening and were performed in some cases.

It is important to emphasize that 50% of the victims could not reach hospital, since they died instantaneously or en route to medical assistance. Helmets and other safety equipment sometimes have showed efficacy in reducing deaths or serious injuries, but solely, they are not sufficient to save lives [17,19]. When dealing with victims who suffer very severe and life-threatening injuries (80% of cases) and considering that half of those victims die before reaching hospital, it must be made clear that prevention is the most important action. Regarding this, laws regulating the use of helmets and the ingestion of alcohol are the most efficient prevention methods available and have had a notable impact on the numbers of accident and deaths. Another important point to note is that in areas in which there is no

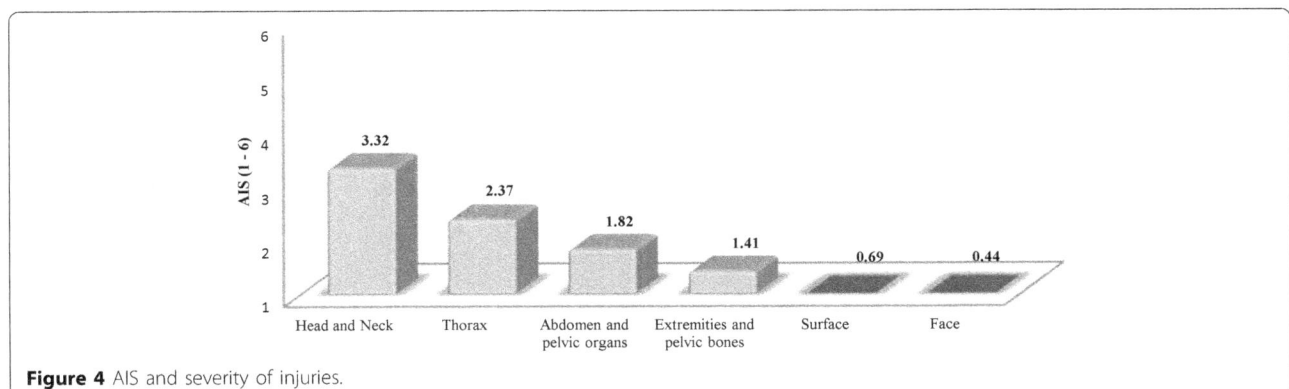

Figure 4 AIS and severity of injuries.

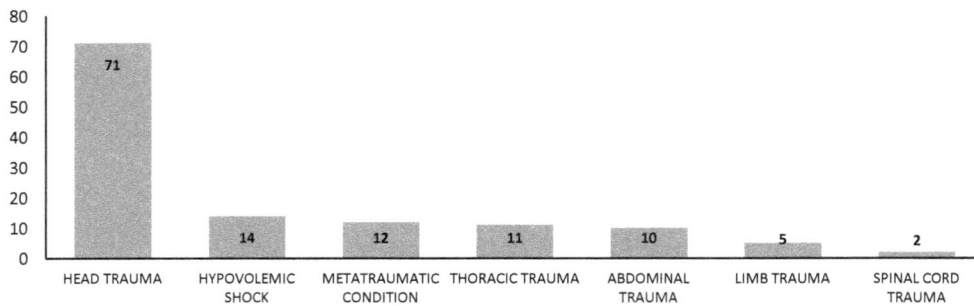

Figure 5 Causes of death of casualties with ISS 9-24.

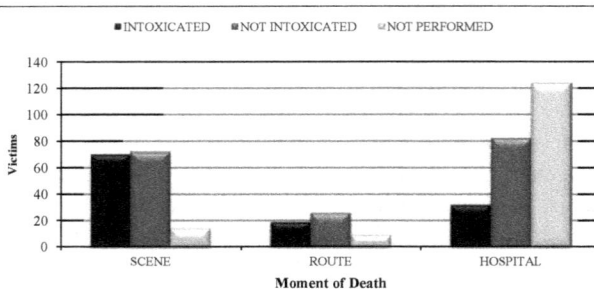

Figure 6 Relation of alcohol intoxication to moment of death.

regular patrolling, even if mandatory laws exist, accidents have been increasing and hence the need for traffic control is urgent [20].

In Campinas, the number of deaths from traffic accidents has already exceeded that of homicides and other external causes of death, and motorcycles play a significant role in these statistics. Motorcycles are being used more and more all over the world and these concerns do not respect borders or private interests. Both developed and underdeveloped countries suffer the same results and therefore should work together, putting in practice appropriate actions to avoid those preventable deaths.

In conclusion, collisions involving motorcyclists frequently result in death. Young men are the most vulnerable group and there is a significant association with alcohol consumption, whose effects usually result in even more severe consequences. Most accidents take place in urban areas, but highways witness the most severe. Despite laws obligating the use of helmets and safety equipment, head trauma is the most frequent and severe injury for motorcyclists. Half of the victims die before reaching hospital, demonstrating the seriousness of the consequences of such accidents and not many victims, once in hospital, survive until surgery. Prevention programs and actions must be put in place, since solely a medical approach is insufficient to save many of these lives.

Acknowledgments
This study has been financed by the Foundation of Support to the Research of the State of São Paulo (FAPESP).
This article has been published as part of *World Journal of Emergency Surgery* Volume 7 Supplement 1, 2012: Proceedings of the World Trauma Congress 2012. The full contents of the supplement are available online at http://www.wjes.org/supplements/7/S1.

Author details
[1]Faculty of Medical Sciences, University of Campinas (FCM / UNICAMP) Campinas, SP, Brazil. [2]Division of Trauma Surgery, Department of Surgery, Faculty of Medical Sciences, University of Campinas (FCM/UNICAMP), Campinas, SP, Brazil. [3]Department of Public Health, Faculty of Medical Sciences, University of Campinas (FCM/UNICAMP), Campinas, SP, Brazil. [4]Departments of Surgery and Critical Care Medicine, Sunnybrook Health Sciences Centre, University of Toronto, Canada.

Competing interests
The authors declare that they have no competing interests.

References
1. Pan American Health Organization: **Deaths from motor vehicle traffic accidents in selected countries of the Americas, 1985-2001.** *Epidemiol Bull* 2004, **25**(1):2-5.
2. Leong QM, Shyen KGT, Appasamy V, Chiu MT: **Young adults and riding position: factors that affect mortality among impatient adult motorcycle casualties: a major trauma center experience.** *World J Surg* 2009, **33**(4):870-873.
3. Latorre G, Bertazzoni G, Zotta D, Van Beeck E, Ricciardi G: **Epidemiology of accidents among users of two-wheeled motor vehicles – A surveillance study in two Italian cities.** *Eur J Public Health* 2002, **12**(2):99-103.
4. Savolainen P, Mannering F: **Probabilistic models of motorcyclists' injury severities in single- and multi-vehicle crashes.** *Accid Anal Prev* 2007, **39**(5):955-963.
5. O'Keeffe T, Dearwater SR, Gentilello LM, Cohen TM, Wilkinson JD, McKenney MM: **Increased fatalities after motorcycle helmet law repeal: is it all because of lack of helmets?** *J Trauma* 2007, **63**:1006-1009.
6. Ankarath S, Giannoudis PV, Barlow I, Bellamy MC, Matthews SJ, Smith RM: **Injury patterns associated with mortality following motorcycle crashes.** *Injury* 2002, **33**:473-477.
7. Zargar M, Khaji A, Karbakhsh M: **Pattern of motorcycle-related injuries in Tehran, 1999 to 2000: a study in 6 hospitals.** *East Mediterr Health J* 2006, **12**(1/2):81-7.
8. Mau-Roung L, Hei-Fen H, Nai-Wen K: **Crash severity, injury patterns, and helmet use in adolescent motorcycle riders.** *J Trauma* 2001, **50**:24-30.
9. Montenegro MMS, Duarte EC, Prado RR, Nascimento AF: **Mortality of motorcyclists in traffic accidents in the Brazilian Federal District from 1996 to 2007.** *Rev Saúde Pública* 2011, **45**(3):1-9.
10. Nunn S: **Death by motorcycle: background, behavioral and situational correlates of fatal motorcycle collisions.** *J Forensic Sci* 2011, 1-9.

11. Barros AJD, Amaral RL, Oliveira MSB, Lima SC, Gonçalves EV: **Motor vehicle accidents resulting in injuries: underreporting, characteristics, and case fatality rate.** *Cad Saúde Pública* 2003, **19**(4):979-986.
12. Scalassara MB, Souza RKT, Soares DFPP: **Characteristics of mortality in traffic accidents in an area of southern Brazil.** *Rev Saúde Pública* 1998, **32**(2):125-132.
13. Jorge MHPM, Gotlieb SLD, Laurenti R: **The National Mortality Information system: problems and proposals for solving them – II – Deaths due to external causes.** *Rev Bras Epidemiol* 2002, **2**:212-223.
14. Empresa Municipal para o Desenvolvimento de Campinas: **Acidentes de trânsito em Campinas 2009 (Traffic Accidents in Campinas 2009).** Campinas: EMDEC; 2010.
15. Marin León L, Belon AP, Barros MBA, Almeida SM, Restitutti M: **Trends in traffic accidents in Campinas, São Paulo State, Brazil: the increasing involvement of motorcyclists.** *Cad Saúde Pública* 2012, **28**(1):39-51.
16. Baker SP, O'Neill B, Haddon W Jr., Long WB: **The Injury Severity Score: a method for describing patients with multiple injuries and evaluating emergency care.** *J Trauma* 1974, **14**:187-196.
17. Lin MR, Kraus JF: **A review of risk factors and patterns of motorcycle injuries.** *Accid Anal Prev* 2009, **41**:710-722.
18. Richter M, Otte D, Lehmann U, Chinn B, Schuller E, Doyle D: **Head injury mechanisms in helmet-protected motorcyclists: prospective multicenter study.** *J Trauma* 2001, **51**:959-958.
19. Mayrose J: **The effects of a mandatory motorcycle helmet law on helmet use and injury patterns among motorcyclist fatalities.** *J Safety Research* 2008, **39**:429-432.
20. Ledesma RD, Peltzer RI: **Helmet use among motorcyclists: observational study in the city of Mar del Plata, Argentina.** *Rev Saúde Pública* 2008, **42**(1):143-5.

12

Analysis and injury paterns of walnut tree falls in central anatolia of turkey

Suleyman Ersoy[1]*, Bedriye Müge Sonmez[2], Fevzi Yilmaz[2], Cemil Kavalci[3], Derya Ozturk[4], Ertugrul Altinbilek[4], Fatih Alagöz[5], Fatma Cesur[2], Ali Erdem Yildirim[5], Ozhan Merzuk Uckun[5] and Tezcan Akin[6]

Abstract

Introduction: Falls are the second most common cause of injury-associated mortality worldwide. This study aimed to analysis the injuries caused by falls from walnut tree and assess their mortality and morbidity risk.

Methods: This is a retrospective hospital-based study of patients presenting to emergency department (ED) of Ahi Evran Univercity between September and October 2012. For each casualty, we computed the ISS (defined as the sum of the squares of the highest Abbreviated Injury Scale (AIS) score in each of the three most severely injured body regions). Severe injury was defined as ISS ≥ 16. The duration of hospital stay and final outcome were recorded. Statistical comparisons were carried out with Chi-Square test for categorical data and non-parametric spearman correlation tests were used to test the association between variables. A p value less than 0.05 was considered to be statistically significant.

Results: Fifty-four patients admitted to our emergency department with fall from walnut tree. Fifty (92.6%) patients were male. The mean age was 48 ± 14 years. Spinal region (44.4%) and particularly lumbar area (25.9%) sustained the most of the injuries among all body parts. Wedge compression fractures ranked first among all spinal injuries. Extremities injuries were the second most common injury. None of the patients died. Morbidity rate was 9.25%.

Conclusion: Falls from walnut trees are a significant health problem. Preventive measures including education of farmers and agricultural workers and using mechanized methods for harvesting walnut will lead to a dramatic decrease in mortality and morbidity caused by falls from walnut trees.

Keywords: Emergency, Falls, Walnut

Introduction

Falls are the second most common cause of injury-associated mortality worldwide and an important type of blunt trauma which form a significant percentage of traumatic accidents and emergency department admissions [1,2]. Injuries due to falls are largely affected by the height of fall since the velocity and mass of the object determine the kinetic energy which the object gains during fall and is in turn converted to action-reaction forces at the time of impact so as the height increases injury of trauma due to falls becomes more severe although much lesser degree of fall injuries may lead to serious morbidity and mortality [3].

In rural areas where the agriculture is at the forefront, falls from trees constitute a different form of falls from height and as some trees possess unique biological features the severity of injury gains intensity like walnut trees [4,5].

Despite the fact that Turkey is one of the countries considered the homeland of walnut, there is only one study from our country about traumas associated with falls from walnut tree [6] and curiously enough, there were only a few studies in the literature worldwide about this topic (Table 1).

This study aimed to analysis the injuries caused by falls from walnut tree and assess their mortality and morbidity risk.

Materials and methods

This is a retrospective hospital-based study of patients presenting to emergency department (ED) of Ahi Evran

* Correspondence: ersoydr@hotmail.com
[1]Emergency Department, Ahi Evran Univercity Training and Research Hospital, Kırsehir (40100), Turkey
Full list of author information is available at the end of the article

Table 1 Details of the studies about falls from walnut tree in literature

	n	Spinal N (%)	Chest N (%)	Abdominal N (%)	Head N (%)	Extremity N (%)	Mortality (%)
Fracture patterns resulting from falls from walnut trees in Kashmir By D.G. Nabi et al.	120	45 (37.5)	1 (0.8)	1 (0.8)	13 (9)	75 (52.9)	
Fall from walnut tree: an occupational hazard by Syed Amin et al.	87	39 (44.8)	21 (24.1)	15 (17.2)	41 (47.1)	23 (26.4)	24.13
Pattern of spine fractures after falling from walnut trees by Seyyed Amirhossein et al.	50	50 (100)					5 (10)
Walnut tree falls as a cause of musculoskeletal injury- a study from a tertiary care center in Kashmir by Asif Nazir et al.	115	52 (45.2)	10 (8.6)	14 (12.1)	34 (29.5)	91 (79)	
Abdominal injury from walnut tree fall. Scientific reports by Imtiaz Wani et al	72	13 (18)	5 (6.9)	17 (23.6)	7 (9.7)	40 (55.5)	5.5
Pattern of trauma related to walnut harvesting and suggested preventive measures by Mudassir M. Wani et al	106	28 (26)	22 (20.7)	8 (7.5)	12 (11.3	90 (84)	5.6

University between September and October 2012. The hospital records of all such patients who were admitted to the ED were studied in detail with regard to patient profile, description and location of the injury, associated injuries, delay in referral, vital signs, labarotory parameters, treatment and survey. For each casualty, we computed the ISS (defined as the sum of the squares of the highest Abbreviated Injury Scale (AIS) score in each of the three most severely injured body regions). Severe injury was defined as ISS $\geq$ 16. The duration of hospital stay and final outcome were recorded.

All data were analyzed with IBM SPSS software, version 19.0. Results were expressed as mean-standard deviation (SD) or percentage. Statistical comparisons were carried out with Chi-Square test for categorical data and nonparametric spearman correlation tests were used to test the association between variables. A p value less than 0.05 was considered to be statistically significant.

Results

Falls from walnut trees are a significant health problem owing to being an important source of morbidity and disability from spinal injury, and also a substantial social and economic burden due to labor force loss.

Demographic data

Fifty-four patients admitted to our emergency department with fall from walnut tree. Of these, 52 were adult and 2 were in pediatric age group. Fifty (92.6%) patients were male and 4 (7.4%) were female. The age range was 14 to 83 years (mean 48 ± 14 years). The earliest admission after the incident occurred at 25th minute and the latest occurred at 24th hour, and the mean delay was 77.96 ± 189.54 minute (Table 2).

Injury patterns

Spinal region (44.4%) and particularly lumbar area (25.9%) sustained the most of the injuries among all body parts.

Wedge compression fractures ranked first among all spinal injuries in which 6 were simple of 15 (27.8%) cases. Other types of spinal injuries were as follows: 1 joint dislocation at C3-C4 level, 3 thoracic and 3 lumbar burst fractures, 1 transverse process fracture, and 1 lumbar spinal listhesis. Fourteen patients were exposed to isolated spinal column injuries (SCI), of whom 10 sustained spinal cord injuries leading to 5 paraplegias, 3 paresthesias, 2 quadriparesis, and 1 paraparesis. Neurological complications occurred the most with lumbar region injuries (40%) and with burst fractures (50%). Spinal trauma was most commonly accompanied by cranial injuries (20.8%). Fracture fixation was carried out in 16 patients and 24 patients underwent a conservative management.

Table 2 Demographycal and clinical characteristics of patient

Characteristics		n (%)
Gender	Male	50 (72.6)
	Female	4 (7.4)
Age	Pediatric	2 (3.7)
	Adult	52 (96.3)
Emergency admission time	25 minute (minimum)	
	24 hour (maximum)	
Iinjury severity score (ISS)	1-9	44 (81.5)
	10-15	4 (7.5)
	16-25	9 (11.1)
	25-75	-
Survey	Discharged	19 (35.2)
	Hospitalized	26 (48.1)
	Referred	9 (16.7)
Duration of hospitalization	2 days (minimum)	
	30 days (maximum)	
Clinical outcome	Morbidity (9.25)	
	Mortality (-)	

Extremities were the second most common (41.7%) injury site after spinal region. Of these, 12 (22.2%) were lower and 10 (18.5%) were upper extremity trauma. While femur and pelvis fractures were the most common injuries among lower extremity traumas, in upper extremity traumas radius fractures were the first (9.3%, 9.3%, and 7.4%, respectively). Eight (36%) of the patients were managed surgically and the other fractures were managed according to the routine orthopedic principles of fracture management. Spinal region injuries, especially the dorsal area, were the most common injuries accompanying both upper and lower extremities (5.3% and 3.1%, respectively).

Fourteen (25.9%) patients had head and neck traumas. No primer traumatic brain injury was observed in any of the patients except for three patients with pneumocephalus. Only 1 patient had a compression fracture in the frontal region and this patient was discharged after a 4-day monitorization period at the neurosurgery department. Spinal injuries were the most common concomitant injury (6.2%).

Eleven (20.4%) patients sustained thoracic trauma and the most common injury specific to this region was rib fractures (16.7%). One patient with multiple rib fractures and hemothorax who underwent tube thoracostomy at the emergency department was operated with urgent thoracotomy as a part of hemorrhagic shock protocol upon drainage of 1300 cc fluid from the chest tube at initial and development of tachycardia (heart rate: 125 bpm) and hypotension (BP: 60/40 mmHg). One patient with pneumomediastinum developed no complication at a 2-week follow-up and was discharged upon regression of the pathology. Yet spinal region injuries were the most common injuries accompanying thoracic injuries (4.9%).

Only 1 patient had maxillofacial trauma. Abdominal trauma was not observed in any patient. Thirteen (24%) patients had injuries to more than one anatomical region.

Details of the injury paterns were shown on Figures 1 and 2.

Injury severity score (ISS)

The range of the injury severity score (ISS) was between 1 and 25 (mean 7.4 ± 6 and median 5). Forty-four (81.5%) cases had minor injuries (ISS = 1-9), 4 (7.5%) had moderate injuries (ISS = 10-15), and 9 (11.1%) had severe injuries (ISS = 16-25). There were no critical injuries (ISS = 26-75). The correlation between ISS and duration of hospital stay was strongly positive, linear, and statistically significant ($r_s = 0.818$, $p < 0.05$). The duration of hospital stay was prolonged as ISS increased (Table 2).

Survey

Nineteen (35.2%) patients were discharged from emergency department while 26 (48.1%) were hospitalized and 9 (16.7%) were referred to a tertiary center. Department of neurosurgery hospitalized the highest number of patients

(33.3%). The mean duration of hospital stay was 6 days (2-30 days) and this duration was ≥10 days in spinal injury patients. Of the hospitalized patients, 14 (40%) were managed surgically and 21 (60%) medically. None of the patients died. Five patients recovered with sequelae and the morbidity rate was 9.25%. Morbidity rate was highest with thoracolumbar injuries (40%) and with burst fractures (40%) (Table 2).

Discussion

Walnut tree is a species with a great economic importance. The fruit of the walnut tree is used both in food and drug industry, its wood is widely used in furniture sector, and its leaves and roots are utilized in dye manufacturing [7]. The province of Kırşehir located in the Central Anatolian Region and one of its counties, Kaman, has a reputation for its walnut [8].

Although walnut has a great importance in terms of national economy in countries like China, USA, Iran, Turkey and India walnut tree has some unfavorable properties for climbers, including a slippery surface, a substantially tall shaft with a maximum height of 15-30 m and the nuts largely cumulated to distal parts of its branches which are franagible due to the hollow structure [4,9-11]. As falls from heights exceeding 15 meters are accepted high-energy traumas walnut tree falls may result potentially severe injuries [12].

Despite the fact of harvesting walnut by walnut tree machine which shakes the branches of the walnut and eliminate the need to climb the tree, the people of our region continue to harvest walnut by climbing the tree. Falls occur due to the slipping during climbing the tree or while kicking the branches with their foot which breaks them or slipping their feet.

Literature data suggest that males more commonly suffered falls from walnut trees [5,9,13,14]. Our study similarly demonstrated that males more commonly were subjected to injuries (92.6%). The reason of this gender predilection is that the task of walnut harvesting is traditionally fulfilled by males. The injury rate (29.8%) was highest between 51-60 years of age. This has probably stemmed from the fact that the majority of the young population living in this region studied in non-agricultural occupations and choose to live in cities than rural areas.

Patients who fall from walnut tree commonly suffer spine injuries particularly in the form of burst and compression wedge fractures. Spinal injuries have a more destructive influence on clinical outcomes, long-term disability and life quality of patient among all major organ systems although they have a less frequency in trauma victims and especially compression fractures are frequently associated with neurological sequela with increased mortality and long-term morbidity rates [9,14,15]. Our study also demonstrated that the injuries most commonly occurred in the spinal region

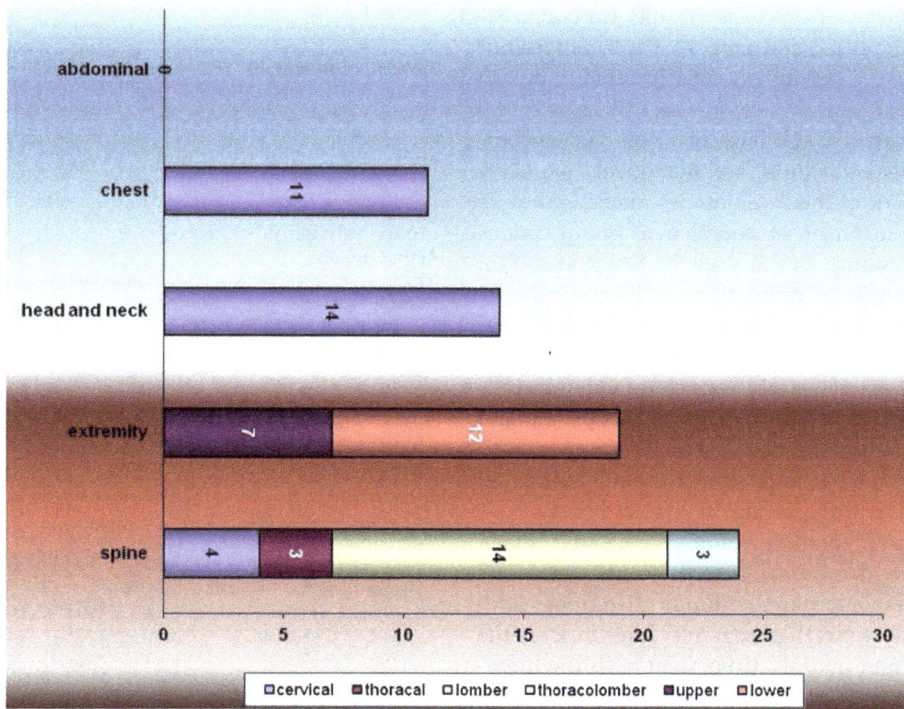

Figure 1 Characteristics of injury paterns.

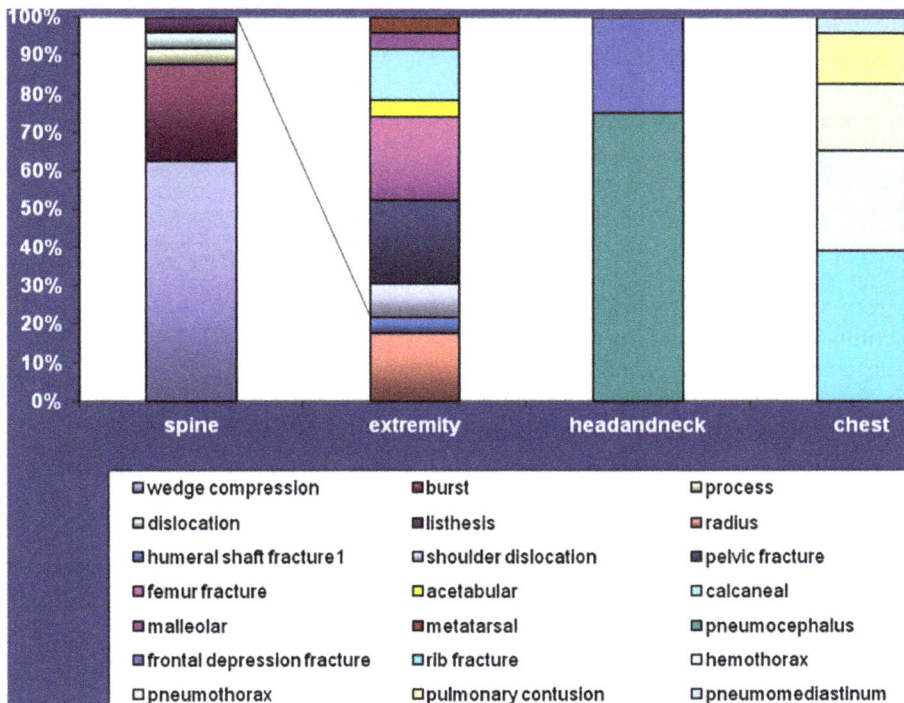

Figure 2 Details of the injury paterns.

(44.4%) and wedge compression fractures were the most common spinal injuries (27.8%). Our results were consistent with the literature [9,14] and supports the fact of walnut tree related falls have a serious potential morbidity due to spinal injuries.

Cervical spine injuries at the level of C3-C4 are uncommon, associated bony fractures are infrequent and early agressive management of this level injuries maintain a more favorable outcome in terms of neurological complications [16]. Despite the literature, in the study by Seyed et al. [13] fractures were accompanied dislocations at the cervical level spinal injuries and entirely responsible from all mortality and the results were consistent with the finding of dislocation and fracture at the level of C3-C4 in our study. Quadriparesis was the concomitant neurological deficit in this patient and despite the surgical stabilization patient recovered with sequelae which puts a large social and economic burden on his quality of life as he was a young 35 years old man.

Extremity and head traumas come second after spinal traumas in injuries due to falls from walnut trees and lower limb fractures were more common than upper limb [2,5,14]. We also observed that extremity injuries were the second most common injuries. Consistent with the literature, lower extremity traumas were more common than upper extremity traumas (22.2% and 18.5%, respectively).

In previous studies the mortality rate associated with falls from walnut trees have ranged between 10% to 24.13%, with the majority being due to cervical injuries but on the other hand, we observed no death in our study and this is possibly due to the absence of abdominal injury and existing a few number of head, thoracic and only one cervical trauma patients unlike the literature [5,10,13,14]. Considering the importance of ISS in showing the trauma severity, observing no deaths is consistent with the higher number of patients, 44 (81.5%), with an ISS score of equal to or less than 9. Of 5 patients with sequelae, 3 had an ISS score equal to or greater than 10 and 2 had an ISS score of 9.

Conclusion

Falls from walnut trees are a significant health problem owing to being an important source of morbidity and disability so are a substantial social and economic burden due to labor force loss. Traditional outdated methods employed in our region for harvesting walnut trees lead to a higher rate of falls from these trees. Preventive measures including education of farmers and agricultural workers and using mechanized methods for harvesting walnut will lead to a dramatic decrease in mortality and morbidity caused by falls from walnut trees.

Limitations of study

The limitation of our study is related to its duration. The study data were obtained from injuries that took place only during September to October 2012.

Competing interests

The authors declare that they have no competing interests.

Authors' contributions

SE was the lead investigator, BMS carried out the data analysis and writing the manuscript; FY, CK, DO, EA and FA participated in reviewing the manuscript, FC carried out the data analyses; AEY,OMU and TA participated in reducting the language in English. All authors read and approved the final manuscript

Author details

[1]Emergency Department, Ahi Evran Univercity Training and Research Hospital, Kırsehir (40100), Turkey. [2]Emergency Department, Ankara Numune Training and Research Hospital, Talatpaşa Bulvarı, Ankara (06100), Turkey. [3]Emergency Department, Baskent Univecity, Taşkent caddesi, Ankara (06490), Turkey. [4]Emergency Department, Şişli Etfal Training and Research Hospital, Halaskargazi caddesi, İstanbul (34371), Turkey. [5]Neurosurgery Department, Ankara Numune Training and Research Hospital, Talatpaşa Bulvarı, Ankara (06100), Turkey. [6]General Surgery Department, Ankara Numune Training and Research Hospital, Talatpaşa Bulvarı, Ankara (06100), Turkey.

References

1. Thierauf A, Preuss J, Lignitz E, Madea B: **Retrospective analysis of fatal falls.** *Forensic Sci Int* 2010, **198**(1–3):92–96.
2. Goren S, Subasi M, Tiraşçi Y, Gurkan F: **Fatal falls from heights in and around Diyarbakir.** *Turkey Forensic Sci Int* 2003, **137**(1):37–40.
3. Petaros A, Slaus M, Coklo M, Sosa I, Cengija M, Bosnar A: **Retrospective analysis of free-fall fractures with regard to height and cause of fall.** *Forensic Sci Int* 2013, **226**(1–3):290–295.
4. Barss P, Dakulala P, Dolan M: **Falls from trees and tree associated injuries in rural Melanesians.** *Br Med J (Clin Res Ed)* 1984, **289**(6460):1717–1720.
5. Tabish SA, Jan RAFA, Rasool T, Geelani I, Farooq BM: **Fall from walnut tree: an occupational hazard.** *Inj Extra* 2004, **35**:65–67.
6. Özkan S, Duman A, Durukan P, Avşaroğulları L, İpekci A, Mutlu A: **Features of injuries due to falls from walnut trees.** *Turk J Emerg Med* 2010, **10**(2):51–54.
7. General Directorate of Forestry: *2012-2016 Walnut Action Plan*; www.ogm. gov.tr/ekutuphane/Yayinlar/ webcite.
8. Kırşehir Governorship Provincial Directorate of Food, Agriculture and Livestock: http://www.kirsehirtarim.gov.tr/teknik-bilgiler/56-bahce-bitkileri/90-kaman-cevizi.html website.
9. Nabi DG, Tak Shafaat R, Kangoo KA, Dar Fiaz A: **Fracture patterns resulting from falls from walnut trees in Kashmir.** *Injury* 2009, **40**(6):591–594.
10. Wani I, Khan NA, Thoker M, Shaha M, Mustafa A: **Abdominal injury from walnut tree fall.** *Sci Rep* 2013, **2**(3):691. doi:10.4172/scientificreports.691/ open Access scientific reports.
11. Wani MM, Bali R, Mir IS, Hamadani N, Wani M: **Pattern of trauma related to walnut harvesting and suggested preventive measures.** *Clin Rev Opinions* 2013, **5**(1):8–10.
12. Demetriades D, Murray J, Brown C, Velmahos G, Salim A, Alo K, Rhee P: **High-level falls: type and severity of injuries and survival outcome according to age.** *J Trauma* 2005, **58**(2):342–345.
13. Javadi SA, Naderi F: **Pattern of spine fractures after falling from walnut trees.** *World Neurosurg* 2013, **80**(5):41–43.
14. Baba AN, Paljor SD, Mır NA, Maajıd S, Wanı NB, Bhat AH, Bhat JA: **Walnut tree falls as a cause of musculoskeletal injury- a study from a tertiary care center in Kashmir.** *Ulus Travma Acil Cerrahi Derg* 2010, **16**(5):464–468.
15. Leucht P, Fischer K, Muhr G, Mueller EJ: **Epidemiology of traumatic spine fractures.** *Injury* 2009, **40**:166–172.
16. Torg JS, Sennett B, Vegso JJ, Pavlov H: **Axial loading injuries to the middle cervical spine segment. An analysis and classification of twenty-five cases.** *Am J Sports Med* 1991, **19**(1):6–20.

13

Challenges of the management of mass casualty: lessons learned from the Jos crisis of 2001

Kenneth N Ozoilo[1*], Ishaya C Pam[2], Simon J Yiltok[1], Alice V Ramyil[3] and Hyacinth C Nwadiaro[1]

Abstract

Background: Jos has witnessed a series of civil crises which have generated mass casualties that the Jos University Teaching Hospital has had to respond to from time to time. We review the challenges that we encountered in the management of the victims of the 2001 crisis.

Methodology: We reviewed the findings of our debriefing sessions following the sectarian crisis of September 2001 and identified the challenges and obstacles experienced during these periods.

Results: Communication was a major challenge, both within and outside the hospital. In the field, there was poor field triage and no prehospital care. Transportation and evacuation was hazardous, for both injured patients and medical personnel. This was worsened by the imposition of a curfew on the city and its environs. In the hospital, supplies such as fluids, emergency drugs, sterile dressings and instruments, splints, and other consumables, blood and food were soon exhausted. Record keeping was erratic. Staff began to show signs of physical and mental exhaustion as well as features of anxiety and stress. Tensions rose between different religious groups in the hospital and an attempt was made by rioters to attack the hospital. Patients suffered poor subsequent care following resuscitation and/or surgery and there was neglect of patients on admission prior to the crisis as well as non trauma medical emergencies.

Conclusion: Mass casualties from disasters that disrupt organized societal mechanisms for days can pose significant challenges to the best of institutional disaster response plans. In the situation that we experienced, our disaster plan was impractical initially because it failed to factor in such a prolongation of both crisis and response. We recommend that institutional disaster response plans should incorporate provisions for the challenges we have enumerated and factor in peculiarities that would emanate from the need for a prolonged response.

Keywords: Challenges, Crisis, Disaster, Mass casualty, Trauma

Introduction

In a mass casualty situation, there is a sudden presentation of large numbers of injured people at a rate that exceeds the capacity of the institution to cope [1]. Traditional institutional response to such situations involves expanding of the surge capacity by mobilizing additional resources from within the hospital to provide care for the injured patients [2]. This involves mobilization of staff from other parts of the hospital to the accident and emergency department and a call out system for staff that are outside the hospital [3]. A slight diminution in standard of care will also be endured in which trauma care assets are

diverted from less critically injured patients to more critically injured, but salvageable patients [4]. Sometimes help might be sought from other hospitals within and outside the region [2]. This works well when there is a one-off event, and preservation of organized societal mechanisms permitting flow of supplies, personnel and other aid to and from the hospital. When there is ongoing hostility, involving the whole city, and lasting several days, new challenges emerge which interfere with this mobilization of resources from within and outside the hospital. This undermines efforts at mounting an effective response to the disaster situation. On the 7th of September 2001, Jos, the capital Plateau state of Nigeria witnessed a sectarian crisis which lasted for five days and generated several injured patients which presented to our hospital the Jos University

* Correspondence: drkenozoilo@yahoo.com
[1]Surgery Department, Jos University Teaching Hospital, Jos, Nigeria
Full list of author information is available at the end of the article

Teaching Hospital as mass casualties. We present challenges faced in the management of this mass casualties.

Methodology

Following the resolution of the crisis we held debriefing sessions to assess our overall response to the crisis and identify challenges that were encountered. Participants at each session included all heads of departments and units involved in the response. All doctors and nurses who were part of the effort were also present as were key staff especially those who had been trapped in the hospital for days at a stretch.

We examined patient records from case notes, Accident and Emergency unit records, operating theatre records and our crisis registry. We also gathered information from the firsthand account of those who were actively involved in the response.

The challenges encountered were catalogued and possible solutions were suggested. The summary of the sessions was compiled and referred to the hospital disaster committee for incorporation into the hospital disaster plan.

Results

Available records showed that 463 patients were registered in the hospital over four days giving an average of about 115 patients per day. They presented in surges however and the highest surges were on days 2 and 3 with fewer patients seen on days 1 and 4. Some patients were attended to without being registered. Of those that were registered, the records of 74 were not available, leaving that of only 389 for analysis. There were 348 (89.5%) males and the median age was 26 years.

Table 1 shows the mechanisms of injury with the most common being gunshot in 203 patients (52.2%) and cuts from machetes and knives in 161 patients (41.4%). Table 2 shows the distribution of the injuries by body part, the most frequently affected being the head and neck in 171 patients (44.0%) and the extremities 168

Table 1 Mechanisms of injury

Mechanism		No	%
Penetrating			
	Gunshot	203	52.2
	Machete/knife cuts	161	41.4
	Arrow impalements	14	3.6
Blunt			
	Clubs/sticks	44	11.3
Burns			
	Flame	7	1.8
Total		429	100*

*: Some patients had injury by multiple mechanisms.

Table 2 Body parts injured

Body part	No	%
Head/neck	171	44.0
Extremity	168	43.2
Abdomen/pelvis	65	16.7
Chest	30	7.7
Total	434	100*

*: Some patients had injury to multiple body parts.

patients (43.2%). Some patients had injury by multiple mechanisms and sustained injuries to multiple body parts.

Table 3 summarizes the challenges encountered in the response to the crisis. Communication was a major challenge, both within and outside the hospital and for collaboration with other agencies responding to the crisis. Field challenges included the violence on the streets, the lack of field triage and the absence of pre-hospital care. Within the hospital, supplies of consumables were quickly exhausted, record keeping was poor, and exhausted staff began to show signs of strain. Hospital safety became threatened at a point both from rising tensions within the premises and from threat of attack from outside. Some patients suffered suboptimal care for reasons ranging from exhaustion of hospital supplies to being forgotten in the heat of the crisis response.

Discussion

The lack of communication between our hospital and the field meant that we were totally caught unawares at the onset of the crisis. Our first inkling was in the arrival of the first surge of wounded patients. Normal hospital response to severe trauma begins with trauma team activation following advance notification. This is the ideal in isolated trauma scenarios but is even more imperative in mass casualty scenarios. Communication has been identified as a key component of disaster preparedness and response. An analysis of the response to three sequential aircraft crashes in Texas, found communication to be one of the major problems encountered in the implementation of the community and hospital disaster plan [5]. Its total absence meant that we were completely unprepared to receive the first surge of casualties and each subsequent surge was without advance warning. Communication was also needed for mobilizing personnel and other resources from within and outside the hospital, and for information and media management as well as the coordination of response efforts between medical personnel and other agencies of government involved in the disaster response such as the police, military, Red Cross, and other voluntary organizations. The lack of this communication made the overall response

Table 3 Challenges encountered

Communication			
	Internal		
	External		
	With other agencies		
Field challenges			
	No triage		
	No pre-hospital care		
	Hazard to medical personnel		
Hospital challenges			
	Exhaustion of supplies		
		Intravenous fluids	
		Drugs	
		Sterile dressings	
		Sterile instruments	
		Blood	
	Poor record keeping		
		Non registration	
		Non documentation	
		Incomplete documentation	
	Staff exhaustion		
		From fatigue/overwork	
		Anxiety/tension	
	Hospital safety		
		Rising tensions within	
		Threat of attack from outside	
	Suboptimal patient care		
		From exhaustion of supplies	
		Forgotten patients	
		Non trauma patients	
		Patients on admission prior to onset of crisis	

efforts disjointed and uncoordinated. The crisis took place before the introduction of mobile telephony in our city and we do not have pagers or two way radios. The existing hospital intercom system and the fixed lines proved grossly inadequate for the internal and external communication needs respectively.

Field triage was crude and did not follow any organized systems. Injured patients were merely conveyed to the hospital if they were fortunate enough to chance upon a military patrol, aid workers and volunteers, or other good Samaritans who were willing and able to help. The aim of triage is to identify that minority of critically injured patients, out of the large pool of patients with less severe injuries so that trauma care assets can be prioritized in favor of the former. Effective triage is necessary to screen out the majority of non critically injured survivors, and results are best when performed by a trained physician in the field [6]. A change in philosophy occurs in the approach to the management of mass casualty: the goal is to do the 'greatest good for the greatest number' and not the greatest good for the individual [2,7]. Most effective triage systems accept an overtriage rate of up to 50%, i.e. patients who have been triaged as having critical injuries when in fact they had less severe injuries. This high rate is necessary to reduce the undertriage rate to below 0.5%, i.e. the proportion of patients who were triaged as having non critical injuries when in fact they had critical injuries [7]. In the absence of systematic field triage, a high proportion of patients brought to our facility had non critical injuries as every injured patient was evacuated to the hospital. Higher overtriage rates paradoxically, increase the critical mortality by putting an avoidable strain on the resources needed to manage the critically injured and is therefore undesirable [8].

The absence of a trauma system in our setting meant that there was no prehospital care. It is therefore reasonable to expect that preventable deaths must have occurred in the field. Chances of survival following injuries depend on how fast the patient can be evacuated to a facility that is able to provide treatment for their injuries.

Movement in the field was hazardous for victims, medical personnel and even the military. For this reason, it was extremely difficult to mobilize staff to the hospital to relieve those that were over-worked; in any case, it was not possible for staff that had been at work for several hours at a stretch to go home for the same reason. Some personnel were on ground for 72 to 96 hours without relief. Evacuation of the casualties was left mainly to security personnel. Non military personnel who carried out rescue did so at great personal risk. Some medical personnel who braved the streets were attacked, and when a 24 hour curfew was imposed on the city and its environs, such attacks were as likely to come from military personnel enforcing the curfew as they were to come from rioting civilians breaking it.

There was a lag in the take off of the hospital response, due to lack of prior warning. Once it started however, it was efficient in the first 24 to 48 hours. Subsequently supplies began to run out with a resultant dip in the standard of care. Intravenous fluids, dressing material, splints, essential drugs, sterile instruments and blood soon ran out. We noted particularly that patients requiring large volumes of blood transfusion for resuscitation in the ER often depleted the blood bank reserves without surviving, in the process putting a huge strain on the availability of the product for those that required it for surgical operations. This explains why some protocols urge that serious consideration be given to avoiding blood transfusion in such situations [9].

Supplies had been mobilized from other parts of the hospital as the ER reserves ran low, but it was not possible to replenish these sources as they became exhausted. Even when certain supplies were available in the main hospital store, the myriad of challenges made their availability impossible. For example, while the ER and wards had run out of supplies of sterile dressing materials, the main hospital store had enough stock to last 90 days. These were not available however because the head of stores who had access and authority to release them was not on the premises. Communicating with him was a challenge. When contact was established, he could not come because of the violence in his neighborhood. There was a pool of duty vehicles to convey him, but most drivers were not on the premises and couldn't come in either. When a driver was mobilized, he required security personnel for protection. The mandate, and preoccupation, of the security personnel of course, was maintenance of law and order, not escort. Such was the nature of the largely logistic problems encountered. The food supplies of the hospital were soon depleted too because not only patients had to be fed, but all people taking refuge in the hospital.

Record keeping was haphazard. Some patients had no medical records. Some had but these were incomplete. Personnel who attended to patients with trivial injuries often moved on to other patients without documenting. Only those who went on to have surgery had detailed and accurate documentation of their treatment. Poor record keeping is ubiquitous in the management of mass casualties but accurate record keeping ensures continuity of care, avoids duplication of efforts, and allows a retrospective analysis of the response effort at debriefing [2,7]. It is recommended that tags (which may be laminated) should be used for identification and teams trained to use short forms and concise writing in keeping patient records under such situations [1,7].

Hospital personnel who were trapped in the hospital for over 72 hours soon began to manifest features of physical and mental stress. Overwork was a major factor, but in addition, there was anxiety for personal safety, fear for the lives of loved ones, and worry over the eventual outcome of the crisis. The sight of severely injured casualties often with grotesque wounds, and the charred, dismembered corpses deposited on the floor outside the morgue (the morgue itself was filled beyond capacity) contributed to the stress. Some people too had narrowly escaped death at the hands of rampaging mobs, prior to finding refuge in the hospital. Acute stress disorders and have been known to accompany the experiencing of such traumatic events and could be a forerunner of Post Traumatic Stress Disorder (PTSD). Although more commonly described among survivors (direct victims) of

disasters [2], it has been found among indirect victims such as first responders and the general public [10] and the need for disaster plans to incorporate provisions for emotional evaluation and rehabilitation of casualties is increasingly advocated [2,7].

The Jos crisis of 2001 was in part a religious one. Tensions flared periodically between Christians and Muslims on the premises, due to the mixed composition of the large numbers of people seeking refuge there. Most people, including personnel invariably found their sentiments swayed to on one side of the divide or the other and the ensuing tension threatened to degenerate into violence. It took the dexterity of top management and senior staff to douse the tensions and focus all efforts on the emergency response while emphasizing the need to maintain neutrality in the hospital. Despite this, rumors that victims identified with a particular section were being discriminated against led to an attempt by some rioters to attack the hospital. The perimeter fence of the hospital was already breached before attack was repelled by military personnel guarding the premises. Work place violence is a well documented phenomenon even in peacetime [11-13]. Whether caused by the strain of the ER environment on the staff, or unmet patient expectations, aggression is ultimately fuelled by perception, intolerance, misunderstanding and loss of control [12]. Some patient expectations maybe unrealistic in the ER environment and some of it may be caused by the media. In our case some of the perceptions about the crisis were due to rumours, inaccurate information and faulty reportage by the media. Eruption of violence in the hospital would have brought all response efforts to a halt. Such a situation where the hospital is unable to render any meaningful care to casualties, either because it is itself, consumed by the event (such as war, earthquake or nuclear disaster) or because it is overwhelmed by the sheer volume of casualties, has been termed a Major Medical Disaster [2] and is a situation best prevented.

In the heat of the response, patients who had been transferred to the wards following resuscitation in the ER or operation in the OR often had suboptimal subsequent care. This was because attention was focused on the fresh casualties from the continuing influx in the ER at the expense of those said to have been already "stabilized". The trickle of personnel who were mobilized from outside the hospital as the crises progressed were directed to the ER and OR, leading to neglect of those in the wards. Some of such patients missed their antibiotics, fluids and wound reviews. Some carried nasogastric tubes and catheters for too long and went for unnecessarily long periods on *nil per os*. There was near total neglect of patients who were on admission in the wards for other reasons prior to the onset of the crisis. Initial response involved mobilization of personnel from the wards to the ER and this did not begin to reverse till near the end of the crisis, five days later.

A unique, if rare category of patients who suffered suboptimal care during this crisis were patients who, developing a medical emergency at home, were able to get to the hospital. Examples include patients with diabetic crises, hypertensive emergencies and other medical emergencies. The care of the trauma patients was prioritized above these patients even when the injuries were not nearly as life threatening. A major contributory factor was the near total absence of internists as part of the disaster response in the erroneous belief that a mass casualty situation called for the mobilization of only surgeons. Some protocols propose that hospital call-in plans should focus on doctors in the surgical specialties and that the inclusion of internists should only occur as a last resort [14]. While this is certainly reasonable, we found we had occasional need for the services of internists because of prolonged duration of the disaster and therefore, response. Emergencies arising from the (internal) medical wards, in patients on admission prior to the crisis were also another instance that required the expertise of internists. Institutional response to a mass casualty situation is an effort that involves the entire hospital. Even non medically trained personnel could be utilized for simple interventions for patients with less severe injuries that would allow the experts to concentrate on those with critical injuries. Yasin et al. [15] found the mobilization of medical students as well as trained and untrained volunteers to be very useful in their response efforts to the mass casualty from the Pakistani earthquake of 2005 and that was our experience. These have to be properly supervised and guided otherwise it could introduce additional chaos that would be detrimental to the response effort [16].

Conclusion

Frykberg points out that because of the rarity of true mass casualty incidents, experience from an actual event is the only reliable way to prepare for and implement the many unique elements of disaster response [17]. We have since incorporated most of the lessons learned from the Jos crisis of 2001 into our institutional preparedness for disaster response and indeed these have improved our response to three subsequent major crises in November 2008, January 2010 and December 2010. We point out that the plan should be tailored to the peculiarities of the environment and should anticipate the challenges posed by a crisis of prolonged duration. Fortunately, we have not had a crisis of similar duration or as destabilizing of organized societal mechanisms as this one since then, but we are guided by the dictum that *anything can happen anywhere, at any time.*

Competing interests
Te authors declare that they have no competing interests.

Authors' contributions
KNO was involved in the mass casualty response, debriefings and drafted the manuscript. ICP was involved in the debriefings and conceptualization of the study. SJY was involved in the mass casualty response, debriefings, study design and literature search. AVR was involved in the debriefings and data collection. HCN was involved in the mass casualty response, debriefings and literature search. All authors read and approved the final manuscript.

Author details
[1]Surgery Department, Jos University Teaching Hospital, Jos, Nigeria.
[2]Obstetrics and Gynaecology Department, Jos University Teaching Hospital, Jos, Nigeria. [3]Ophthalmology Department, Jos University Teaching Hospital, Jos, Nigeria.

References
1. Levi L, Michaelson M, Admi H, Bregman D, Bar-Nahor R: **National strategy for mass casualty situations and its effects on the hospital.** *Prehosp Dis Med* 2002, **17**(1):12–16.
2. Hirschberg A, Stein M: **Trauma care in mass casualty incidents.** In *Trauma.* 6th edition. Edited by Feliciano DV, Mattox KL, Moore EE. New York: McGraw-Hill; 2008:141–155.
3. Nwadiaro HC, Yiltok SJ, Kidmas AT: **Immediate management of mass casualty. A successful trial of the Jos protocol.** *WAJM* 2000, **19**(3):230–234.
4. Hirschberg A, Holcomb JB, Mattox KL: **Hospital trauma care in multiple-casualty incidents: a critical review.** *Ann Emerg Med* 2001, **37**:647.
5. Klein JS, Weigelt JA: **Disaster management: lessons learned.** *Surg Clin North Am* 1991, **71**:17–21.
6. Champion HR, Sacco WJ, Gainer PS, *et al*: **The effect of medical direction on trauma triage.** *J Trauma* 1988, **28**:235–239.
7. Frykberg ER: **Medical management of disasters and mass casualties from terrorist bombings: how can we cope?** *J Trauma* 2002, **53**:201–212.
8. Frykberg ER, Tepas JJ: **Terrorist bombings: lessons learned from Belfast to Beirut.** *Ann Surg* 1988, **208**:569–576.
9. Stein M, Hirschberg A: **Medical consequences of terrorism: the conventional weapon threat.** *Surg Clin North Am* 1999, **79**:1537–1552.
10. Neria Y, Nandi A, Galea S: **Post traumatic stress disorders following disasters: a systematic review.** *Psychol Med* 2008, **38**:467–480.
11. Gulap B, Karcioglu O, Koseoglu Z, Sari A: **Dangers faced by emergency staff: experience in urban centers in southern turkey.** *Turkish J Trauma Emerg Surg* 2009, **15**(3):239–242.
12. Morrison LJ: **Abuse of emergency department workers: an inherent risk or a barometer of the evolving health care system.** *JAMC* 1999, **161**(10):1262–1263.
13. Kowalenko T, Walters BL, Khare RK, Compton S: **Workplace violence: a survey of emergency physicians in the state of Michigan.** *Ann Emerg Med* 2005, **46**(2):142–147.
14. Lynn M, Gurr D, Memon A, Kaliff J: **Management of conventional mass casualty incidents: ten commandments of hospital planning.** *J Burn Care Res* 2006, **27**(5):649–658.
15. Yasin MA, Malik SA, Nasreen G, Safdar CA: **Experience with masss casualties in a subcontinent earthquake.** *Turkish J Trauma Emerg Surg* 2009, **15**(5):487–492.
16. Halpern P, Tsai M, Arnold JL, Stock E, Esroy G: **Mass casualty, terrorist bombings: Implications for emergency department and hospital response (Part II).** *Pre Hosp Dis Med* 2003, **18**(3):235–241.
17. Frykberg ER: **Principles of mass casualty management following terrorist disasters.** *Ann Surg* 2004, **239**(3):319–321.

14

Nonoperative management for patients with grade IV blunt hepatic trauma

Thiago Messias Zago[1*], Bruno Monteiro Tavares Pereira[1], Thiago Rodrigues Araujo Calderan[1], Mauricio Godinho[1], Bartolomeu Nascimento[2], Gustavo Pereira Fraga[1]

From World Trauma Congress 2012
Rio de Janeiro, Brazil. 22-25 August 2012

Abstract

Introduction: The treatment of complex liver injuries remains a challenge. Nonoperative treatment for such injuries is increasingly being adopted as the initial management strategy. We reviewed our experience, at a University teaching hospital, in the nonoperative management of grade IV liver injuries with the intent to evaluate failure rates; need for angioembolization and blood transfusions; and in-hospital mortality and complications.

Methods: This is a retrospective analysis conducted at a single large trauma centre in Brazil. All consecutive, hemodynamically stable, blunt trauma patients with grade IV hepatic injury, between 1996 and 2011, were analyzed. Demographics and baseline characteristics were recorded. Failure of nonoperative management was defined by the need for surgical intervention. Need for angioembolization and transfusions, in-hospital death, and complications were also assessed

Results: Eighteen patients with grade IV hepatic injury treated nonoperatively during the study period were included. The nonoperative treatment failed in only one patient (5.5%) who had refractory abdominal pain. However, no missed injuries and/or worsening of bleeding were observed during the operation. None of the patients died nor need angioembolization. No complications directly related to the liver were observed. Unrelated complications to the liver occurred in three patients (16.7%); one patient developed a tracheal stenosis (secondary to tracheal intubation); one had pleural effusion; and one developed an abscess in the pleural cavity. The hospital length of stay was on average 11.56 days.

Conclusions: In our experience, nonoperative management of grade IV liver injury for stable blunt trauma patients is associated with high success rates without significant complications.

Introduction

The treatment of complex liver injuries remains a challenge for surgeons despite the last decade's advances in diagnostic and therapeutic techniques. The mortality rate for liver injuries grade IV (parenchymal disruption involving 25–75% of hepatic lobe or 1–3 Coinaud's segments in a single lobe) in the literature varies from 8% to 56%. [1-4].

The nonoperative treatment for such injuries in hemodynamically stable patients with blunt abdominal trauma

admitted with no signs of peritonitis is being progressively more utilized as the initial therapeutic approach in many designated trauma centers. Although some studies have demonstrated that the nonoperative treatment is safe for selected patients, many surgeons still choose to operate high-grade hepatic injuries solely according to the grade of the injury [5-8].

One of the most significant advances in the management of trauma patients in recent years was the introduction of Computed Tomography (CT) scan for stable patients. The recommendations on the use of CT for hemodynamically stable patients are well established, as outlined by the manual of the Advanced Trauma Life Support (ATLS®) of the American College of Surgeons.

* Correspondence: thiagomzago@hotmail.com
[1]Rua Alexander Fleming, 181 Zip code: 13.083-970, Cidade Universitaria "Prof. Zeferino Vaz, Campinas – SP, Brazil
Full list of author information is available at the end of the article

CT scan allows detection and classification of hepatic lesions and excludes the presence of associated injuries; especially injuries to hollow viscera, although in some cases it underestimates the findings. CT scan, due to its high sensitivity, specificity and accuracy, is an important screening and diagnostic tool for intra-abdominal injuries in hemodynamically stable patients; patients with altered level of consciousness; and those with difficult clinical examination or associated pelvic fractures [9-12].

The goal of this study was to determine the effectiveness of nonoperative management of grade IV liver injuries evaluating failure rates; need for angioembolization and blood transfusions; and in-hospital morbidity and mortality.

Methods

Our University teaching hospital is one of the referral trauma centers in a metropolitan area of approximately 2.8 million people. This study included patients admitted to our trauma center from 1996 through 2011. The study protocol was reviewed and approved by our institution's research ethics board.

Patients were eligible for this analysis if they were adult (15 years or more); sustained grade IV hepatic injury, classified according to the American Association for the Surgery of Trauma Organ Injury Scale (grade IV hepatic trauma corresponds to parenchymal disruption involving 25–75% of hepatic lobe or 1–3 Coinaud's segments in a single lobe) [1]; and were initially managed nonoperatively as per our hospital guidelines for hepatic injury. We excluded all patients who did not meet the aforementioned inclusion criteria.

All patients were initially resuscitated in accordance to the Advanced Trauma Life Support (ATLS®) and were submitted to CT scan examination. Selection criteria for nonoperative liver injuries management were hemodynamic stability after initial resuscitation with crystalloid and no need for blood transfusion, absence of clinical signs of peritonitis, and no bowel injuries shown on CT scan.

The nonoperative treatment protocol adopted in our trauma division is described in Table 1.

Until March 2009 helical CT scan was used as a diagnostic tool. After this period, multi-slice CT became routine for all admitted trauma patients in our hospital. For the CT scan evaluation, the patient must be hemodynamically stable, or remain stable after adequate fluid replacement. According to this protocol, Glasgow Coma Score wasn't an exclusion criterion. The presence of contrast extravasation has usually indicated embolization through arteriography prior to surgery indication.

Study variables and outcome measures

Age, gender, mechanism of injury, systolic blood pressure (SBP), Revised Trauma Score (RTS), Injury Severity Score (ISS), CT scan findings, presence of associated abdominal injuries, need for surgical intervention, need for blood transfusions, complications related to liver (re-bleeding of the liver, biliary fistula, biliar peritonitis, liver abscess and intra-abdominal abscess) and non-liver related complications (pneumonia, empyema, atelectasis, Adult Respiratory Distress Syndrome, kidney failure, intestinal fistulae, urinary tract infections, sepsis and brain injury), mortality and length of stay in the hospital, were analyzed [13,14].

Statistical analysis

Discrete variables are summarized as frequency and percentages. Summary data for continuous variables is presented as means and standard deviations, or medians and ranges depending on the distribution.

Results

During the study period, 754 patients with hepatic trauma were admitted in our service. This total included 294 (39%) patients with blunt hepatic trauma. Eighty patients (27.2%) of this total met the criteria and were treated nonoperatively. Eighteen (22.5%) out of these 80 patients were classified as having a grade IV hepatic injury; and thus constitute the study cohort. Of the 18 admitted patients with AAST-OIS grade IV blunt hepatic trauma, six patients (33.3%) were women and 12 patients (66.7%) were men. The mean age of patients was 34.22 ± 13.02 years, ranging from 20 to 59 years.

The mechanisms of injury are distributed as follows: 11 patients were involved in motor vehicle crashes; 7 (38.9%) in motorcycle collisions; and 4 (22.2%) in small utility car crashes. Two (11.1%) were pedestrians hit by a car and 5 patients (27.8%) suffered other types of blunt trauma.

The mean systolic blood pressure on admission was 116.76 ± 28.33 mmHg. The only patient admitted with hypotension remained stable after 2000 ml crystalloid infusion. The mean Revised Trauma Score was 7.60 ± 0.58. The average Injury Severity Score of these patients was 24.11 ± 8.73.

Twelve patients (66.7%) required blood transfusion, with a mean of 2.26 ± 1.57 packed red blood cells per patient.

Additional abdominal injuries were found in four patients (22.2%). Kidney was the most affected organ (all 4 patients), and the spleen was affected in one patient. None of the patients developed complications related to the liver injury. Complications unrelated to the liver occurred in 3 patients (16.7%); 1 developed a tracheal stenosis (secondary to tracheal intubation); 1 had a pleural effusion; and 1 an abscess in the pleural cavity. Patient characteristics evaluated are described in Table 2.

Table 1 Protocol of nonoperative management in AAST-OIS grade IV blunt hepatic trauma.

Protocol of nonoperative management in AAST-OIS grade IV blunt hepatic trauma - Division of Trauma Surgery - University of Campinas

Criteria for patient selection:
1- Abdominal blunt trauma
2- Hemodynamic stability after initial resuscitation with no need for blood:
  a. Systemic blood pressure > 90 mmHg
  b. Initial hemoglobin level > 8
3- Evaluation by Computed Tomography with:
  a. Absence of associated injuries on hollow viscus and pneumoperitonium
  b. Absence of contrast blush (evidence of active arterial bleeding is indication for angiography and embolization)
4- Clinical evaluation with no signs of peritonitis

Monitorization of patients undergoing nonoperative management: 1- Hemoglobin/ Hematocrit measurement every 6 hours or more frequently if any clinical deterioration 2- ABG measurements every 6 hours or more frequently if any clinical deterioration 3- ICU (Intensive Care Unit)

Criteria for failure of nonoperative management:
1- Need for surgical intervention determined by:
  a. Hemodynamic instability
  b. Failure of angioembolization to control active bleeding
  c. Progressive fall of hemoglobin/ hematocrit levels with recurrent blood transfusion
  d. Clinical signs of peritonitis

Regarding the CT scan findings, seven patients (38.8%) had isolated hepatic injury with perihepatic fluid and 11 patients (61.1%) had liver injury and free fluid in the abdominal cavity (Figures 1 and 2). Ten patients (55.5%) had helical CT evaluation while 8 (44.5%) had multi-slice CT scans. Six patients (33.3%) had repeated follow-up scans, on average 5 days after the initial CT. None of the follow-up CTs demonstrated progression of the injury. Nonoperative management failed in a single patient (5.5%) that had a progression of the free fluid (hemoperitoneum) in the abdomen along with peritonitis. The patient was operated 4 days after admission when a large hemoperitoneum was found but no active bleeding from the liver. Thus nonoperative hepatic trauma management as per our protocol resulted in an overall success rate of 94.5%. No patient died and the mean hospital stay was 11.56 ± 5.3 days (Table 3).

Discussion

Since 1980 several studies have proposed that nonoperative treatment of blunt liver injuries be considered the

treatment of choice for patients with hemodynamic stability. The great capacity of the liver for regenerating, the pattern of venous bleeding, and the high rate of spontaneous hemostasis, may explain and be responsible for high success rates associated with nonoperative treatment. Pachter et al, in a multicenter study with 13 Level I Trauma Centers in the USA, reported a 98.5% rate of success in nonoperative treatment for selected patients [7,8,12,15-18].

Severe liver injuries (grade III, IV and V) have higher morbidity and mortality. In a study with 170 patients with hepatic trauma, Rizoli et al observed a total of 10 deaths, all with grade IV and V injuries. Many surgeons choose to operate complex lesions of the liver even in patients admitted with hemodynamic stability, fearing a

Table 2 Evaluated aspects of patients with grade IV blunt hepatic trauma undergoing nonoperative management.

Demographics and baseline characteristics Aspect evaluated	N=18 Frequence / mean (n/SD)
Male	66.7% (12)
Age	34 (± 13)
Systolic Blood Pressure on admission	117 (± 28)
RTS	7.6 (± 0.58)
ISS	24 (± 9)
Blood transfusion	66.7% (12)
Packed red blood cell transfused	2.26 ± 1.57
Associated abdominal injuries	22.2% (4)

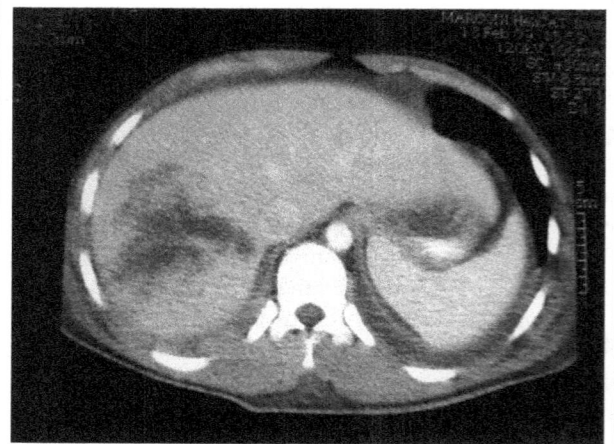

Figure 1 Pedestrian hit by a car; multislice CT showing abdominal free fluid and intraparenchymal hematoma in the right lobe (grade IV hepatic injury), no blush of contrast in the arterial phase.

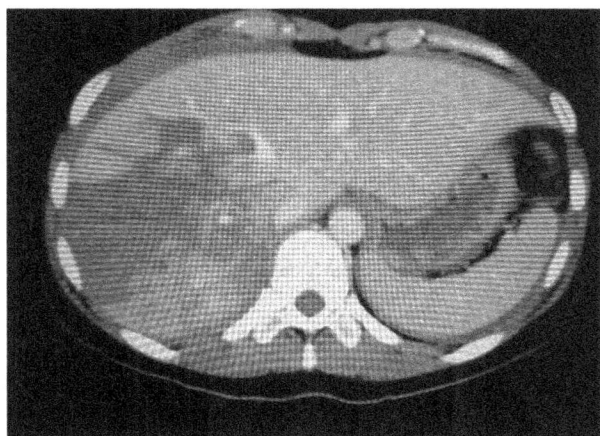

Figure 2 Bicycle crash; multisclice CT showing the presence of abdominal free fluid, with intraparenchymal hematoma in the right lobe (grade IV hepatic injury), no blush of contrast in the arterial phase.

possible rebleeding of liver injury. It is known that the liver rebleeding in patients admitted with hemodynamic stability and with no blush on CT scan, is a rare event [2,6,16,19].

Patients admitted with severe liver injuries tend to be more critical. The average ISS of patients in this study was 24.1. Kozar et al found an average of ISS 28 for patients with grade IV blunt hepatic trauma. In other studies involving patients with blunt or penetrating liver trauma with grade IV and V injuries, submitted to surgical treatment or non-surgical, the average ISS was 25, 33, 34 and 36 respectively [2,6,20-22].

None of the patients in our study died, in agreement with other studies showing that nonoperative treatment for grade IV blunt hepatic trauma is safe for selected patients [5,22].

In this study we observed that none of the 18 patients developed any complications related to the liver and three patients developed non-liver related complications. Kozar et al found complications in 19 of 92 patients (21%) with grade IV injuries treated nonoperatively. Of these patients, less than a half needed some kind of surgical intervention. Duane et al reported a complication

Table 3 Outcome of patients with grade IV blunt hepatic trauma undergoing nonoperative management.

Outcome Aspect evaluated	N=18 Frequence / mean (n/SD)
Complications related to the liver	0
Non -liver related complications	16.7% (3)
Failure of nonoperative management	5.5% (1)
In-hospital Mortality	0
Length of hospital stay	11.56 ± 5.3

rate of 0% for patients with grade IV blunt liver injury that did not undergo surgery or angioembolization [6,22].

Only one of the 18 patients studied herein required surgical conversion secondary to abdominal pain, showing a success rate of 94.5% of nonoperative treatment. In a study with patients with grades III and IV hepatic trauma Coimbra et al, related that 22% of patients undergoing nonoperative treatment needed surgical intervention. In another study with 230 patients with grades III, IV and V blunt hepatic trauma treated nonoperatively, Kozar et al had 12 patients (5.2%) who failed with nonoperative management and required surgical intervention [5,6].

The abdominal CT scan is the diagnostic modality of choice for hemodynamically stable patients with suspected abdominal injuries. CT scan has some advantage over ultrasound exam. CT is less operator-dependent and is not limited by the abdominal wall, subcutaneous emphysema, obesity or intestinal distention. CT is very important to diagnose abdominal injuries in patients with neurological damage, since physical examination is feasible in no more than 16% of these patients [12,22-27].

CT scan allows visualization of hemoperitoneum, one of the most obvious signs of the presence of abdominal injury. Usually the hemoperitoneum is seen in the Morison pouch, perihepatic space and in the right paracolic gutter and is reabsorbed after 5 to 10 days after injury. The amount of hemoperitoneum have previously been considered an indicator of liver trauma severity, but some recent studies have indicated that the amount of hemoperitoneum does not correlate with failure of nonoperative management [12,17,24,28,29]. Besides hemoperitoneum, CT allows the visualization of contusions, subcapsular hematomas, intraparenchymal hematomas and lacerations to the liver parenchyma [30,31].

An important role of the CT scan is to detect active extravasation of contrast, indicating the presence of active bleeding. With this information, an angiography should be performed even in hemodinamically stable patients due to the risk of bleeding and subsequent failure of the nonoperative management. Angiographic embolization is a safe strategy in the management of hepatic arterial hemorrhage in patients with blunt trauma. It was demonstrated to reduce the amount of transfusions, the need for further liver-related surgeries and the mortality in high-grade liver injuries. Almost all patients in this series were evaluated by helical CT scan, which has a low accuracy to identify extravasation of contrast. This explains the fact that no patient underwent angiographic embolization in the present study [21,32-36].

Besides the diagnostic capacity, CT also has an important role in monitoring patients treated nonoperatively.

In this study, the follow-up CT did not have an important role. Six patients were submitted to follow-up CT, which never demonstrated worsening in the injuries or contributed for the indication of any intervention. In a study with 74 patients with grade IV blunt liver trauma treated nonoperatively and with repeated performance of CT, only three patients required another therapeutic procedure. Of these three patients, two underwent angiography and one drainage of a bilioma. However, these three patients had strong clinical signs of changes in the clinical course as tachycardia, abdominal pain and elevated enzymes. Another study concluded that repeated CT scan matters in patients with clinical deterioration and signs of peritonitis or sepsis [18,24,37,38].

Conclusions

In our experience, the nonoperative treatment can be performed in trauma centers with protocols in place; 24-hour operating rooms; trained surgical teams; blood banks; critical care support; and image diagnosing methods available, such as mult-islide or helical CT scan. Although AAST-OIS grade IV blunt hepatic trauma patients are critical, nonoperative approach can be adopted in hemodynamically stable patients safely and with high success rates.

Acknowledgements
This article has been published as part of *World Journal of Emergency Surgery* Volume 7 Supplement 1, 2012: Proceedings of the World Trauma Congress 2012. The full contents of the supplement are available online at http://www.wjes.org/supplements/7/S1.

Author details
[1]Rua Alexander Fleming, 181 Zip code: 13.083-970, Cidade Universitaria "Prof. Zeferino Vaz, Campinas – SP, Brazil. [2]2075 Bayview Ave., Room B5 12, Toronto, Ontario, M4N 3M5 Canada.

Authors' contributions
TMZ participated in the conception, design and intellectual content, collection, analysis and interpretation of data. *BMTP* participated in the intellectual content; revision of the manuscript, figures and tables. *TRAC* participated in the revision of the manuscript, figures and tables. *MG* participated in the revision of the manuscript, figures and tables. *BN* participated in the revision of the manuscript, figures and tables. *GPF* had overall responsibility for the study including conception, design and intellectual content, collection, analysis and interpretation of data.

Authors' information
Thiago Messias Zago. Medical student of Faculty of Medical Sciences (FCM) – University of Campinas (Unicamp).
Bruno Monteiro Tavares Pereira. Assistant Surgeon of Division of Trauma Surgery, FCM - Unicamp.
Thiago Rodrigues Araujo Calderan. Assistant Surgeon of Division of Trauma Surgery, FCM - Unicamp.
Mauricio Godinho. Assistant Surgeon of Division of Trauma Surgery, FCM - Unicamp.
Bartolomeu Nascimento. Fellow, Trauma Program, Sunnybrook Health Sciences Centre, University of Toronto and Visiting Professor of the Division of Trauma Surgery, FCM - Unicamp.
Gustavo Pereira Fraga. Professor of Surgery and Coordinator of Division of Trauma Surgery, FCM - Unicamp.

Competing interests
Sources of funding: Fundação de Amparo à Pesquisa do Estado de São Paulo (FAPESP). Grant number 12698/2010.

References
1. Moore EE, Cogbill TH, Jurkovich GJ, Shackford SR, Malangoni MA, Champion HR: **Organ injury scaling: spleen and liver (1994 revision).** *J Trauma* 1995, **38**(3):323-4.
2. Asensio JA, Demetriades D, Chahwan S, Gomez H, Hanpeter D, Velmahos G, Murray J, Shoemaker W, Berne TV: **Approach to the management of complex hepatic injuries.** *J Trauma* 2000, **48**(1):66-9.
3. Cogbill TH, Moore EE, Jurkovich GJ, *et al*: **Severe hepatic trauma: a multi-center experience with 1,335 liver injuries.** *J Trauma* 1988, **28**:1433-38.
4. Cue JI, Cryer HG, Miller FB, *et al*: **Packing and planned reexploration for hepatic and retroperitoneal hemorrhage: critical refinements of a useful technique.** *J Trauma* 1990, **30**:1007-13.
5. Coimbra R, Hoyt DB, Engelhart S, Fortlage D: **Nonoperative management reduces the overall mortality of grades 3 and 4 blunt liver injuries.** *Int Surg* 2006, **91**(5):251-7.
6. Kozar RA, Moore JB, Niles SE, Holcomb JB, Moore EE, Cothren CC, *et al*: **Complications of nonoperative management of high-grade blunt hepatic injuries.** *J Trauma* 2005, **59**(5):1066-71.
7. Norrman G, Tingstedt B, Ekelund M, Andersson R: **Nonoperative management of blunt liver trauma: feasible and safe also in centres with a low trauma incidence.** *HPB (Oxford)* 2009, **11**(1):50-6.
8. Pachter HL, Knudson MM, Esrig B, Ross S, Hoyt D, Cogbill T, *et al*: **Status of nonoperative management of blunt hepatic injuries in 1995: a multicenter experience with 404 patients.** *J Trauma* 1996, **40**(1):31-8.
9. Committee on Trauma, American College of Surgeons: **Advanced Trauma Life Support Instructor's Manual.** Chicago, IL: American College of Surgeons; 1997.
10. Mullinix AJ, Foley WD: **Multidetector computed tomography and blunt thoracoabdominal trauma.** *J Comput Assist Tomogr* 2004, **28**(Suppl 1): S20-S27.
11. Croce MA, Fabian TC, Kudsk KA, Baum SL, Payne LW, Mangiante EC, *et al*: **AAST organ injury scale: correlation of CT-graded liver injuries and operative findings.** *J Trauma* 1991, **31**(6):806-12.
12. Wolfman NT, Bechtold RE, Scharling ES, Meredith JW: **Blunt upper abdominal trauma: evaluation by CT.** *AJR Am J Roentgenol* 1992, **158**(3):493-501.
13. Champion HR, Sacco WJ, Copes WS, Gann DS, Gennarelli TA, Flanagan ME: **A revision of the Trauma Score.** *J Trauma* 1989, **29**(5):623-9.
14. Baker SP, O'Neill B, Haddon W Jr, Long WB: **The injury severity score: a method for describing patients with multiple injuries and evaluating emergency care.** *J Trauma* 1974, **14**(3):187-96.
15. Feliciano DV, Mattox KL, Jordan GL Jr, Burch JM, Bitondo CG, Cruse PA: **Management of 1000 consecutive cases of hepatic trauma.** *Ann Surg* 1986, **204**(4):438-45.
16. Velmahos GC, Toutouzas K, Radin R, Chan L, Rhee P, Tillou A, Demetriades D: **High success with nonoperative management of blunt hepatic trauma: the liver is a sturdy organ.** *Arch Surg* 2003, **138**(5):475-80.
17. Croce MA, Fabian TC, Menke PG, Waddle-Smith L, Minard G, Kudsk KA, *et al*: **Nonoperative management of blunt hepatic trauma is the treatment of choice for hemodynamically stable patients. Results of a prospective trial.** *Ann Surg* 1995, **221**(6):744-53.
18. Cox JC, Fabian TC, Maish GO 3rd, Bee TK, Pritchard FE, Russ SE, *et al*: **Routine follow-up imaging is unnecessary in the management of blunt hepatic injury.** *J Trauma* 2005, **59**(5):1175-80.
19. Rizoli SB, Brenneman FD, Hanna SS, Kahnamoui K: **Classification of liver trauma.** *HPB Surg* 1996, **9**(4):235-8.
20. Asensio JA, Petrone P, García-Núñez L, Kimbrell B, Kuncir E: **Multidisciplinary approach for the management of complex hepatic injuries AAST-OIS grades IV-V: a prospective study.** *Scand J Surg* 2007, **96**(3):214-20.
21. Asensio JA, Roldán G, Petrone P, Rojo E, Tillou A, Kuncir E, *et al*: **Operative management and outcomes in 103 AAST-OIS grades IV and V complex hepatic injuries: trauma surgeons still need to operate, but angioembolization helps.** *J Trauma* 2003, **54**(4):647-53.

22. Duane TM, Como JJ, Bochicchio GV, Scalea TM: **Reevaluating the management and outcomes of severe blunt liver injury.** *J Trauma* 2004, **57**(3):494-500.

23. Jacobs DG, Sarafin JL, Marx JA: **Abdominal CT scanning for trauma: how low can we go?** *Injury* 2000, **31**(5):337-43.

24. Becker CD, Mentha G, Terrier F: **Blunt abdominal trauma in adults: role of CT in the diagnosis and management of visceral injuries. Part 1: liver and spleen.** *Eur Radiol* 1998, **8**(4):553-62.

25. Schurink GW, Bode PJ, van Luijt PA, van Vugt AB: **The value of physical examination in the diagnosis of patients with blunt abdominal trauma: a retrospective study.** *Injury* 1997, **28**(4):261-5.

26. Röthlin MA, Näf R, Amgwerd M, Candinas D, Frick T, Trentz O: **Ultrasound in blunt abdominal and thoracic trauma.** *J Trauma* 1993, **34**(4):488-95.

27. Ferrera PC, Verdile VP, Bartfield JM, Snyder HS, Salluzzo RF: **Injuries distracting from intraabdominal injuries after blunt trauma.** *Am J Emerg Med* 1998, **16**(2):145-9.

28. Romano L, Giovine S, Guidi G, Tortora G, Cinque T, Romano S: **Hepatic trauma: CT findings and considerations based on our experience in emergency diagnostic imaging.** *Eur J Radiol* 2004, **50**(1):59-66.

29. Hiatt JR, Harrier HD, Koenig BV, Ransom KJ: **Nonoperative management of major blunt liver injury with hemoperitoneum.** *Arch Surg* 1990, **125**(1):101-3.

30. Federle MP, Crass RA, Jeffrey RB, Trunkey DD: **Computed tomography in blunt abdominal trauma.** *Arch Surg* 1982, **117**(5):645-50.

31. Moon KL Jr, Federle MP: **Computed tomography in hepatic trauma.** *AJR Am J Roentgenol* 1983, **141**(2):309-14.

32. Fang JF, Chen RJ, Wong YC, Lin BC, Hsu YB, Kao JL, Kao YC: **Pooling of contrast material on computed tomography mandates aggressive management of blunt hepatic injury.** *Am J Surg* 1998, **176**(4):315-9.

33. Ciraulo DL, Luk S, Palter M, Cowell V, Welch J, Cortes V, *et al*: **Selective hepatic arterial embolization of grade IV and V blunt hepatic injuries: an extension of resuscitation in the nonoperative management of traumatic hepatic injuries.** *J Trauma* 1998, **45**(2):353-9.

34. Wahl WL, Ahrns KS, Brandt MM, Franklin GA, Taheri PA: **The need for early angiographic embolization in blunt liver injuries.** *J Trauma* 2002, **52**(6):1097-101.

35. Mohr AM, Lavery RF, Barone A, Bahramipour P, Magnotti LJ, Osband AJ, *et al*: **Angiographic embolization for liver injuries: low mortality, high morbidity.** *J Trauma* 2003, **55**(6):1077-82.

36. Letoublon C, Morra I, Chen Y, Monnin V, Voirin D, Arvieux C: **Hepatic arterial embolization in the management of blunt hepatic trauma: indications and complications.** *J Trauma* 2011, **70**(5):1032-7.

37. Becker CD, Gal I, Baer HU, Vock P: **Blunt hepatic trauma in adults: correlation of CT injury grading with outcome.** *Radiology* 1996, **201**(1):215-20.

38. Sharma OP, Oswanski MF, Singer D: **Role of repeat computerized tomography in nonoperative management of solid organ trauma.** *Am Surg* 2005, **71**(3):244-9.

15

Occupational Injury Patterns of Turkey

Kaan Celik[1], Fevzi Yilmaz[1], Cemil Kavalci[2*], Miray Ozlem[1], Ali Demir[1], Tamer Durdu[1], Bedriye Müge Sonmez[1], Muhittin Serkan Yilmaz[1], Muhammed Evvah Karakilic[1], Engin Deniz Arslan[1] and Cihat Yel[1]

Abstract

Introduction and aim: Each year, a significant number of people die or become handicapped due to preventable occupational accidents or occupational diseases. The aim of this study was to investigate socio-demographic features, mechanism, causes, injury area, and sectoral features of occupational accidents in patients presented to our department.

Materials and methods: The study was carried out retrospectively after local ethics committee approval. Age and sex of the patients, mechanism of injury, type and exact location of injuries were all evaluated. The groups were compared using Chi-Square test, Student's T test and Kruskall-Wallis test. p value <0.05 was accepted as statistically significant.

Results: Totally 654 patients were included in the study. 93.4% of patients were male, and mean age was 32.96 ± 5.97 (18–73) years. Sectoral distribution of accidents was statistically significant and mostly occurred in industrial and construction workers ($p < 0.05$, respectively). There is a statistically significant relationship between educational level and sector of the worker ($p < 0.05$). While the most frequent cause of admission to emergency department was penetrating injuries (36.4%), the least was due to multiple traumas (0.5%). Distribution of occupational accidents according to injury type was statistically significant ($p < 0.05$). The mean Injury Severity Score (ISS) was 9.79 ± 8.1. The mean cost of occupational injury was $\$1729.57 \pm 8178.3$. There was statistically significant difference between the sectors with respect to cost. Seventy-one patients (10.9%) recovered with permanent sequel and two (0.3%) died in hospital.

Conclusion: Occupational accidents are most commonly seen in young males, especially in primary school graduated workers, and during daytime period.

Keywords: Emergency department, Occupational accident, Work, Cost

Introduction

World Health Organization (WHO) has defined occupational accident as "an unplanned event commonly leading to personal injury, damage to machinery and working equipment, and temporary halt of production" [1]. 270 million occupational injuries occur each year throughout the world, resulting 1.1 million deaths [2]. A considerable high number of people die or become handicapped each year due to preventable occupational accidents or occupational diseases [3-5].

Ankara is the second largest city of Turkey and has a population of 4.890.000 million. There are 10 organized industrial zone and since December 31, 2011 a total of

1,843 industrial companies have been registered in Ankara Chamber of Industry and a total of 286,860 workers have been employed in their establishments [6]. Small and Medium Industrial Enterprises (SMEs) account for the majority of industry in Ankara, Ankara is the 3rd largest industrialized province in Turkey (7% of total industrial enterprises) and today, 40% of industrial establishments in the area of production are machinery and metal industries [6]. According to the Health and Safety Executive Statistics 2011/12 of European Agency for Safety and Health, 173 workers were killed at work, a rate of 0.6 fatalities per 100,000 workers and 111,164 other injuries to employees were reported in United Kingdom [7]. Looking at the 2011 statistics of the Ministry of Labor and Social Security of Turkey, totally 62,903 occupational accidents were occurred and 2715 of these were in Ankara [8]. Due

* Correspondence: cemkavalci@yahoo.com
[2]Baskent University Faculty of Medicine, Emergency department, Ankara, Turkey
Full list of author information is available at the end of the article

to proximity of our hospital to industrial zones, occupational accidents occurring in these areas are primarily admitted to our emergency department.

We aimed to investigate the socio-demographic features, mechanism, causes, and site of injury, and sectoral features in occupational accidents in patients presenting to Ankara Numune Training and Research Hospital emergency department.

Materials and methods

This study enrolled 654 patients over the age of 18 years and admitted to Ankara Numune Training and Research Hospital emergency department with occupational accident between the dates 1 January 2011 and 31 December 2011. Patient files in hospital records system, patient assessment forms and judicial case reports prepared in emergency department were evaluated retrospectively after obtaining local ethics committee approval. Age and sex of the patients, mechanism of injury, cause of emergency department admissions, educational level and sector of worker, month of injury, hour of accident during the day, length of working hours, social security status, injured organ, state of preventive measures, disabled workers, injury severity score (ISS), hospital cost of occupational injuries, and site and healing status of injury were examined.

Collected data were analyzed using SPSS 19.0 software package programme. Normal distribution of descriptive statistical data was analyzed with Kolmogorov Smirnov test. The groups were compared using Chi-Square test, Student's t test or Kruskall-Wallis test. The results were evaluated in a confidence interval of 95% and at a significance level of $p < 0.05$.

Results

Among 654 patients admitted to Ankara Numune Training and Research Hospital due to occupational injury, 611 (93.4%) were male. Mean age of male and female patients were 32.9 ± 9.7 and 32.8 ± 9 years, respectively. There was no significant difference between both sexes with respect to age ($p > 0.05$) (Table 1). The number of occupational accidents increased in 26–35 age groups (37%). There was a significant difference between age groups with respect to occupational accident rate ($p < 0.05$) (Figure 1).

Monthly distribution of occupational accidents demonstrated that these accidents mostly occurred in May (12%) and least in February (4.9%). This distribution of occupational accidents was statistically significant ($p < 0.05$) (Figure 2).

The most occupational injury occurred in construction sector (28.7%). Sectoral distribution of accidents was statistically significant ($p < 0.05$) (Table 2). Analysis of occupational accidents with respect to educational level revealed that 251 (38.4%) were primary school graduate, 249 (38.1%) were high school graduate (Table 2).

Median working duration was 5.97 years (1 days-42 years). Most patients had a working duration of 1–5 years. Distribution of occupational accidents by working duration was statistically significant ($p < 0.05$). No significant difference was detected between male and female patients with respect to working duration ($p > 0.05$) (Table 1).

Time intervals of occupational accidents were as follows: 24^{00}-08^{00} in 44 (6.7%) patients, 08^{00}-16^{00} in 419 (64.1%) patients. The hourly distribution of occupational accidents was statistically significant ($p < 0.05$) (Figure 3).

The most common cause of admissions was cuts (36.4%). The distribution of occupational accidents by injury type was statistically significant ($p < 0.05$) (Table 3).

The most frequent mechanism of occupational accidents was blunt object traumas in 158 (24.2%) cases. Distribution of patients according to mechanism of injury was given on Table 3. The mean ISS was 9.79 ± 8.1. Distribution of ISS score according to sector is summarized on Table 4.

The most commonly affected body parts were upper extremities (53.7%, n = 351). Second most common region involved was lower extremities (15.3%, n = 100). Other data regarding affected body parts by occupational accidents are given on Table 1. No statistically significant difference was detected between males and females with respect to trauma region ($p > 0.05$).

The mean cost of occupational injury was 1729.57 ± 8178.3. Distribution of hospital cost according to sector was summarized on Table 4.

Of the patients, 549 (83.9%) were discharged after emergency department evaluation and treatment, while 105 (16.1%) patients were hospitalized. Two patients died at the admission ward. While 581 (88.8%) patients recovered without a sequel, 71 (10.9%) with sequel.

Discussion

According to Social Security Institution statistics, the number of deaths due to occupational accidents in recent years are as follows: 1043 deaths in 80,602 occupational accidents in 2007, 865 deaths in 72,693 occupational accidents in 2008, 1171 deaths in 64,316 occupational accidents in 2009, and 1444 deaths in 62,903 occupational accidents in 2010. Moreover, hundreds of people have become handicapped each year [9]. These data indicate the importance of occupational accidents.

It has been reported that occupational accidents are more common in males (84-86%) [10-13], and our results correlate with the literature. More participation of males in work life possibly contributes to this finding. It has also been reported that occupational accidents are more common in 25–34 age group [9,10,12,14]. Majority of our study population were also in that age group. This may have been resulted from the fact that people from

Table 1 Demographic characteristics according to gender

Variable		Gender				p value
		Male		Female		
		n	%	n	%	
Age (mean ± year)		611	32.9 ± 9.7	43	32.8 ± 9	0.934
Working experience (years)	0-1	131	96.3	5	3.7	
	1-5	297	92.2	25	7.8	
	5-10	79	91.9	7	8.1	0.366
	10+	104	94.5	6	5.5	
Mechanism	Machine Induced Hand Trauma	60	93.8	4	6.2	
	Glass Cut	43	89.6	5	10.4	
	Penetrating or Sharp Object Trauma	112	99.1	1	0.9	
	Blunt Object Trauma	150	94.9	8	5.1	0.04
	Foreign Object	11	100	0	0	
	Squeezing	35	100	0	0	
	Falls	139	89	17	11	
	Burns	44	91.7	4	8.3	
	Electric Injury	13	86.7	2	13.3	
	İntoxication	4	93.6	2	6.6	
Trauma region	Head & Neck	59	95.2	3	4.8	
	Face	25	100	0	0	
	Thorax	5	83.3	1	16.7	
	Abdomen	1	100	0	0	
	Pelvis	3	75	1	25	0.141
	Arm-Shoulder	70	93.3	5	6.7	
	Hand-Finger	264	95.7	12	4.3	
	Lower Extremity		90		10	
	Skin	22	84.6	4	15.4	
	Back-Vertebrae	27	87.1	4	12.9	

this age group belong to the productive population segment, and at the same time they are employed in more risky and hard jobs.

Karakurt et al. [15] reported that most occupational accidents occurred in December whereas Dizdar et al. [3]

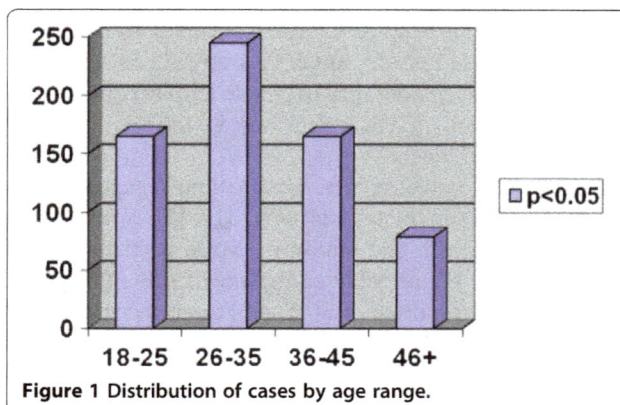

Figure 1 Distribution of cases by age range.

and Satar et al. [16] reported that occupational accidents increased in June, July and August. We observed that occupational accidents increased in May, June and July possibly because of air warming with resulting increase in volume of construction and agriculture sectors, with a parallel increase in manufacture of goods.

Previous studies showed that occupational accidents mostly occur with workers having less than 10 working years [12,17]. We found that rate of occupational accidents was the highest in workers with working years between 1–5 years, possibly because beginner workers are more careful at the beginning due to fear of making mistakes, but they may be progressively more careless as they gain experience.

Sayhan et al. [12] reported that occupational accidents occur mostly between 08.00-16.00 hours. Serinken et al. reported that the highest frequency of occupational accidents was observed between 08.00-12.00 hours [18]. We also found that most occupational accidents (64.1%) were

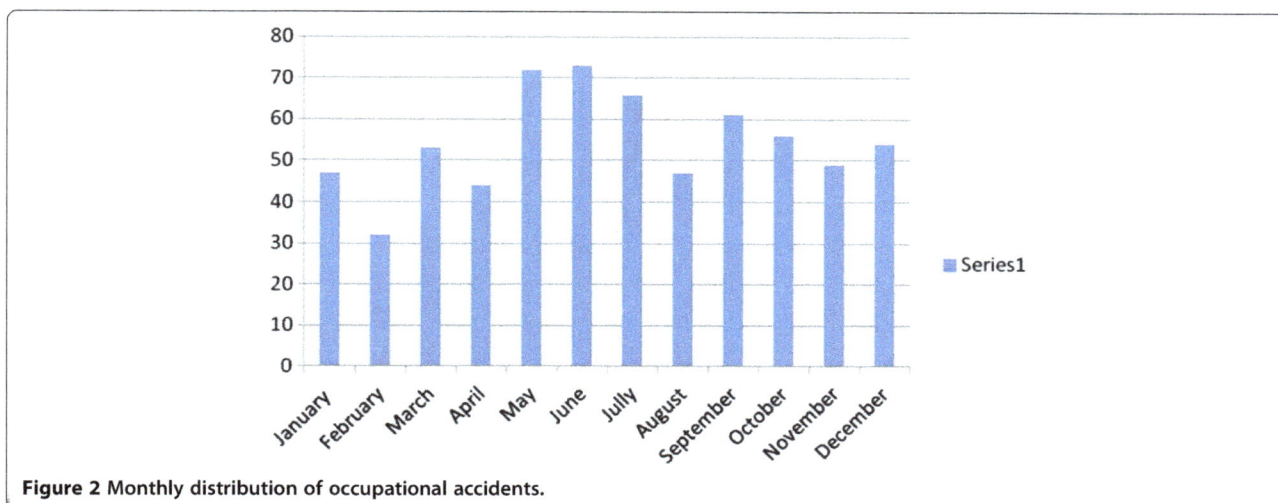

Figure 2 Monthly distribution of occupational accidents.

seen between 08.00-16.00 hours. The frequency of occupational accidents increased during the day, gradually decreased at evening, and became minimized at night, possibly because only those working in night shifts remain at work at those hours. Another reason for the tendency of occupational accidents to occur more frequently during the first hours of a workday may be the fact that the workers begin to work without enough focus or adaptation to working environment.

Ozkan et al. [2] reported that majority of victims of occupational accidents worked in manufacturing and construction sectors (60%, 24%). In our study, 28.7% of the occupational accident cases worked in construction sector, 10.2% in manufacturing sector. Regional differences also brought about sectoral variations.

Serinken et al. [18] reported that cuts and lacerations had the highest rate with 40.1% followed by fractures-dislocations with a rate of 25.8%. In the study by Ozkan et al. [2], on the other hand, soft tissue injuries ranked

first with a rate of 36.7% followed by cuts and fractures-dislocations with rates of 26.3% and 11.2%, respectively. Statistical data from Social Security Institution show that accidents related with sharp or penetrating objects ranked first with a rate of 13.3%, followed by falling from a height with 11.7% and machinery-related accidents with a rate of 10.6% [9]. We also detected that cuts had the highest rate of 36.4% followed by soft tissue trauma. The reason of a higher rate of cuts and soft tissue traumas may be increased safety level of the newly introduced machinery devices, an advanced level of alertness of workers while performing tasks that have a potential to cause a severe trauma, or carelessness of workers while performing tasks that have a potential to cause small traumas.

Ozkan et al. [2] reported that injuries due to penetrating objects/machinery had the highest rate (48.5%) followed by blunt object traumas (21.5%) and falls (18.9%). Jackson et al. [19] found that 54% of cases were due to penetrating

Table 2 Relationship between sectoral distribution and education level

Sector (n)	Education				p value
	İlliterate	Primary-Secondary school	High school	College	
Industry	35	75	60	0	p < 0.001
Manufacturing	11	16	36	4	p < 0.001
Building	45	88	54	1	p < 0.001
Food	18	27	29	1	p < 0.001
Service	6	8	23	11	p < 0.001
Agriculture	2	1	1	0	p < 0.05
Transportation	5	5	15	0	p < 0.001
Woodwork	9	25	15	0	p < 0.001
Electricity	0	1	10	1	p < 0.001
Other	3	5	6	2	p < 0.001
Total	134	251	249	20	p < 0.001

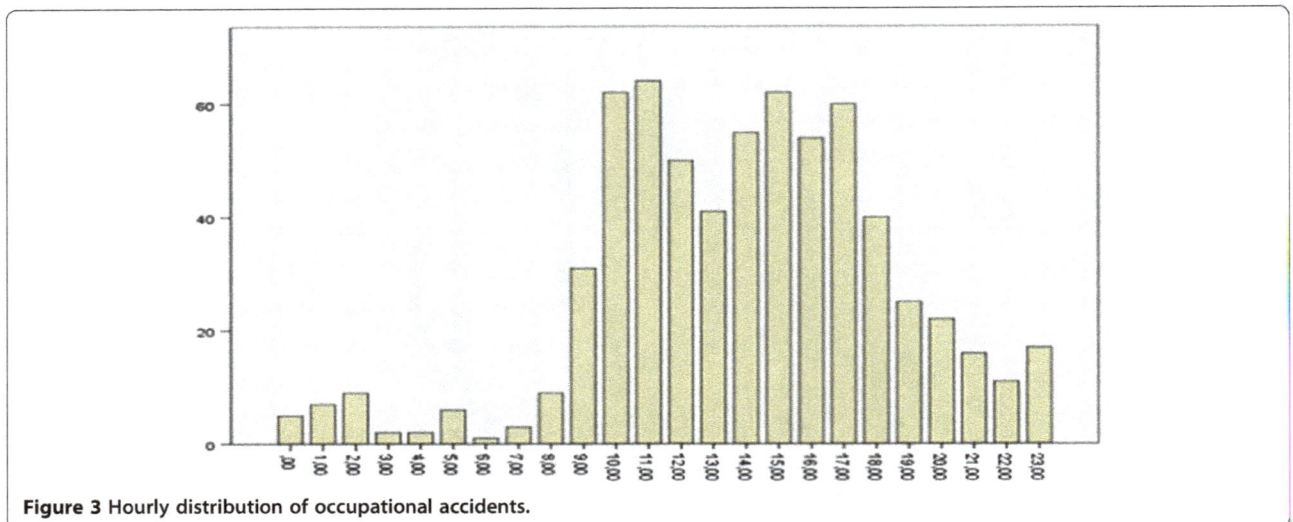

Figure 3 Hourly distribution of occupational accidents.

objects/machinery. Our data indicate that 39.8% of the cases were due to penetrating objects/machinery followed by blunt object traumas (24.2%) and falls (23.9%). The primary reason responsible for the differences among these studies is the principle sector in the region of study. Some trauma mechanisms may be lower in women as a result of a negligible ratio of female workers to males in some sectors, as in the case of transportation and construction sectors. Thus, there may have been a significant difference between the trauma mechanism and sex.

Anders et al. reported a mean ISS of 19.2 for patients having a work accident [20]. Our patients had a mean ISS of 9.79 ± 8.1. We suggest that our patients had a low ISS since they sustained accidents of very low energy levels.

Anders et al. reported a mean hospital cost of €35.661 [20] while Asfaw et al. gave a figure of $2,328 [21]. Our patients had a mean cost of occupational injury of $1729.57 ± 8178.3. These costs don't include the money

spent for rehabilitation. If labor force loss and rehabilitation expenses are added, the cost exceeds millions of dollars. We believe that the hospital cost was lower in our study as a result of our patients' lower ISS score and cross-national differences of prices. Highest costs were observed in accidents of agriculture and transportation sectors. We think that accidents and costs can be reduced if universal safety measures are followed in construction sector and traffic rules observed in transportation sector.

It has previously been reported that the rate of occupational accidents increases when the educational level decreases [2,12]. Our results are consistent with the literature. Possible reasons of decreased occupational accident rate with increased educational level include the following: Educated persons may do their jobs more seriously; and they may take care of warning signs more compared to less educated people. In addition, educated persons may work in administrative positions, potentially avoiding dangerous jobs.

Table 3 The distribution of occupational accidents by inury type

Injury type	Frequency (n)	(%)
Cuts	238	36.4
Soft tissue trauma	152	23.2
Amputation	51	7.8
Crush	66	10.1
Fracture-Dislocation	77	11.8
Burns	48	7.3
Electric Injury	10	1.5
Intoxication	1	0.2
Ocular Injury	8	1.2
Multiorgan Injury	3	0.5
Total	654	100

Table 4 Distrubition of ISS score and cost according to sector

Sector (n)	Cost (mean ± SD) ($)	p value	ISS	p value
Industry	1427.5 ± 3443		11.83 ± 9.2	
Manufacturing	732.16 ± 1657.2		8.26 ± 6.1	
Building	2836.44 ± 14039.7		9.17 ± 8	
Food	1547.68 ± 6055.3		7.82 ± 6.3	
Service	739.3 ± 2184.7		7.22 ± 5.3	
Agriculture	870.5 ± 651.6	p < 0.01	15.75 ± 10.8	p < 0.001
Transportation	2077.32 ± 5997.2		9.2 ± 8.3	
Woodwork	1458.06 ± 2677.8		10.51 ± 6.7	
Electricity	1523.08 ± 2805.5		17.25 ± 15.3	
Other	591.37 ± 574.1		10.18 ± 6.9	
Total	1729.57 ± 8178.3		9.79 ± 8.1	

In our study, examination of injured body parts revealed that upper extremity injuries were at the top point with a rate of 53.7%. They were followed by, in descending order, lower extremity injuries (15.9%) and head-neck injuries (9.5%). Previous studies from our country have also revealed similar results [2-4]. Upper extremity injuries were the most common injuries since hands are intensely used at work.

It has been reported that 62-90% of patients admitting with occupational accident are discharged after first medical care at emergency departments [2,3,15,18]. In this study, 83.9% of cases were discharged after first medical care at emergency department, and 16.1% were hospitalized. No patients were referred to another health-care facility as our center is a tertiary care center with all trauma-related surgical branches and a burn center readily available.

Limitation of the study
A major limitations of the study was a retrospectiveness of it.

Conclusion
Occupational accidents most commonly occur in young male workers, during daytime and primary school graduates.

Competing interests
The authors declare that they have no competing interests.

Author contributions
KC: conception and design, or acquisition of data, or analysis and interpretation of data, have given final approval of the version to be published. FY, MO, MEK: acquisition of data, MMS: revising it critically for important intellectual content; CK: analysis and interpretation of data or revising it critically for important intellectual content; AD, TD, EDA: have made substantial contributions to conception and design. MSY: have made substantial contributions to conception and design. All authors read and approved the final manuscript.

Author details
[1]Numune Training and Research Hospital, Emergency department, Ankara, Turkey. [2]Baskent University Faculty of Medicine, Emergency department, Ankara, Turkey.

References
1. Ince H, Ince N, Ozyildirim BA: Occupational accidents and Forensic Medicine in Turkey. *J Clinb Forensic Med* 2006, 13:326–30.
2. Ozkan S, Kilic S, Durukan P, Akdur O, Vardar A, Geyik S, *et al*: Occupational injuries admitted to the emergency department. *Ulus Travma Acil Cerrahi Derg* 2010, 16:241–247.
3. Dizdar MG, Asirdizer M, Yavuz MS: Evaluation of the ocular trauma cases applied to emergency service of Celal Bayar University hospital. *Adli Tip Dergisi* 2008, 22:14–20.
4. Yardim N, Cipil Z, Vardar C, Mollahaliloglu S: Mortality rates due to occupational accidents and diseases between 2000–2005 in Turkey. *Dicle Tip Derg.* 2007, 34:264–71.
5. Kalemoglu M, Keskin O, Yildirim I, Ersanli D: Analysis of traumatic occupational accidents admitted to the emergency department. *Nobel Medicus* 2006, 2:21–23.
6. 81 City Status Report: *Republic of Turkey Ministry of Science, Industry and Technology.* http://www.sanayi.gov.tr/Files/Documents/81-il-durum-raporu-2012-11052012113452.pdf.
7. *European Agency for Safety and Health at Work.* https://osha.europa.eu/en. last avaliable date 07.10.2013.
8. *Republic of Turkey Ministry of Labour and Social Security, Labour Statistics.* http://www.csgb.gov.tr/csgbPortal/ShowProperty/WLP%20Repository/csgb/dosyalar/istatistikler/calisma_hayati_2011. last avaliable date 07.10.2013.
9. *Employment Injury and Occupational Diseases Statistics*; 2012. http://www.sgk.gov.tr/wps/portal/tr/kurumsal/istatistikler/sgk_istatistik_yilliklari/!ut/p/b1/hdLJkqJAEIDhZkHsCm2Ao7FIhQCKggCFwJEEKEEIdWnH6enr92Tt4z48_JFUjEVUvEtHasy7av2IjZ_9xgmOq3rkkwjIHoAAEwzXAC8Pa2r3Dulfg4wB_53f6RCN1pmtbXLNZKTbg9tXmVq3M7OBWZd8BjLqFcq00NzWeS8RFbDXgOzbwAYMJsNdkgEi9GESbOPJbEiuniYYGMQsR1cw05NOW5q9TgCBVk4T3jbINbsxB2m6ESUtdgUrDLRyUmFEu4b4ukQvJs2drG0TXZoOvaYeWlgHgn96wFgzOwNITeNtvBum20uIlzM7QdpxC6QE6J5r3x7gh0H_9TCpuMrI53QinCTZYElaA4yLAN4RoA8FVwjKKhPPGnITS7neMPdx4uK8q1SusqnsvFJmPNsvKSS9d0U-3TdSrMx07vzy2sCrTVLMUHvVqS1xpO9IGokcbP7IgeouHY7NISx9sIbx. last avaliable date 07.09.2013.
10. Dagli B, Serinken M: Occupational injuries admitted to the emergency department. *JAEM* 2012, 11:167–70.
11. Forst LS, Hryhorczuk D, Jaros M: A state trauma registry as a tool for occupational injury surveillance. *J Occup Environ Med* 1999, 41:514–520.
12. Sayhan MB, Sayhan ES, Yemenici S, Oguz S: Occupational injuries admitted to the emergency department. *J Pak Med Assoc* 2013, 63:179–84.
13. Holizki T, McDonald R, Foster V, Guzmicky M: Causes of work related injuries among young workers in British Columbia. *Am J Ind Med* 2008, 51:357–63.
14. Breslin FC, Smith P: Age-related differences in work injuries: a multivariate, population-based study. *Am J Ind Med* 2005, 48:50–6.
15. Karakurt U, Satar S, Acikalın A, Bilen A, Gulen M, Baz U: Analysis of Occupational Accidents Admitted to the Emergency Medicine Department. *JAEM.* 10.5152/jaem.2012.031.
16. Satar S, Kekec Z, Sebe A, Sarı A: Analysis of Occupational Accidents Admitted to the Cukurova University faculty of Medicine Emergency Department. *Cukurova Universitesi Tip Fakultesi Dergisi* 2004, 29:118–27.
17. Kumar SG, Rathnakar U, Harsha KH: Epidemiology of accidents in tile factories of mangalore city in Karnataka. *Indian J Community Med* 2010, 35:78–81.
18. Serinken M, Karcioglu O, Sener S: Occupational Hand Injuries Treated at a Tertiary Care Facility in Western Turkey. *Ind Health* 2008, 46:239–246.
19. Jackson LL: Non-fatal occupational injuries and illnesses treated in hospital Emergency Departments in the United States. *Inj Prev* 2001, 7:21–6.
20. Anders B, Ommen O, Pfaff H, Lüngen M, Lefering R, Thüm S, *et al*: Direct, indirect, and intangible costs after severe trauma up to occupational reintegration – an empirical analysis of 113 seriously injured patients. *GMS Psycho-Soc-Med* 2013, 10:1–15.
21. Asfaw A, Pana-Cryan R, Bushnell PT: Incidence and costs of family member hospitalization following injuries of Workers' Compensation Claimants. *Ind Med* 2012, 55:1028–1036.

16

Alcohol acute intoxication before sepsis impairs the wound healing of intestinal anastomosis: rat model of the abdominal trauma patient

Pedro Henrique Alves de Morais[1], Vinícius Lacerda Ribeiro[1], Igor Eduardo Caetano de Farias[1], Luiz Eduardo Almeida Silva[1], Fabiana Pirani Carneiro[2], Joel Paulo Russomano Veiga[2], João Batista de Sousa[1,3*]

Abstract

Introduction: Most trauma patients are drunk at the time of injury. Up to 2% of traumatized patients develop sepsis, which considerably increases their mortality. Inadequate wound healing of the colonic repair can lead to postoperative complications such as leakage and sepsis.

Objective: To assess the effects of acute alcohol intoxication on colonic anastomosis wound healing in septic rats.

Methods: Thirty six Wistar rats were allocated into two groups: S (induction of sepsis) and AS (alcohol intake before sepsis induction). A colonic anastomosis was performed in all groups. After 1, 3 or 7 days the animals were killed. Weight variations, mortality rate, histopathology and tensile breaking strength of the colonic anastomosis were evaluated.

Results: There was an overall mortality of 4 animals (11.1%), three in the group AS (16.6%) and one in the S group (5.5%). Weight loss occurred in all groups. The colon anastomosis of the AS group didn't gain strength from the first to the seventh postoperative day. On the histopathological analysis there were no differences in the deposition of collagen or fibroblasts between the groups AS and S.

Conclusion: Alcohol intake increased the mortality rate three times in septic animals. Acute alcohol intoxication delays the acquisition of tensile strength of colonic anastomosis in septic rats. Therefore, acute alcohol intoxication before sepsis leads to worse prognosis in animal models of the abdominal trauma patients.

Introduction

Abdominal trauma patients are often acutely intoxicated with alcohol, and one of the injuries they can suffer is the rupture of the colon. This injury leads to leakage of feces into the abdominal cavity, and has as consequences peritonitis and sepsis. After surgery, the prognosis of the patient depends to a large extent on the wound healing of the colon.

Healing is a sequential and organized biological process which aims to repair damaged tissue and reunite the edges of the wound, to finally restore both the organ's physiological functions and the barrier that separates the external and internal environments [1]. It can be divided into four sequential steps: hemostasis, inflammation, proliferation and remodeling [1].

Inadequate wound healing is responsible for postoperative colonic repair complications such as dehiscence and leakage. The postoperative rate of anastomotic leakage in abdominal trauma patients varies from 7% to 14% in low risk patients, and can be as high as 40% in higher risk patients [2]. These complications are responsible for longer hospital stay, reoperation and increased morbidity and mortality [2,3].

* Correspondence: sousajb@unb.br
[1]Medical School, Academic League of Emergency and Trauma, University of Brasilia, Brasilia, Brazil
Full list of author information is available at the end of the article

Studies have shown that up to 2% of traumatized patients develop sepsis, which considerably increases the mortality if compared to non-septic individuals [4].

Sepsis was the 11th leading cause of death in the U.S. in 2003 and in Brazil the prevalence and mortality are high, with up to 60% of mortality in septic chock [5].

Alcohol is the most consumed drug in the world [6]. Epidemiological data of the emergency units and intervention studies indicate that most patients seen by some traumatic disorder were drunk [7-9].

Over 50% of the beds for trauma are occupied by patients who were acutely intoxicated by alcohol at the time of injury [10]. The intake of alcohol contributes to worsen the injuries caused by trauma and can complicate the management of these patients.

The aim of this study was to assess the impact of acute alcohol intoxication on colonic anastomosis wound healing in rats under sepsis in an experimental model of the abdominal trauma patient.

Materials and methods

This randomized blinded experimental study was performed after the consent of the Ethics Committee of Animal Usage (CEUA), University of Brasilia. All procedures were guided by ethical standards proposed by the Brazilian College of Animal Experimentation (COBEA).

The study was designed with 36 male Wistar rats, which were randomly allocated into two groups of 18 animals each:

◊ GROUP S (Sepsis): anesthesia, sepsis induction, segmental colectomy, colonic anastomosis, wound healing evaluation.

◊ GROUP AS (Alcohol and Sepsis): alcohol intake, anesthesia, sepsis induction, segmental colectomy, colonic anastomosis, wound healing evaluation.

Each group was subdivided into three subgroups of six animals, to be euthanized after 1, 3 or 7 days postoperatively (POD), named as:

◊ GROUP S: S1, S3 and S7;

◊ GROUP AS: AS1, AS3 and AS7;

On the operation day the rats were fasted for one hour. The animals of the AS group were alcoholized with ethanol diluted in saline to a concentration of 40% with a standard dose of 2 ml of solution. This dose is equivalent to a 480mL spirits intake or approximately 10 shots, in a young adult male of 75kg of weight. Half of the dose (1ml) was administered by mouth, using the gavage method. Another 1ml was given one hour later also by mouth, immediately before anesthesia. The surgeons were blinded to whether the rats had received alcohol or not.

The anesthetic induction was performed with xylazine in a dose of 10 mg / kg, and ketamine at a dose of 75 mg / kg, both intramuscularly. Then the abdomen was cleaned with iodinated detergent.

A midline abdominal incision that began one centimeter cranial to the pubis symphysis, with a length of approximately 4.5 cm, was performed. One centimeter of the left colon was resected, and an end-to-end anastomosis was performed with single layer running sutures, with 6-0 polypropylene (Figure 1). The abdominal wall closure was performed with running sutures, in two layers, using 3-0 polypropylene. Postoperative analgesia was done with tramadol in a dose of 0,72 mg / kg at every 12 hours.

Peritonitis was induced, in all groups, by the method of Wichterman *et al.* [11] consisting of a partial ligation of the cecum with cotton suture, immediately below the triangular ileocecal fold to increase the pressure within that segment of the intestine without causing ischemia and allowing free passage of the contents of the small intestine into the large intestine. Then the cecum was perforated in 10 random points with a 40x12mm needle, followed by its compression for fecal leakage (Figure 2).

At 1, 3, or 7 post operative days (POD) the animals were weighed, anesthetized, re-operated and killed with an overdose of thionembutal intravenously.

The anastomotic breaking strength (ABS) was evaluated with a vertical test apparatus called Versa Test (Mecmesin Versa Test, United Kingdom), coupled to a portable digital dynamometer in which the colonic anastomosis samples were attached and pulled with a speed of 25mm/min [12].

The maximum traction force value that the tissue endured before rupture was measured in Newtons.

A sample of the anastomotic scar was collected for histopathological analysis, fixed in formalin and stained by hematoxylin and eosin. The amount of collagen,

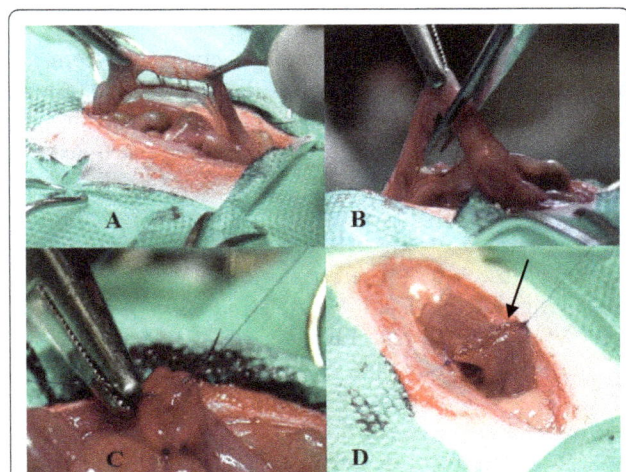

Figure 1 Segmental colectomy and colonic anastomosis in the rat. **A**: identification of the segment of the colon to be resected. **B**: segmental colectomy. **C**: running suture of the posterior anastomotic lip. **D**: colon transit restored by end to end anastomosis, the arrow indicates the suture line.

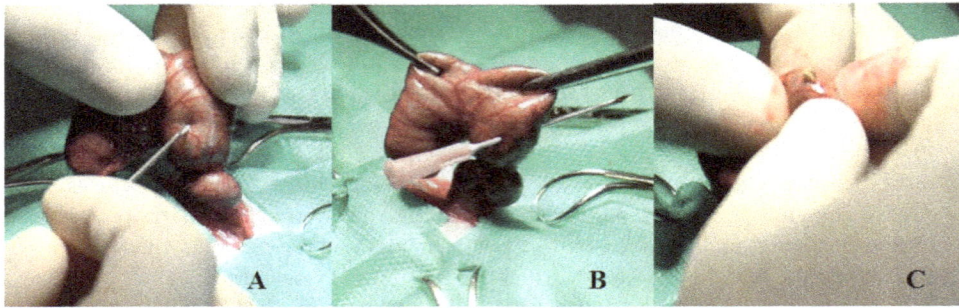

Figure 2 Wichterman sepsis induction method. A and B the cecum is perforated. C the cecum is squeezed to leak feces and induce the sepsis.

fibroblast, mononuclear and polymorphonuclear infiltrations and neovascularization were marked with values 0, 1, 2 or 3 each, in which 0 means nothing and 3 a large amount. The parameters of abscess, bacterial colony, foreign body, crust and fibrin were signalized as 0 or 1, meaning absent or present, respectively.

The results were analyzed using SPSS software (Special Package for Social Sciences) version 18.0. Parametric and nonparametric tests were performed, according to the nature of the variables. The paired samples t test was used for the weight variations and Kruskal-Wallis test for anastomotic breaking strength. The Fisher exact test was used to perform the statistical analysis of all histopathological variables. Significance was set at a value of p <0.05.

Results

There was an overall mortality of four deaths (11,11%). Three animals from the group AS died (16,6%), one of them in the subgroup AS1 and two in the AS7. In the S group only an animal died, in the S3 group, a death rate of 5,5%. (Figure 3).

There was weight loss in almost every group, from the operation day to the day of euthanize (p < 0,05), as shown in the Table 1. The average preoperative weight of all groups was 321,05 grams, and the post operative weight was 299,6 grams.

The anastomotic breaking strength (ABS) was not different between groups AS and S, from the first to the third day (p > 0.05). There was no statistical difference between groups AS1 and S1, AS3 and S3 or AS7 and S7 (p > 0.05), Figure 4 and Table 2.

There was no difference between the groups AS1, AS3 and AS7 (p > 0,05). The S7 group had a higher anastomotic breaking strength than S1 and S3 (p < 0,05). The AS group anastomotic breaking strength (ABS) had a sharper decline than the S group from the first to the third day, and at the seventh day the AS group ABS was not recovered (Figure 5).

On the histopathological evaluation there was no difference of any of the analyzed parameters between

groups AS and S (Table 3). There was no difference of collagen between the groups AS7 and S7 (p>0.05).

Discussion

The aim of this study was to evaluate the effects of acute ethanol exposure at single high dose just before an injury in rats with fecal sepsis. To evaluate that, we have analyzed the death rate, weight variations, anastomosis breaking strength and histopathology.

Both alcohol and sepsis are known to lead to weight loss after surgery, and their combination diminished the post-operative body mass in this study, and even at the 7 POD that weight wasn't recovered [13,14]. Sepsis leads to a consumptive syndrome due to the inflammation and alcohol intake is responsible for malnutrition because of intestinal malabsorption and is also responsible for body fat reduction [13,14].

Sepsis is an important cause of death in trauma patients. It was the cause of 9% of deaths in a level I trauma centre in USA in 2003 [15]. Alcohol is also a

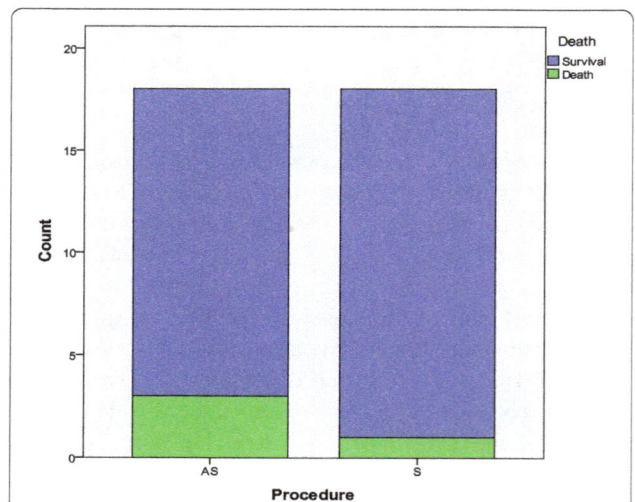

Figure 3 Number of animals that died are in green and those that survived are in blue.

Table 1 Preoperative and postoperative average weight of each group. The statistically significant differences were signaled.

Weight per group			
	Preoperative	Postoperative	P
AS1	320,2	309,7	<0,05*
AS3	326,0	291,3	<0,05*
AS7	292,6	269,4	<0,05*
S1	351,6	348,3	>0,05
S3	308,9	272,1	<0,05*
S7	313,8	292,6	<0,05*

Table 2 Minimum, Maximum, median, mean and standard deviation for the colonic anastomosis breaking strength at each group and subgroups. Values measured in Newtons.

	Anastomosis Breaking Strength					
	AS1	S1	AS3	S3	AS7	S7
n (survived)	5	6	6	5	4	6
Minimum	0,03	0,15	0,09	0,07	0,31	0,25
Maximum	0,37	0,41	0,31	0,29	0,49	0,52
Median	0,23	0,22	0,14	0,19	0,31	0,42
Mean	0,20	0,24	0,17	0,18	0,35	0,40
Std. Deviation	0,14	0,09	0,08	0,08	0,09	0,09

risk factor for death in animal models and human patients [13,16,17]. This study showed that the combination of alcohol and sepsis have an even greater impact on postoperative mortality, since the group AS had a death rate three times greater the S group.

The scar tissue healing can be mechanically evaluated by both longitudinal anastomotic breaking strength (ABS) used in our study and radial bursting strength [13,18]. Longitudinal breaking strength is the measure of intestinal wall resistance to forces applied on its longitudinal direction while bursting pressure measures the resistance to intraluminal elevated preassures [19]. The ABS measures the risk for total dehiscence, because it measures the strength of the scar's strongest bit, while the bursting pressure evaluates the risk of leakage, because it measures the strength of the weakest segment of the scar.

The AS group colon surgical wound didn't became stronger by day 7, because it was not different from the 3AS or the 1AS groups (p> 0,05). The acquisition of

tensile strength of the wound is due to the deposition and organization of the collagen, and an impaired wound healing is responsible not only for the lack of collagen, but also for disorganized collagen [1]. It is possible that the alcohol intake was responsible for an impaired inflammation stage of the wound healing and magnified the deleterious effects of sepsis, such as disorganized deposition of collagen and excessive activity of matrix metalloproteases [1,20-22].

The effects of alcohol on wound healing are dependent to the pattern of the alcohol exposure: chronic or acute abuse, the dose intake, duration of consumption, time from alcohol exposure to injury, alcohol withdrawal and associated factors such as infection, sepsis, smoking, usage of medication, obesity, diabetes, and other comorbidities [1]. Acute ethanol exposure in non-septic patients can

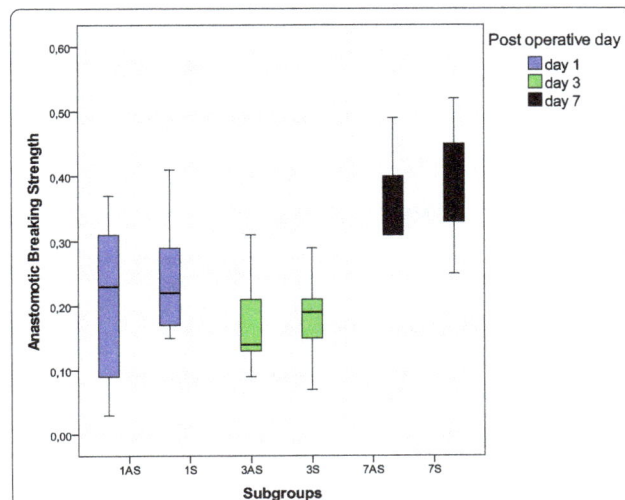

Figure 4 Anastomotic breaking strength distribution in Newtons: superior and inferior limits, interquartils interval and the median in the central part of the boxes. All groups have been displayed.

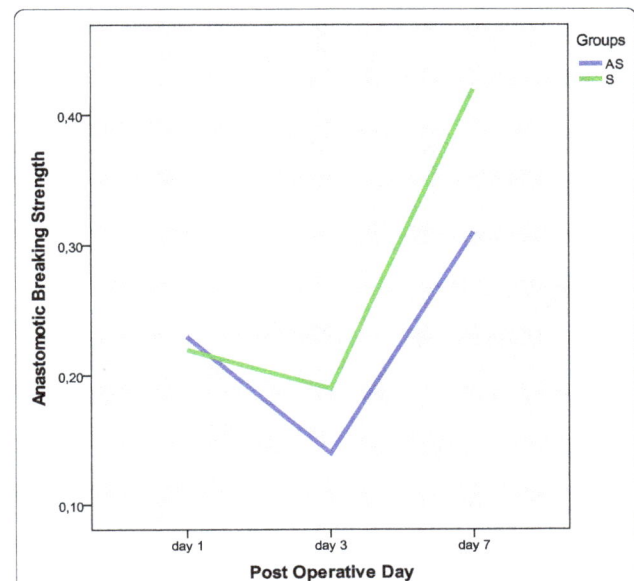

Figure 5 Median of the anastomotic breaking strength, in Newton, one, three and seven post-operative days. Even after 7 days the AS group (blue) colonic anastomosis did not become stronger (p>0,05) while the S group (green) did (p<0,05).

Table 3 Sum of the values of all animals of the groups due to the analyzed histopathological parameters. The amount of collagen, fibroblast, mononuclear and polymorphonuclear infiltrations and the neovascularization were marked with values from 0 to 3 each, in which 0 means nothing and 3 a large amount. The parameters of abscess, bacterial colony, foreign body, crust and fibrin were signalized as 0 or 1, meaning absent or present respectively.

	Histopathological Analysis					
	AS1	S1	AS3	S3	AS7	S7
	n=5	n=6	n=6	n=5	n=4	n=6
Collagen	0	0	0	0	4	6
Fibroblast	0	0	6	5	12	18
Neovascularization	0	0	6	5	8	12
Mononuclear	0	0	6	5	8	12
Polymorphonuclear	7	6	15	13	9	13
Abscess	1	0	4	4	1	1
Bacterial Colony	1	1	2	5	2	1
Foreign Body	1	0	2	3	4	5
Crust	5	6	4	5	3	4
Fibrin	4	5	6	5	0	0

lead to inadequate wound healing, by impairing the early inflammatory response, inhibiting wound closure, angiogenesis and collagen production, and changing the protease balance at the wound site [1], although we didn't observe this in the septic conditions of this study.

Inflammation is a normal part of the wound healing process, and is important to the removal of contaminating micro-organisms [1]. In the absence of effective decontamination, such as in fecal sepsis, inflammation may be prolonged, thus the next steps in wound healing, the inflammation and remodeling, can be prolonged or impaired, but not always [1]. Both bacteria and endotoxins can lead to prolonged elevation of pro-inflammatory cytokines such as interleukin-1 (IL-1), IL-6, IL-10, TNF-α, and increased levels of matrix metalloproteases (MMP) [1,20-22].

Conclusions

Sepsis and its association with ethanol led to weight loss postoperatively. Alcohol intake increased the mortality rate three times in septic animals. Acute alcohol intoxication delays the acquisition of tensile strength of colonic anastomosis in septic rats. Therefore, acute alcohol intoxication before sepsis leads to worse prognosis in animal models of abdominal trauma patients.

Acknowledgements
This research was only possible through the support from the following institutions: 2nd/2010 grants of FINATEC (Foundation of Scientific and Technological Developments), supply of Wistar rats by the Labocien of UniCEUB (University Center of Brasilia), scientific initiation scholarships from the University of Brasília (UnB) and CNPq (National Council of Research and Development).
Also thanks to Gabizao Alves for the high quality professional photos, displayed as Figures 1 and 2.
Finally we must thank the Academic League of Emergency and Trauma of the University of Brasilia (LETUnB) for supporting us and supplying our minds with curiosity and curiosity for trauma, emergency and surgery.
This article has been published as part of World Journal of Emergency Surgery Volume 7 Supplement 1, 2012: Proceedings of the World Trauma Congress 2012. The full contents of the supplement are available online at http://www.wjes.org/supplements/7/S1.

Author details
[1]Medical School, Academic League of Emergency and Trauma, University of Brasilia, Brasilia, Brazil. [2]Medical School, University of Brasilia, Brasilia, Brazil. [3]Campus Universitário Darcy Ribeiro, Prédio da Reitoria, 2° pavimento, sala B2-16, 70910-900 Brasília – DF Brasil, Brazil.

Authors' contributions
PHAM did the project design and coordination, surgical and technical work, statistical analysis, data acquisition and interpretation and manuscript writing. VLR, IECF and LEAS all did the project design, surgical and technical work, data acquisition and interpretation. FPC was responsible for the histopathological work and data interpretation. JPRV helped with the project design, technical work and data interpretation. JBS did the data interpretation, critical review and manuscript writing. All authors read and approved the final manuscript.

Competing interests
The authors declare that they have no competing interests of any kind.

References
1. Guo S, Dipietro LA: Factors affecting wound healing. J Dent Res 2010, 89:219-29.
2. Miller PR, Fabian TC, Croce MA, Magnotti LJ, Pritchard FE, Minard G, Stewart RM: Improving outcomes following penetrating colon wounds: application of a clinical pathway. Ann Surg 2002, 235:775-81.
3. Ott MM, Norris PR, Diaz JJ, Collier BR, Jenkins JM, Gunter OL, Morris JA: Colon anastomosis after damage control laparotomy: recommendations from 174 trauma colectomies. The Journal of Trauma 2011, 70:595-602.
4. Osborn TM, Tracy JK, Dunne JR, Pasquale M, Napolitano LM: Epidemiology of sepsis in patients with traumatic injury. Crit Care Med 2004, 32:2234-40.
5. Rangel-Frausto MS: Sepsis: still going strong. Arch Med Res 2005, 36:672-81.
6. Lieber CS: Medical disorders of alcoholism. N Engl J Med 1995, 333:1058-65.
7. Smith GS, Brenas CC, Miller TR: Fatal Nontraffic Injuries Involving Alcohol: A Metanalysis. Annals of emergency medicine 1999, 33:659-668.
8. Gazal-Carvalho C, Carlini-Cotrima B, Silvab OA, Sauaia N: Blood alcohol content prevalence among trauma patients seen at a level 1 trauma Center. Rev Saúde Pública 2002, 36:47-54.
9. Gentilello LM, Rivara FP, Donovan DM, Jurkovich GJ, Daranciang E, Dunn CW, Villaveces A, Copass M, Ries RR: Alcohol Interventions in a Trauma Center as a Means of Reducing the Risk of Injury Recurrence. Ann of Surg 1999, 230:473-483.
10. Spies CD, Rommelspacher H: Alcohol Withdrawal in the Surgical Patient: Prevention and Treatment. Anesth Analg 1999, 88:946-54.
11. Wichterman KA, Baue AAAE, Chaudry IH: Sepsis and septic shock - a review of laboratory models and a proposal. J Surg Res 1980, 29:189-201.
12. Morais PH, Farias IC, Duraes LC, Carneiro FP, Oliveira PG, Sousa JB: Evaluation of the effects of carbon dioxide pneumoperitoneum on abdominal wall wound healing in rats undergoing segmental resection and anastomosis of the left colon. Acta Cir Bras 2012, 27:63-70.
13. Pereira RSC, Hasimoto CN, Pelafsky L, Llanos JC, Cataneo DC, Spadella CT, Minossi JG: Intestinal healing in rats submitted to ethanol ingestion. Acta Cir Bras 2012, 27:236-43.
14. Silva SM, Oliveira MVM, Brandao AM, Carneiro FP, Ferreira VMM, Parra RS, Feres O, Sousa JB: Study on adhesion formation and the healing of colon anastomosis in rats with induced peritoneal sepsis. Acta Cir Bras 2011, 26:100-5.

13. Stwart RM, Myers JG, Dent DL, Ermis P, Gray GA, Villarreal R, Blow O,
     Woods B, McFarland M, Garavaglia J, Root HD, Pruitt BA Jr: **Seven hundred
     fifty-three consecutive deaths in a level I trauma center: the argument
     for injury prevention.** *J Trauma* 2003, **54**:66-71.
15. Tonnesen H, Kehlet H: **Preoperative alcoholism and postoperative
     morbidity.** *Br J Surg* 1999, **86**:869-74.
17. Radek KA, Matthies AM, Burns AL, Heinrich SA, Kovacs EJ, DiPietro LA: **Acute
     alcohol exposure impairs angiogenesis and the proliferative phase of
     wound healing.** *Am J Physiol Heart Circ Physiol* 2005, **289**:H1084-90.
18. Thompson SK, Chang EY, Jobe BA: **Clinical Review: healing in
     gastrointestinal anastomosis.** *Microsurgery* 2006, **26**:131-6.
19. Mansson P, Zhang XW, Jeppsson B, Thorlaciuss H: **Anastomotic healing in
     the rat colon: comparison between a radiological method, breaking
     strength and bursting pressure.** *Int J Colorectal Dis* 2002, **17**:420-5.
20. Ishimura K, Tsubouchi T, Okano K, Maeba T, Maeta H: **Wound Healing after
     digestive surgery under septic conditions: participation of local
     interleukin-6 expression.** *World J Surg* 1998, **22**:1069-76.
21. Ishimura K, Moroguchi A, Okano K, Maeba T, Maeta H: **Local expression of
     tumor necrosis factor and interleukin-10 on wound healing of intestinal
     anastomosis during endotoxemia in mice.** *J Surg Res* 2002, **108**:91-97.
22. Teke Z, Sacar S, Yenisey C, Atalay AO: **Role of activated protein C on
     Wound Healing process in left colonic anastomoses in presence of intra-
     abdominal sepsis induced by cecal ligation and puncture: an
     experimental study in rat.** *World J Surg* 2008, **32**:2434-43.

17

Non-operative management attempted for selective high grade blunt hepatosplenic trauma is a feasible strategy

Ting-Min Hsieh[1], Tsung Cheng Tsai[2], Jiun-Lung Liang[3] and Chih Che Lin[4*]

Abstract

Background: There is growing evidence of clinical data recently for successful outcomes of non-operative management (NOM) for blunt hepatic and spleen injuries (BHSI). However, the effectiveness of NOM for high-grade BHSI remains undefined. The aim of the present study was to review our experience with NOM in high-grade BHSI and compare results with the existing related data worldwide.

Methods: In this retrospectively protocol-driven study, 150 patients with grade 3–5 BHSI were enrolled during a 3-year period. Patients were divided into immediate laparotomy (immediate OP) and initial non-operative (initial NOM) groups according to hemodynamic status judged by duty trauma surgeon. Patients who received initial NOM were divided into successful NOM (s-NOM) and failed NOM (f-NOM) subgroups according to conservative treatment failure. We analyzed the clinical characteristics and the outcomes of patients.

Results: Twenty-eight (18.7%) patients underwent immediate operations, and the remaining 122 (81.3%) were initially treated with NOM. Compared with the initial NOM group, the immediate OP group had significantly lower hemoglobin levels, a higher incidence of tube thoracostomy, contrast extravasation and large hemoperitoneum on computed tomography, a higher injury severity score, increased need for transfusions, and longer length of stay (LOS) in the intensive care unit (ICU) and hospitalization. Further analysis of the initial NOM group indicated that NOM had failed in 6 (4.9%) cases. Compared with the s-NOM subgroup, f-NOM patients had significantly lower hemoglobin levels, more hospitalized transfusions, and longer ICU LOS.

Conclusions: NOM of high-grade BHSI in selected patients is a feasible strategy. Notwithstanding, patients with initial low hemoglobin level and a high number of blood transfusions in the ICU are associated with a high risk for NOM failure.

Keywords: Non-operative management, Blunt hepatic injury, Blunt splenic injury, Blunt hepatic and splenic injuries

Introduction

Blunt abdominal trauma (BAT) resulting from a traffic accident, fall, assault, or occupational accident is not unusual in the emergency room. The prevalence of intra-abdominal injury after BAT has been reported to be high at 12-15% [1]. The liver and spleen are the most commonly injured organs in BAT, accounting for up to 70% of all visceral injuries [2,3]. Since the 1980s, there had been a paradigm shift from surgical to nonsurgical

treatment for blunt hepatic and/or splenic injuries (BHSI). Many authors published their experiences showing satisfactory results [4,5]. Computed tomography (CT), which can accurately assess the severity of organ injury, hemoperitoneum, presence of contrast extravasation, viscus injury, and can predict the necessity for prompt intervention, is the diagnostic modality of choice for hemodynamically stable patients. Routine follow-up CT is no longer suggested for NOM of patient with solid organ injury because it has poor ability to detect unidentified injuries [4-6]. Contrast-enhanced ultrasound (CEUS), which can provide a safe and accurate alternative to CT [7], and

* Correspondence: immunologylin@gmail.com
[4]Division of General Surgery, Kaohsiung Chang Gung Memorial Hospital and Chang Gung University College of Medicine, 123 Ta Pei Road, Niao-Sung District, Kaohsiung, Taiwan
Full list of author information is available at the end of the article

can guide a percutaneous treatment, is a save adjunct to observation in NOM [8]. An increasing body of literature emphasizing promising results, the wide use of CT, and the emergence of CEUS promoted the acceptance of non-operative management (NOM) as the standard therapeutic strategy. In fact, with numerous recent studies have shown success rates > 90% and failure rates < 11% [9-11]. Moreover, high success rates with NOM have been in pediatric patients [3]. Additionally, some studies [12,13] have documented the feasibility and safety of NOM in patients with advanced age, or neurologic impairment, which were not recommended for NOM before. As the concept of NOM is now established, there is a growing concern regarding its morbidity and drawbacks of angio-embolization, which are especially prevalent in high-grade injuries [14-18]. Moreover, the effectiveness of NOM in high-grade injuries is still under scrutiny. On the other hand, some authors suggested that surgeons should temper enthusiasm for NOM despite advances in the quality of critical care and radiological intervention [8,19,20]. Because few studies have focused exclusively on high-grade BHSI, the present study aimed to investigate the efficacy of NOM for complex BHSI in the setting of a tertiary care center.

Methods

Setting, study protocol

Patients admitted to Kaohsiung Chang Gung Memorial Hospital with BHSI between January 2010 to December 2012 were retrospectively reviewed. All patients were initially assessed and resuscitated at the emergency room (ER) according to the advanced trauma life support (ATLS) guidelines. The selection of patients for a nonsurgical management protocol [21] was based on the following criteria: hemodynamic stability on admission or shortly after initial resuscitation, maintenance of hemodynamic stability [systolic blood pressure (SBP) > 90 mmHg] without the need for excessive blood transfusion, no obvious peritonitis, and no associated multiple traumas requiring immediate operation. Indication signs for angiography were: significant hemoperitoneum (>1000 mL) with episode of hypotension (SBP < 90 mmHg) or contrast extravasation on CT scan, recurrent hypotension despite fluid resuscitation, grade 4–6 hepatic or grade 4–5 splenic injuries, and falling hemoglobin level (<8 g/dL) with progressive need for blood transfusions. We determined that angiography should be performed early after initial stabilization if the criteria were met. In the case of rapid clinical deterioration, the procedure was abandoned, and the patient underwent immediate emergency surgery.

Data collection, definitions and exclusion criteria

Although this was a retrospective study, data on age, gender, mechanism of blunt trauma, initial vital signs [i.e. SBP, heart rate (HR), respiratory rate (RR)], hemoglobin level, Glasgow coma scale (GCS), alcohol intoxication, incidences of endotracheal intubation and tube thoracostomy, CT findings, Injury Severity Score (ISS), blood transfusion at ER and during admission, length of stay (LOS) at intensive care unit (ICU), duration of hospitalization, and outcomes, including morbidities and mortalities, were prospectively collected. ER transfusions included units of blood transfused during resuscitation at ER or before transfer from a local clinic, whereas admission transfusions referred to all units administered during hospitalization, except resuscitation at ER. The severity of BHSI was graded according to the classification of the American Association for the Surgery of Trauma (1994 revision). Patients with concomitant liver and spleen injuries were assigned to either liver or splenic injury group according to the organ with higher injury grading. The presence of intra-abdomen fluid was determined using CT. The amount of hemoperitoneum was quantified as follows: minimal, perihepatic blood in subphrenic or subhepatic space or perisplenic fossae (<500 mL); moderate, minimal plus blood along paracolic gutter (500-1000 mL); and large, moderate plus blood accumulating in pelvic cavity (>1000 mL). Patients who died at ER, those without available abdominal CT, and those with CT findings consistent with grade I or II injuries were excluded from the present study. High-grade injury referred grade III-VI in blunt hepatic injurIES (BHI) and grade III-V in blunt spleinc injuries (BSI).

Study population and grouping

The patients were initially categorized into two groups: those initially treated non-operatively were included in the initial NOM group and those receiving early laparotomy at ER because of hemodynamic instability or suspected peritonitis were included in the immediate OP group. Patients in the initial NOM group were admitted to ICU for close monitoring and were further divided into two subgroups, the s-NOM included patients that treated successfully with conservative methods and the f-NOM included those who eventually required laparotomy according to the judgment of trauma surgeons after observation in ICU.

Statistical analysis

Data are presented as percentages for categorical data, and means ± SE for ordinal and continuous data. Statistical analyses were performed using the chi-square test or Fisher's exact test for discrete variables and the Mann Whitney U test for continuous variables. All differences at the $p < 0.05$ level were considered statistically significant.

Table 1 Correlations between severity of hemoperitoneum and grading of liver/spleen injuries on computed tomography

Severity of hemoperitoneum	Grade of liver/spleen laceration					Total no. of patients
	I	II	III	IV	V	
Nil to minimal	2/3	49[3]/14	52[2]/17	12/0	4/1	119/35
Moderate	0/0	1/0	2/7[1]	4/1	1/2	8/10
Large	0/0	0/4	4[1]/11	7/10	5*/10[2]	16/35
Total	2/3	50/18	58/35	23/11	10/13	143/80

*Including a grade VI liver laceration with large hemoperitoneum, parentheses: means including patient number of concomitant liver and spleen injuries.

Results

Patient characteristic, trauma mechanisms

During the 3-year study period, 150 patients presented with high-grade BHSI, of whom 91 and 59 had BHI and BSI, respectively. The relationship between the severity of hemoperitoneum and CT grading is shown in Table 1.

The majority of the study subjects were men (62%), with a mean age of 31.9 ± 16.3 years (range, 3–77).

The most common causes of high-grade BHI were motorcycle collision (n = 55, 60.4%), motor vehicle collision (n = 18, 19.8%), falls from greater height (n = 7, 7.7%) or from own height (n = 4, 4.4%), pedestrian struck (n = 3, 3.3%), assaults (n = 2, 2.2%), and bicycle collision (n = 2, 2.2%). In high-grade BSI, motorcycle collisions were responsible for most injuries (n = 46, 78%), while other causes included motor vehicle collision (n = 4, 6.8%), assaults (n = 3, 5.1%), falls from own height (n = 2, 3.4%) and from greater height (n = 1, 1.7%), bicycle collision (n = 2, 3.4%), and pedestrian struck (n = 1, 1.7%) (Tables 2, 3 and 4).

Patient management algorithm, final outcomes

The patient population, morbidity, mortality, and management algorithm are described in Figure 1. The causes of

Table 2 Comparisons between initial NOM group and immediate OP group

	Initial NOM	Immediate OP	p
Number of patients (n)	122	28	-
Gender (male)	73 (59.8%)	20 (71.4%)	0.25
Age (years)	32.52 ± 16.73	29.64 ± 14.47	0.40
SBP (mmHg)	118.68 ± 29.32	107.36 ± 28.85	0.06
HR (beats/min)	98.13 ± 20.31	105.11 ± 25.94	0.12
RR (breaths/min)	20.06 ± 3.65	21.82 ± 6.36	0.16
Hemoglobin (g/dL)	11.94 ± 2.34	10.46 ± 3.09	0.005
Endotracheal intubation (%)	13 (10.7%)	5 (17.9%)	0.33
Tube thoracostomy (%)	18 (14.8%)	10 (35.7%)	0.01
CT extravasation (%)	30 (24.6%)	16 (57.1%)	0.001
Large hemoperiotneum (%)	28 (23.0%)	19 (67.9%)	<0.001
Alcohol intoxication (%)	85 (69.7%)	24 (85.7%)	0.08
GCS	13.78 ± 2.73	13.11 ± 3.42	0.26
ISS	19.78 ± 10.35	26.30 ± 11.55	0.004
Mechanism:			0.45
Motorcycle	84 (69%)	17 (61%)	
Motor vehicle	15 (12%)	6 (21%)	
others	21 (19%)	5 (18%)	
Emergency room BT (U)	1.48 ± 2.05	5.14 ± 5.26	0.001
Hospitalization BT(U)	2.41 ± 4.98	10.86 ± 11.95	0.001
BT requirement (%)	73 (59.8%)	26 (92.9%)	0.001
Hospitalization LOS(day)	13.66 ± 10.20	21.64 ± 14.75	0.01
ICU LOS(day)	4.57 ± 4.45	8.68 ± 9.17	0.02
Patients with associated injury (%)	96 (78.7%)	23 (82.1%)	0.684
Patients with complication(s) (%)	14 (11.4%)	6 (21.4%)	0.12
Mortality (%)	6 (4.9%)	4 (14.3%)	0.09

NOM: Non-operative management; OP: Operation; SBP: Systolic blood pressure; CT: Computed tomography; GCS: Gasglow coma scale; ISS: Injury severity score; BT: Blood transfusion; ICU: Intensive care unit; LOS: Length of stay.

Table 3 Comparisons between patients with s-NOM and f-NOM

	Non-operative (s-NOM)	f-NOM	P
Number of patients (n)	116	6	-
Gender (male)	69 (59.5%)	4 (66.7%)	1.00
Age (years)	32.34 ± 16.21	36.00 ± 26.69	0.69
SBP (mmHg)	119.44 ± 29.37	104.00 ± 26.35	0.25
HR (beats/min)	98.13 ± 20.13	98.17 ± 25.66	0.74
RR (breaths/min)	20.03 ± 3.59	20.67 ± 5.00	0.95
Hemoglobin (g/dL)	12.11 ± 2.27	8.67 ± 0.51	0.001
Endotracheal intubation (%)	11 (9.5%)	2 (33.3%)	0.12
Tube thoracostomy (%)	16 (13.8%)	2 (33.3%)	0.21
CT extravasation (%)	29 (25.0%)	1 (16.7%)	1.00
Large hemoperiotneum (%)	25 (21.6%)	3 (50.0%)	0.13
Alcohol (%)	79 (68.1%)	6 (100.0%)	0.17
GCS	13.88 ± 2.55	11.83 ± 5.15	0.44
ISS	19.36 ± 10.24	27.83 ± 9.80	0.06
Mechanism:			0.47
Motorcycle	79 (68%)	5 (83%)	
Motor vehicle	14 (12%)	1 (17%)	
Others	23 (10%)	0 (0%)	
Emergency room BT (U)	1.43 ± 2.05	2.33 ± 1.96	0.12
Hospitalization BT (U)	2.01 ± 4.15	10.17 ± 11.35	0.001
BT requirement (%)	67 (57.8%)	6 (100.0%)	0.08
Hospitalization (days)	13.22 ± 9.28	22.17 ± 21.12	0.33
ICU LOS (days)	4.19 ± 3.60	12.00 ± 10.60	0.02
Patients with associated injury (%)	91 (78.4%)	5 (83.3%)	1.00
Patients with complication(s) (%)	8 (6.8%)	0 (0.0%)	1.00
Mortality (%)	4 (3.4%)	2 (33.3%)	0.02

s-NOM: Successful non-operative management; f-NOM: Failed non-operative management; SBP: Systolic blood pressure; CT: Computed tomography; GCS: Gasglow coma scale; ISS: Injury severity score; BT: Blood transfusion; ICU: Intensive care unit; LOS: Length of stay.

failure of NOM included complications in 14 patients in the initial NOM group (11.4%, 14/122). The f-NOM group included 6 patients, and the s-NOM group included 8 patients. Of the 6 patients in the f-NOM, 1 presented with BSI with persistent hemorrhage and atrial fibrillation attack, 1 with a history of liver cirrhosis showing re-bleeding after splenic angioembolization, 1 had splenic abscess with profound sepsis after splenic angioembolization, 2 showed reduced hemoglobin levels despite active resuscitation and hepatic angioembolization, and 1 showed unstable hemodynamics with concomitant BHSI and lung contusion. Complications, including re-bleeding (n = 2), liver abscess (n = 2), empyema (n = 1), intra-abdominal abscess (n = 2), and intestinal obstruction (n = 1), were successfully treated conservatively in the remaining 8 patients in the s-NOM group. Six patients in the immediate OP group developed complications, including sepsis (n = 1), the formation of

intra-abdominal abscess (n = 3), hepatic abscess (n = 1), and biloma (n = 1), which were also successfully treated conservatively.

In addition, there were 10 deaths, including 4 in the s-NOM group, 2 in the f-NOM group, and 4 in the immediate OP group. Of the 4 patients in the s-NOM group, 3 died of intracranial hemorrhage and 1 died of severe lung contusion. Of the 4 patients in the immediate OP, 1 with grade V BHI died of persistent shock postoperatively, 1 with BHI and pelvis fracture died of massive transfusion-related coagulopathy, 1 with BHI and mesentery tear died of liver cirrhosis, and 1 with BSI died of intracranial hemorrhage. Of the 2 patients in the f-NOM group, 1 with concomitant BHSI died of severe lung contusion (ISS:34) on the second postoperative day, and 1 with grade IV BSI (ISS:38) and post angioembolization re-bleeding died of liver cirrhosis 6 days postoperatively.

Table 4 Comparisons between patients with and without operations for blunt high-grade liver or spleen injuries

	Non-operative (s-NOM)	Operative (f-NOM + Immediate OP)	P
Number of patients (n)	116	34	-
Gender (male)	69 (59.5%)	24 (70.6%)	0.24
Age (years)	32.34 ± 16.21	30.76 ± 16.89	0.62
SBP (mmHg)	119.44 ± 29.37	106.76 ± 28.06	0.02
HR (beats/min)	98.13 ± 20.13	103.88 ± 25.64	0.23
RR (breaths/min)	20.03 ± 3.59	21.62 ± 6.09	0.15
Hemoglobin (g/dL)	12.11 ± 2.27	10.15 ± 2.89	<0.00⁻
Endotracheal intubation (%)	11 (9.5%)	7 (20.6%)	0.12
Tube thoracostomy (%)	16 (13.8%)	12 (35.3%)	0.005
CT extravasation (%)	29 (25.0%)	17 (50.0%)	0.005
Large hemoperiotneum (%)	25 (21.6%)	22 (64.7%)	<0.001
Alcohol (%)	79 (68.1%)	30 (88.2%)	0.02
GCS	13.88 ± 2.55	12.88 ± 3.72	0.15
ISS	19.36 ± 10.24	26.58 ± 11.13	0.001
Mechanism:			0.41
Motorcycle	79 (68%)	22 (65%)	
Motor vehicle	14 (12%)	7 (21%)	
Others	23 (10%)	5 (15%)	
Emergency room BT (U)	1.43 ± 2.05	4.65 ± 4.94	0.001
Hospitalization BT (U)	2.01 ± 4.15	11.06 ± 11.70	<0.001
BT requirement (%)	67 (57.8%)	32 (94.1%)	<0.001
Hospitalization (days)	13.22 ± 9.28	21.74 ± 15.67	0.004
ICU LOS (days)	4.19 ± 3.60	9.26 ± 9.35	0.004
Patients with associated injury (%)	91 (78.4%)	28 (82.4%)	0.62
Patients with complication(s) (%)	8 (6.8%)	6 (17.6%)	0.27
Mortality (%)	4 (3.4%)	6 (17.6%)	0.01

s-NOM: Successful non-operative management; f-NOM: Failed non-operative management; OP: Operation; SBP: Systolic blood pressure; CT: Computed tomography; GCS: Gasglow coma scale; ISS: Injury severity score; BT: Blood transfusion; ICU: Intensive care unit; LOS: Length of stay.

Initial NOM vs. immediate OP

NOM was initially applied in 81.3% (n = 122) of all patients with high-grade BHSI. Twenty-eight (18.7%) patients underwent emergency laparotomy. The incidences of initial NOM for high-grade BHSI were 88% (80/91) and 71% (42/59), respectively. The comparisons of characteristics of the initial NOM and immediate OP groups are presented in Table 2.

s-NOM vs. f-NOM

Of the 122 patients initially treated with NOM, 116 were treated successfully (95%). Further analysis of the two subgroups of the initial NOM group is presented in Table 3.

Non-operative vs. patients receiving operations

In terms of operative treatment, comparisons between the s-NOM and patients receiving operations (immediate OP + f-NOM) are shown in Table 4.

Discussion

NOM is currently the main treatment for patients with BHSI and has shown excellent results [4,5,8,11,13-15]. This may be partly attributed to the aggressive use of angioembolization in recent years [14,15,17,21,22]. Another factor is that strict use of a protocol based approach and algorithm leads to a significantly expansion of NOM. According to the study of Miller et al. [14], the failure rate of NOM attempted for high-grade BSI improved from 15% to 5% with the incorporation of a protocol. Mitsusada et al. [23] reported that NOM of BHI applied for selected hemodynamically unstable patients (target SBP of 80 mmHg) under a revision protocol can decrease the overall laparotomy rates and transfusion requirements. Accordingly, a protocol based algorithm for the management of BHSI is proposed.

In present study, NOM was applied in 81.3% of high-grade BHSI patients with a failure rate of 3.7% and 7.1%

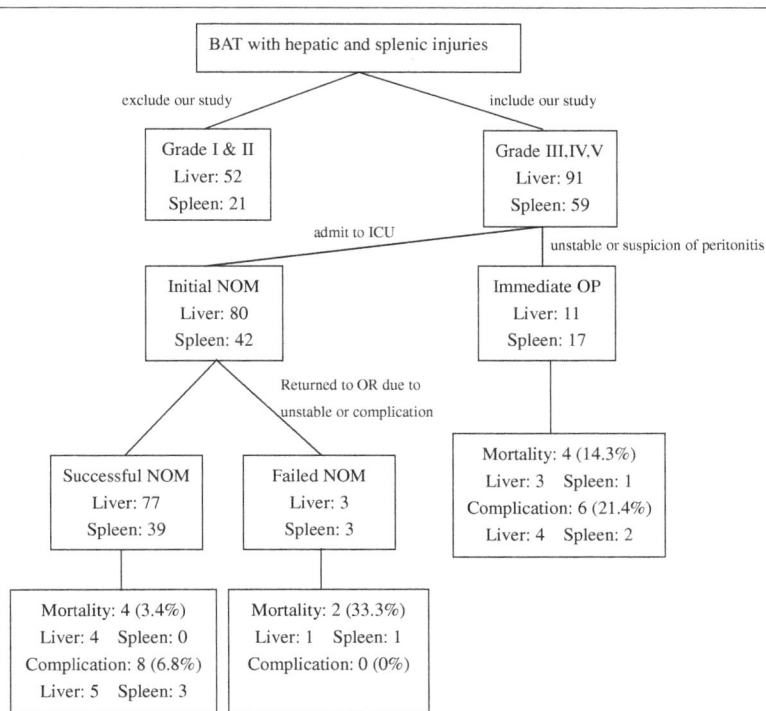

Figure 1 NOM was initially applied in 81.3% of all patients with high-grade blunt hepatic and/or splenic injuries with a failure rate of 4.9%. NOM: non-operative management; BAT: blunt abdominal trauma; ICU: intensive care unit; OR: operation room.

for BHI and BSI, respectively, resulting in an overall failure rate of 4.9%. Our results are comparable to those of prior studies [8,9] showing that 72%-81% of BHSI patients are treated by NOM with a failure rate of 5.2%-5.8%. On the other hand, unlike previous studies [8,9], the present study focused exclusively on high-grade injuries. Accordingly, this could justify NOM is adequate in most high-grade BHSI patients.

Among previous organ-specific studies, those examining high-grade BHI, reported the use of initial NOM in 78%(63/81) of patients with a failure of 3.7%(3/81) [13]. In the present study, 91(60%) patients had high-grade BHI, of which 80(88%) were managed nonoperatively, with 3.7%(3/80) failures. In terms of splenic trauma, one study [10] reported on 324(56%) patients had high-grade BSI, of which 258(79%) were managed nonoperatively, with 18(7%) failures. In present study, 59(74%) patients had high-grade BSI, of which 42(71%) were managed nonoperatively, with 7.1%(3/42) failures. Therefore, compared with previous studies analyzing high-grade injuries in a single specific organ [10,13], our study showed similar results. It may be attributed to the standardized protocol followed at our institute, which emphasizes the early introduction of angioembolization for BHSI, and a dedicated radiology team [21,22].

Most prior studies concluded that the main reason for the failure of NOM is the hemodynamic instability, whereas

this observation was contradicted by Mitsusada et al. [23]. Various predictors of NOM failure have been documented in the literatures [2,9,13,24-26]. Literature review of Bhangu et al. [24] reported AAST grades 4–5, the presence of moderate or large haemoperitoneum, increasing ISS, and increasing age were significantly associated with increased risk factor of NON failure in BSI, which led to significantly longer ICU and overall lengths of stay. Hashemzadeh et al. [25] suggested age, female gender and ISS were significant predictors of NOM failure in BHSI. In another study, Olthof et al. [26] reported age ≥ 40 years, ISS ≥ 25, splenic injury grade ≥ 3 are prognostic factors of NOM failure in BSI. In current study, lower level of hemoglobin, longer ICU LOS, and higher number of hospitalization transfusions were significant risk factors in those patients for whom NOM failed. These observations were similar with previous published studies [2,9,24,27]. Robinson 3ed et al. [9] reported blood transfusion is a predictor of mortality, hospital LOS and NOM failure in BHSI. Additionally, Sartorelli et al. [27] proposed that the failure rate is higher in patients who received more than 4U of blood. In our study, in terms of the overall transfusions in ER and during hospitalization, the overall mean transfusion amounts in the s-NOM and initial NOM groups were within the 4U limit, which was in agreement with the values reported previously [27]. Further prospective study of transfusion practices in treatment algorithms of BHSI is warranted.

Another factor of NOM failure is a concomitant BHSI. In a study of Sharma et al. [28] found a higher failure rate (14.3%) than isolated liver (1.5%) or spleen (5.6%) injury. However, it was contradicted by Robinson III et al. [9]. In our study, there were only 6 patients with combined high-grade BHSI, so it is difficult to compare significance.

A potential drawback of NOM is that hollow viscus injuries are overlooked. Swaid et al. [29] reported a hollow viscus injury rate of 1.5% in a BAT with neither splenic nor hepatic injuries, 3.1% with isolated BSI, 3.1% with isolated BHI, and 6.7% with concomitant BHSI, respectively. Miller et al. [30] found an associated intra-abdominal injury rate of 5% in a NOM liver group and 1.7% in a NOM spleen group, and a missed injury rate of 2.3% and 0%, respectively. On the other hand, the reported rate of hollow organ injury is approximately 0.3% of 227972 BAT admissions with an approximately 0.6-0.8% missed injury rate in patients selected for NOM [27,31,32]. Thus, hollow viscus injury is not unusual in combined BHSI. Although the overall incidence of missed injury is relatively low, we should not abandon the suspicion of peritonitis in every BAT patient. In our series, there was no missed injury in initial NOM group.

Multiple studies have documented that successful NOM not only can increase organ salvage rates, but also can decrease blood transfusions requirements, hospital stays, nontherapeutic laparotomy rates, septic complications, and mortality rates [4,5]. Studies conducted by Schnuriger et al. [13] and Velmahos et al. [15] reported complications rates of approximately 17%-20% in high-grade BHSI with NOM. On the other hand, in a collective review of 1489 non-therapeutic laparotomies, the complication rate was 14.6% [33]. Our data showed that the morbidities of s-NOM (6.8%) and initial NOM (11.4%) were lower than previous studies [13,15,33]. Although our numbers were low, they lend further support to the contention that the complication rate is acceptable to justify this form of therapy.

Of the two mortality cases in f-NOM group, one (ISS:34) died of concomitant severe lung contusion and the other one (ISS:38) died of coexistent liver cirrhosis coagulopathy. Fang et al. [34] considers that cirrhosis is a contraindication for NOM in BSI and suggested early surgery for these patients. Another study of Schnuriger et al. [13] suggested that concomitant injuries, especially extraabdominal lesions, are a major determinant of outcome in patients with high-grade BHI and should be consulted early by trauma surgeon. When NOM for BHSI is often advocated, we should not forget that safe NOM requires adherence to cardinal surgical principles and fastidious clinical decision-making.

The present study had two limitations; one was we put discussions of BHI and BSI together and another was the lower number of cases included in the f-NOM group. Hence, it may not be an accurate reflection of the true results of the applicability of NOM to isolated hepatic or splenic injuries. Despite these limitations, our results provided valid information on the applicability of NOM to high-grade BHSI as the data of the study was collected prospectively with strict protocols.

Conclusions

Parallel to the rapid growth of economics in Taiwan, motor vehicles accidents will continue to contribute significantly to the high-grade BHSI. Our study shows lower morbidities in successful NOM justify further attempts for NOM in high-grade BHSI in selected patients aiming at formulating a specific standardized diagnostic/management algorithm. With the incorporation of a protocol, 95% of hemodynamically stable patients with high-grade BHSI can be managed safely with NOM. This study can help emergency practitioners and trauma surgeons recognize and introduce the practice.

Abbreviations
NOM: Non-operative management; BHSI: Blunt hepatic and/or splenic injuries; OP: Operation; LOS: Length of stay; ICU: Intensive care unit; BAT: Blunt abdominal trauma; CT: Computed tomography; CEUS: Contrast-enhanced ultrasound; ER: Emergency room; SBP: Systolic blood pressure; HR: Heart rate; RR: Respiratory rate; GCS: Glasgow coma scale; ISS: Injury severity score; BHI: Blunt hepatic injuries; BSI: Blunt splenic injuries; BT: Blood transfusion; OR: Operation room.

Competing interests
The authors declare that they have no competing interests.

Authors' contributions
HTM was involved in conception, design, analysis and interpretation of data; drafting the manuscript. TTC was involved in analysis and interpretation of data; performed statistical analysis. LJL was involved in acquisition and analysis of the data. LCC was involved in coordination of the study and revision of the manuscript. All authors read and approved the final manuscript.

Acknowledgements
The authors thank to Dr. Po Ping Liu for the establishment of protocol of blunt hepatic and splenic injuries in our hospital.

Author details
[1]Division of Trauma Surgery, Kaohsiung Chang Gung Memorial Hospital and Chang Gung University College of Medicine, 123 Ta Pei Road, Niao-Sung District, Kaohsiung, Taiwan. [2]Department of Emergency, Kaohsiung Chang Gung Memorial Hospital and Chang Gung University College of Medicine, 123 Ta Pei Road, Niao-Sung District, Kaohsiung, Taiwan. [3]Department of Radiology, Kaohsiung Chang Gung Memorial Hospital and Chang Gung University College of Medicine, 123 Ta Pei Road, Niao-Sung District, Kaohsiung, Taiwan. [4]Division of General Surgery, Kaohsiung Chang Gung Memorial Hospital and Chang Gung University College of Medicine, 123 Ta Pei Road, Niao-Sung District, Kaohsiung, Taiwan.

References
1.   Kendall JL, Kestler AM, Whitaker KT, Adkisson MM, Haukoos JS: Blunt abdominal trauma patients are at very low risk for intra-abdominal injury after emergency department observation. West J Emerg Med 2011, 12(4):496–504.

2. Yanar H, Ertekin C, Taviloglu K, Kabay B, Bakkaloglu H, Guloglu R: Nonoperative treatment of multiple intra-abdominal solid organ injury after blunt abdominal trauma. *J Trauma Acute Care Surg* 2008, **64**(4):943–948.

3   Tataria M, Nance ML, Holmes JH 4th, Miller CC 3rd, Mattix KD, Brown RL, Mooney DP, Scherer LR 3rd, Groner JI, Scaife ER, Spain DA, Brundage SI: Pediatric blunt abdominal injury: age is irrelevant and delayed operation is not detrimental. *J Trauma Acute Care Surg* 2007, **63**(3):608–614.

4. Stassen NA, Bhullar I, Cheng JD, Crandall ML, Friese RS, Guillamondegui OD, Jawa RS, Maung AA, Rohs TJ Jr, Sangosanya A, Schuster KM, Seamon MJ, Tchorz KM, Zarzuar BL, Kerwin AJ: Eastern Association for the Surgery of Trauma: Nonoperative management of blunt hepatic injury: an Eastern Association for the Surgery of Trauma practice management guideline. *J Trauma Acute Care Surg* 2012, **73**(5):S288–293.

5. Stassen NA, Bhullar I, Cheng JD, Crandall ML, Friese RS, Guillamondegui OD, Jawa RS, Maung AA, Rohs TJ Jr, Sangosanya A, Schuster KM, Seamon MJ, Tchorz KM, Zarzuar BL, Kerwin AJ: Eastern Association for the Surgery of Trauma:Selective nonoperative management of blunt splenic injury: an Eastern Association for the Surgery of Trauma practice management guideline. *J Trauma Acute Care Surg* 2012, **73**(5):S294–300.

6. Kuo WY, Lin HJ, Foo NP, Guo HR, Jen CC, Chen KT: Will computed tomography (CT) miss something? The characteristics and pitfalls of torso CT in evaluating patients with blunt solid organ trauma. *Ulus Travma Acil Cerrahi Derg* 2011, **17**(3):215–219.

7. Mihalik JE, Smith RS, Toevs CC, Putnam AT, Foster JE: The use of contrast-enhanced ultrasound for the evaluation of solid abdominal organ injury in patients with blunt abdominal trauma. *J Trauma Acute Care Surg* 2012, **73**(5):1100–1105.

8. Lv F, Tang J, Luo Y, Nie Y, Jiao Z, Li T, Zhou X: Percutaneous treatment of blunt hepatic and splenic trauma under contrast-enhanced ultrasound guidance. *Clin Imaging* 2012, **36**(3):191–198.

9. Malhotra AK, Latifi R, Fabian TC, Ivatury RR, Dhage S, Bee TK, Miller PR, Croce MA, Yelon JA: Multiplicity of solid organ injury: influence on management and outcomes after blunt abdominal trauma. *J Trauma Acute Care Surg* 2003, **54**(5):925–929.

10. Robinson WP 3rd, Ahn J, Stiffler A, Rutherford EJ, Hurd H, Zarzaur BL, Baker CC, Meyer AA, Rich PB: Blood transfusion is an independent predictor of increased mortality in nonoperatively managed blunt hepatic and splenic injuries. *J Trauma Acute Care Surg* 2005, **58**(3):437–444.

11. Sabe AA, Claridge JA, Rosenblum DI, Lie K, Malangoni MA: The effects of splenic artery embolization on nonoperative management of blunt splenic injury: a 16-year experience. *J Trauma Acute Care Surg* 2009, **67**(3):565–572.

12. Myers JG, Dent DL, Stewart RM, Gray GA, Smith DS, Rhodes JE, Root HD, Pruitt BA Jr, Strodel WE: Blunt splenic injuries: dedicated trauma surgeons can achieve a high rate of nonoperative success in patients of all ages. *J Trauma Acute Care Surg* 2000, **48**(5):801–805.

13. Shapiro MB, Nance ML, Schiller HJ, Hoff WS, Kauder DR, Schwab CW: Nonoperative management of solid abdominal organ injuries from blunt trauma: impact of neurologic impairment. *Am Surg* 2001, **67**(8):793–796.

14. Schnüriger B, Inderbitzin D, Schafer M, Kickuth R, Exadaktylos A, Candinas D: Concomitant injuries are an important determinant of outcome of high-grade blunt hepatic trauma. *Br J Surg* 2009, **96**(1):104–110.

15. Miller PR, Chang MC, Hoth JJ, Mowery NT, Hildreth AN, Martin RS, Holmes JH, Meredith JW, Requarth JA: Prospective trial of angiography and embolization for all grade III toV blunt splenic injuries: nonoperative management success rate is significantly improved. *Am Coll Surg* 2014, **218**(4):644–648.

16. Velmahos GC, Zacharias N, Emhoff TA, Feeney JM, Hurst JM, Crookes BA, Harrington DT, Gregg SC, Brotman S, Burke PA, Davis KA, Gupta R, Winchell RJ, Desjardins S, Alouidor R, Gross RI, Rosenblatt MS, Schulz JT, Chang Y: Management of the most severely injured spleen: a multicenter study of the Research Consortium of New England Centers for Trauma (ReCONECT). *Arch Surg* 2010, **145**(5):456–460.

17. Bala M, Gazalla SA, Faroja M, Bloom AI, Zamir G, Rivkind AI, Almogy G: Complications of high grade liver injuries: management and outcome with focus on bile leaks. *Scand J Trauma Resusc Emerg Med* 2012, **20**:20.

18. Skattum J, Naess PA, Eken T, Gaarder C: Refining the role of splenic angiographic embolization in high-grade splenic injuries. *J Trauma Acute Care Surg* 2013, **74**(1):100–103.

19. Di Saverio S, Moore EE, Tugnoli G, Naidoo N, Ansaloni L, Bonilauri S, Cucchi M, Catena F: Nonoperative management of liver and spleen traumatic injuries: a giant with clay feet. *World J Emerg Surg* 2012, **7**(1):3.

20. Peitzman AB, Ferrada P, Puyana JC: Nonoperative management of blunt abdominal trauma: have we gone too far? *Surg Infect* 2009, **10**(5):427–433.

21. Liu PP, Lee WC, Cheng YF, Hsieh PM, Hsieh YM, Tan BL, Chen FC, Huang TC, Tung CC: Use of splenic artery embolization as an adjunct to nonsurgical management of blunt splenic injury. *J Trauma Acute Care Surg* 2004, **56**(4):768–772.

22. Liu PP, Liu HT, Hsieh TM, Huang CY, Ko SF: Nonsurgical management of delayed splenic rupture after blunt trauma. *J Trauma Acute Care Surg* 2012, **72**(4):1019–1023.

23. Mitsusada M, Nakajima Y, Shirokawa M, Takeda T, Honda H: Non-operative management of blunt liver injury: a new protocol for selected hemodynamically unstable patients under hypotensive resuscitation. *J Hepatobiliary Pancreat Sci* 2014, **21**(3):205–211.

24. Bhangu A, Nepogodiev D, Lal N, Bowley DM: Meta-analysis of predictive factors and outcomes for failure of non-operative management of blunt splenic trauma. *Injury* 2012, **43**(9):1337–1346.

25. Hashemzadeh SH, Hashemzadeh KH, Dehdilani M, Rezaei S: Non-operative management of blunt trauma in abdominal solid organ injuries: a prospective study to evaluate the success rate and predictive factors of failure. *Minerva Chir* 2010, **65**(3):267–274.

26. Olthof DC, Joosse P, van der Vlies CH, de Haan RJ, Goslings JC: Prognostic factors for failure of nonoperative management in adults with blunt splenic injury: a systematic review. *J Trauma Acute Care Surg* 2013, **74**(2):546–557.

27. Sartorelli KH, Frumiento C, Rogers FB, Osler TM: Nonoperative management of hepatic, splenic, and renal injuries in adults with multiple injuries. *J Trauma Acute Care Surg* 2000, **49**:56–61.

28. Sharma OP, Oswanski MF, Singer D, Raj SS, Daoud YA: Assessment of nonoperative management of blunt spleen and liver trauma. *Am Surg* 2005, **71**(5):379–386.

29. Swaid F, Peleg K, Alfici R, Matter I, Olsha O, Ashkenazi I, Givon A, Israel Trauma Group, Kessel B: Concomitant hollow viscus injuries in patients with blunt hepatic and splenic injuries: An analysis of a National Trauma Registry database. *Injury* 2014, **45**(9):1409–1412.

30. Miller PR, Croce MA, Bee TK, Malhotra AK, Fabian TC: Associated injuries in blunt solid organ trauma: implications for missed injury in nonoperative management. *J Trauma Acute Care Surg* 2002, **53**(2):238–242.

31. Velmahos GC, Toutouzas KG, Radin R, Chan L, Demetriades D: Nonoperative treatment of blunt injury to solid abdominal organs: a prospective study. *Arch Surg* 2003, **138**(3):844–851.

32. Fakhry SM, Watts DD, Luchette FA: EAST Multi-Institutional Hollow Viscus Injury Research Group: EAST Multi-Institutional Hollow Viscus Injury Research Group: Current diagnostic approaches lack sensitivity in the diagnosis of perforated blunt small bowel injury: analysis from 275,557 trauma admissions from the EAST multi-institutional HVI trial. *J Trauma Acute Care Surg* 2003, **54**(2):295–306.

33. Demetriades D, Velmahos G: Indications for and techniques of laparotomy. In *Trauma*. 6th edition. Edited by Moore, Feliciano, Mattox. New Yourk: McGraw-Hill; 2008.

34. Fang JF, Chen RJ, Lin BC, Hsu YB, Kao JL, Chen MF: Liver cirrhosis: an unfavorable factor for nonoperative management of blunt splenic injury. *J Trauma Acute Care Surg* 2003, **54**(6):1131–1136.

Management of traumatic wounds in the Emergency Department: position paper from the Academy of Emergency Medicine and Care (AcEMC) and the World Society of Emergency Surgery (WSES)

Carolina Prevaldi[1]* , Ciro Paolillo[2], Carlo Locatelli[3], Giorgio Ricci[4], Fausto Catena[5], Luca Ansaloni[6] and Gianfranco Cervellin[7]

Abstract

Traumatic wounds are one of the most common problems leading people to the Emergency Department (ED), accounting for approximately 5,4 % of all the visits, and up to 24 % of all the medical lawsuits. In order to provide a standardized method for wound management in the ED, we have organized a workshop, involving several Italian and European experts. Later, all the discussed statements have been submitted for external validation to a multidisciplinary expert team, based on the so called Delphi method. Eight main statements have been established, each of them comprising different issues, covering the fields of wound classification, infectious risk stratification, tetanus and rabies prophylaxis, wound cleansing, pain management, and suture. Here we present the results of this work, shared by the Academy of Emergency Medicine and Care (AcEMC), and the World Society of Emergency Surgery (WSES).

Keywords: Traumatic wounds, Infection, Foreign body, Tetanus, Rabies, Suture

Introduction

Traumatic wounds are one of the most common problems leading people to the Emergency Department (ED), and account for approximately 5,4 % of all the visits [1, 2]. The ED represents the most available facility for wound care, due to the 24-h free access and the decreasing primary care availability. As such, provision for effective and safe wound care will continue to be a priority for Emergency Physicians (EPs). Moreover, traumatic wounds have been historically a major source of litigation against EPs, accounting for up to 24 % of all the medical lawsuits, mainly due to missed identification and treatment of tendon or nerve injuries, or to infection and/or presence of foreign bodies [2]. Hence, although most wounds will

heal without any treatment, a prompt and careful repair of these injuries reduces infection and scarring, so improving the patient satisfaction and avoiding significant additional costs [1]. However, in current clinical practice several different approaches to traumatic wounds are still practiced, due to cultural gaps, myths and local traditions.

One of the specific goals of the third European Union (EU) program in the health care area, years 2014–2020, is to improve access to a skilled, standardized and safe health care for EU citizens, thus improving the quality of health care and patient safety. According to these objectives we have organized a workshop aimed to share knowledge and experiences in the field of wound care, involving several Italian and European experts. The workshop was settled in Venice, in October 2014. Later, all the discussed statements have been submitted for external validation to a multidisciplinary expert team, as described in the methods. On the basis of the results of this complex and time-consuming work, the Academy of Emergency Medicine and Care (AcEMC), and the World Society of

* Correspondence: cprevaldi@fastwebnet.it
[1]Emergency Department, Hospital of San Donà di Piave VE, Parma, Italy
Full list of author information is available at the end of the article

Emergency Surgery (WSES) have decided to build, write and spread a multidisciplinary position statement on the management of traumatic wounds in the ED.

The main purposes of the present work are:

- To assess the current scientific evidence on the subject.
- To draw up a multidisciplinary consensus document aimed to establish a standardized and correct method of management of traumatic wounds in the ED.
- To help clinicians in the clinical risk stratification, to improve diagnostic and therapeutic appropriateness as well as the cost-benefit ratio, to reduce clinical errors, and to increase patient satisfaction.
- To provide an opportunity for research and educational initiative.

Methods

We have decided to use a modified Delphi method, that is a structured communication technique, originally developed as a systematic, interactive forecasting method which relies on a panel of experts [3, 4]. The experts answer to one ore more questionnaires in two or more rounds. After each round, a facilitator provides an anonymous summary of the experts' forecasts from the previous round as well as the reasons they provided for their judgments. Thus, experts are encouraged to revise their earlier answers in light of the replies of other members of the panel. It is expected that during this process the range of differences of the answers will decrease and the group will converge towards the "correct" answer. Finally, the process is stopped after a pre-defined stop criterion (e.g. number of rounds, achievement of consensus, stability of results) and the mean or median scores of the final rounds determine the results [5].

The Delphi method is based on the principle that forecasts or decisions obtained from a structured group of individuals are more accurate than those from unstructured groups [6]. The name "Delphi" derives from the Oracle of Delphi, thus carrying in itself a somewhat mythical nuance. However, the method was developed at the beginning of the Cold War to forecast the impact of technology on warfare [6]. One of the key characteristics of the method relies on the anonymity of the participants. As such, usually all participants remain anonymous, at least until the completion of the final report. This prevents the authority, personality, or reputation of some participants from dominating others in the process. Another important key characteristic is the regular feedback given to the participants, so that they can know comments on their own forecasts, as well as the responses of others, and the progress of the panel as a whole. The last key characteristic relies on the role of the facilitator, i.e. the person coordinating the group. He/she facilitates the responses of their

panel of experts, collects and analyzes them, thus identifying the conflicting viewpoints. If consensus is not reached, the process continues through thesis and antithesis, to gradually work towards synthesis, and building consensus.

To build this document we have composed a multidisciplinary panel consisting of EPs and Surgeons, as well as other experts in different fields, coming from different countries. The study, which lasted about four months, was divided into two different phases. In both phases a dedicated questionnaire was sent by e-mail to each member of the panel. In the first phase, there were three rounds. After that, consensus was reached in eight of the topics addressed. as such, it was considered as appropriate, in the second step, to repeat the round in order to try to reach consensus on all the addressed issues. The external validation of the document was reached organizing a two days' workshop, inviting a group of European experts to discuss and validate the statements [7, 8]. See Appendix.

As such, the first step was based on a series of key questions, as reported in Table 1.

Results
Definitions

At the end of the work the panel and the referees have reached an agreement on the following definitions of traumatic wounds:

Table 1 The questions submitted to the experts

Can you define "clean" a traumatic wound in the setting of the emergency department?

What is your approach to the prophylaxis of wounds with a high risk of infection (e.g., bites, wounds of the hand/foot...)?

Do exist, and, if yes, how reliable are the signs predictive of risk of infection?

Your opinion on methods of prevention of infection: irrigation, closure technique, antibiotic prophylaxis.

In such wounds do you consider as appropriate to assess the status of immunization against tetanus?

Do you consider appropriate the classification of traumatic wounds "clean wound not tetanigenic"?

Since it has been shown that only about 15 % of patients with traumatic wounds carry with them the documentation on their own tetanus immunization status, as noted by the vaccination status of patients prior to tetanus prophylaxis?

Have you ever had difficulties during the anamnesis to assess the state of tetanus vaccine injured patients who present to the emergency department?

Since only 15 % of patients present with documented data on vaccinations and health registry is rarely accessible from the emergency room, in the absence of data, trusts the patient's history on their vaccination status?

If you had to provide a quick diagnostic test to evaluate immediately and with certainty immunization status of injured patients compared to tetanus, would consider it useful in the emergency department to improve the appropriateness of tetanus immunoprophylaxis and management of his patients?

Traumatic Wound: a wound or laceration of traumatic origin with no evidence of macroscopic contamination or signs of active infection (and likely low probability of infection).

Dirty Traumatic Wound: a wound or laceration of traumatic origin macroscopically contaminated. Among these wounds we include those with simultaneous perforation of a viscus; with presence of devitalized tissues; with foreign bodies; those that occurred in a contaminated environment (dung, marshes); animal bites; puncture wounds; wounds with a delayed treatment.

Infected Traumatic Wound: a wound or laceration of traumatic origin with signs of infection (secretions) [9–13].

After completed that step, the panel reached consensus on a series of statements concerning the management of traumatic wounds. For each statement, selected references are provided. The statements are as follows:

STATEMENT 1
All traumatic wounds are to be considered contaminated at presentation in ED.

STATEMENT 2
It is useful to provide an initial stratification of the risk of infection for all the traumatic wounds.
The risk assessment should be based on both the following: i) type of wound; ii) location of the wound; iii) characteristics of the wounded patient.
With the aim of simplifying and optimizing the management of patients in the ED, the following fields of stratification of the risk of infection was identified: type of wound, location of the wound, characteristics of the patients. In Tables 2, 3, 4 the suggested items for risk assessment are summarized.
- 2A. Avoid antibiotic administration in low risk wounds (for all three variables considered).

Table 2 Infection risk assessment based on type of wound

Straight stab wounds	low risk
Tears/bruises/contusion wounds	high risk
Puncture wounds	high risk
Wound with crush injuries	high risk
Bite wounds	high risk
Wounds contaminated with feces	high risk
Wounds contaminated with soil and dirt, or mineral oil	high risk
Wounds with the presence of foreign bodies	high risk
Wounds with edge diastasis	high risk
Engagement of deep tissues, exposed fracture	high risk

Table 3 Infection risk assessment based on the location of the wound

Well vascularized tissue (head, neck, scalp)	low risk
High concentration of commensal flora (oral mucosa, genitals, armpits)	high risk
Poorly vascularised (hand, foot, lower and upper limb)	high risk

- 2B. Consider antibiotic administration when one or two high risk variables are present.
- 2C. If the decision to avoid antibiotic administration in high risk wounds is made the reason must always be clearly stated.
- 2D. In every wound consider the risk of tetanus according to the patient's immunization status.

STATEMENT 3
Antibiotic prophylaxis (i.e., a preventive administration of an antibiotic before the emergence of an infection with the aim to prevent it). It is desirable to implement prophylactic antibiotics in selected cases of wounds at high risk of infection.
- 3A. Avoid antibiotic prophylaxis in a not macroscopically contaminated wound, well vascularized, at low risk of infection (according to statements 2).
- 3B. Antibiotic prophylaxis should be considered in grossly contaminated wounds and in cases at high risk of infection (according to statement 2) depending on the epidemiological criteria of antibiotic resistance in the area. In high risk wounds (all three variables considered) the EP should explain clearly the reason for avoiding the antibiotic administration [14–19].

STATEMENT 4
The assessment of tetanus immunization status in every traumatic wounded patient who arrive in the ED is desirable.

Table 4 Infection risk assessment based on the characteristics of the patient

Child	low risk
Young	low risk
Adult	low risk
Elderly (>65 years)	high risk
Immunocompromised (treated with steroids, immunosuppressive agents, splenectomised, HIV ...)	high risk
Vascular disease	high risk
Diabetic	high risk

- 5A. All traumatic wounds are potentially at risk for tetanus infection
- 5B. The assessment of tetanus immunization status of patients should be performed through a thorough history and consultation of documentation confirming vaccination/booster, and eventually using a diagnostic quick test in doubtful cases.
- 5C. The following items should be considered as "doubtful" (i.e., cases for which it is not possible to determine the immunization status of the patient):
  a. Patient who does not remember the date of the last booster;
  b. Patient unconscious, intoxicated or cognitively impaired;
  c. Patient who does not understand your language;
  d. Patient who, presumably, has never carried out a complete vaccination course.
- 5D. Access to vaccination data and the availability of a rapid diagnostic test for assessing the status of tetanus immunization permit to streamline costs and to act with greater appropriateness [20–23].

STATEMENT 5

It is desirable that in any ED is available the first administration of rabies vaccine (for at least two patients). Doses sufficient for full courses of rabies immunoglobulin treatment for two patients should be available in Poison Control Centers and in 2nd level EDs (at least 1 for every 5 million inhabitants and at least 1 in each major island) [24, 25].

STATEMENT 6

It is desirable a proper and timely implementation of procedures and methods for preventing infection in any traumatic wound. The identified methods of preventing infection are the following:

- 6A. Irrigation using appropriate security safeguards. Irrigation can be performed with saline (or tap water), with high pressure if necessary, according to the degree of contamination of the wound and the anatomic location.
- 6B. Search for foreign bodies. Beside an accurate visual inspection, X-rays, CT or ultrasound examination should be taken into consideration.
- 6C. Suture technique
  ✓ Avoid shaving of hair
  ✓ With simple stitches, always after irrigation
  ✓ The intradermal suture should be avoided in most cases
  ✓ If the risk of infection is high suture may be delayed [26–28].

STATEMENT 7

All the wounds of the hand should be carefully evaluated, considering them at high risk of error.

- 7A. Any traumatic injury of the hand should be considered for a possible tendon injury, especially if located on the volar or dorsal side.
- 7B. Any traumatic injury of the hand should be considered for a nerve injury, especially if located on the lateral side of the fingers
- 7C. A physical examination should be performed in any traumatic injury of the hand to check for any eventual tendon or nerve damage before performing the anaesthesia.
- 7D. In every traumatic injury of the hand treated in the emergency department the possibility of performing a follow-up should be considered [29–38].

STATEMENT 8

It is a priority to treat pain in traumatic wounds in all patients who attend to the ED. Several different protocols for the pain management are available, both pharmacological and non-pharmacological. Oral, local, intravenous, intra-nasal, and respiratory way (i.e., nitrous oxide) may be taken into consideration [39].

Conclusions

We consider our work as a starting point and networking opportunity for participation in the forthcoming call funding programs in health care. In addition, the shared document (position paper), validated during the workshop with the precious contribution of international experts, intends to contribute to policy and health priorities in the European and international areas.

Appendix

Writing committee members: Francesca Venturi Visconti, Rome; Massimo Pesenti Campagnoni, Aosta; Ivo Casagranda, Alessandria; Pierdante Piccioni, Codogno; Daniele Coen, Milan; Massimo Crapis, Udine; Andrea Rocchetti, Alessandria; Egidio Barbi, Trieste; Augusto Tricerri, Rome; Libero Barozzi, Bologna; Fabio Brunato, Padova; Mario Cavazza, Bologna; Marco Ricca, Cuneo; Massimo Rega, Cuneo; Pasquale Picciano, Jesolo; Stefano M. Calderale, Rome; Alberto Albani, Rome; Donatella Del Gaizo, Neaples; Andrea Drei, Faenza; Fabrizio Giostra, fermo; Franco Laterza, San Donà di Piave; Luigi Zulli, Rome; Maria Giuliano, Neaples; Francesca Velluti, San Donà di Piave; Carlo Manfredi, Firenze; Maria Carolina Barbazza, San Donà di Piave.

External referees: Nikolaos K Paschos, Joannina, Greece; Miguel Angel Bratos, Valladolid, Spain; Federica Norat,

Nice, France; Fabio Toffoletto, San Donà di Piave, Italy; Rodolfo Sbrojavacca, Udine, Italy; Bruno Mégarbane, Paris, France; Biagio Epifani, Mirano, Italy; Camilla Negri, Gorizia, Italy; Matteo Pistorello, Montebelluna, Italy; Michael Espa, Lyon, France; Cavenaile Jean-Christophe, Bruxelles, Belgium; Primo Botti, Firenze, Italy; Paola De Benedictis, Legnaro, Italy; Roberta Aiello, Legnaro, Italy; Marta Mazzoleni, Pavia, Italy; Michele Alzetta, Venezia, Italy; Michele Mitaritonno, Parma, Italy; Arianna Fede Catania, San Donà di. Piave, Italy; Antonella Tonetto, San Donà di. Piave, Italy; Farhadullah Khan, San Donà di. Piave, Italy; Buffolo Gabriella, San Donà di. Piave, Italy; Flavia Gandin, Udine, Italy; Maria Rita Laera, Alessandria, Italy; Cesare Montecucco, Padova, Italy; Lorenzo Calligaris, Trieste, Italy; Peter Heinz, Cambridge, UK; Tiziana Zangardi, Padova, Italy; Maria Paola Saggese, Brescia, Italy; Mario Saia, Venice, Italy; Fabio De Jaco, Imperia, Italy; Francesco Prattico, Verona, Italy; Roberto Lerza, Savona, Italy; Guido Grazie, Savona, Italy; Liviana Da Dalt, Padova, Italy; Almerto De Mas, Pordenone, Italy.

Acknowledgments
The work has been made possible with the contribution of the "Progetto Mattone Internazionale" of the Italian Ministry of Health.

Authors' contribution
CP[1] conceived the study, partecipated in its design and coordination and drafted the manuscrip, CP[2] partecipated in the organization of process and the coordination of the panellists, CL participated in the organization of process and was involved in tetanus and rabies infections statements, GR participated in the organization of the process of external revision of the position paper, FC partecipated in the design of the study, LA partecipated in the design of the study, GC participated in the organization of the process and the drafting of the manuscript. All the authors read and approved the final manuscript.

Competing interests
The authors declare that they have no competing interests.

Author details
[1]Emergency Department, Hospital of San Donà di Piave VE, Parma, Italy. [2]Emergency Department, Academic Hospital of Udine, Parma, Italy. [3]Institute of Toxicology, IRCCS Fondazione Maugeri Pavia, Parma, Italy. [4]Emergency Deparment, Academic Hospital of Verona, Parma, Italy. [5]Emergency Surgery, Academic Hospital of Parma, Parma, Italy. [6]Emergency surgery, Hospital of Bergamo, Parma, Italy. [7]Emergency Department, Academic Hospital of Parma, Parma, Italy.

References
1. Hollander JE, Singer AJ. State of the art laceration management. Ann Emerg Med. 1999;34:356–67.
2. Singer AJ, Hollander JE, Quinn JV. Evaluation and management of traumatic lacerations. N Engl J Med. 1997;337:1142–8.
3. Kung J, et al. Failure of clinical practice guidelines to meet Institute of medicine standards. Two more decades of little, if any, progress. Arch Intern Med. 2012;172:1628–33.
4. Shaneyfekt T. In guidelines we cannot trust. Comment on "failure of clinical practice guidelines to meet Institute of Medicine Standards". Arch Intern Med. 2012;172:1633–4.
5. Rowe G, Wright G. The Delphi technique as a forecasting tool: issues and analysis. Intern J Forecast. 1999;15:353–75.
6. Rowe G, Wright G. Expert opinions in forecasting. Role of the Delphi Technique. In: Armstrong, editor. Principles of forecasting: a handbook of researchers and practitioners. Boston: Kluwer Academic Publishers; 2001.
7. Dalkey N, Helmer O. An Experimental Application of the Delphi Method to the use of experts. Manag Sci. 1963;9:458–67.
8. Linstone HA, Turoff M. The Delphi method: techniques and applicationshttp://is.njit.edu/pubs/delphibook/.
9. Edlich RF, Rodeheaver GT, Thacker JG, et al. Revolutionary advances in the management of traumatic wounds in the emergency department during the last 40 years: Part I. J Emerg Med. 2010;38:40–50.
10. Edlich RF, Rodeheaver GT, Thacker JG, et al. Revolutionary advances in the management of traumatic wounds in the emergency department during the last 40 years: Part II. J Emerg Med. 2010;38:201–7.
11. Quinn JV, Polevoi SK, Kohn MA. Traumatic lacerations: what are the risks for infection and has the 'golden period' of laceration care disappeared? Emerg Med J. 2014;31:96–100.
12. Heggers JP. Assessing and controlling wound infection. Clin Plast Surg. 2003;30:25–35.
13. Lazarus GS, Zenilman GM. Wound microbiology: tabula rosa, a blank slate. Wound Rep Reg. 2011;19:531.
14. Shaw TJ, Martin P. Wound repair at a glance. J Cell Science. 2014;122:3209–13.
15. Hollander JE, Singer AJ, Valentine SM, et al. Risk factors for infection in patients with traumatic lacerations. Acad Emerg Med. 2001;8:716–20.
16. Garcia-Gubern CF, Colon-Rolon L, Bond MC. Essential concepts of wounds management. Emerg Med N Am. 2010;28:951–67.
17. Caldwell MD. Wound surgery. Surg Clin N Am. 2010;90:1125–32.
18. Cooke J. When antibiotics can be avoided in skin inflammation and bacterial colonization: a review of topical treatments. Cur Opin Infect Dis. 2014;27:125–9.
19. Zehtabchi S. The impact of wound age on the infection rate of simple lacerations repaired in the emergency department. Injury. 2012;43:1793–8.
20. Abbate R, Angelillo IF. Appropriate tetanus prophylaxis practices in patients attending Emergency Departments in Italy. Vaccines. 2008;26:3634–9.
21. Talan DA, Abrahamian FM, Moran GJ, et al. Tetanus immunity and physician compliance with tetanus prophylaxis practices among emergency department patients presenting with wounds. Ann Emerg Med. 2004;43:305–14.
22. Elkharrat D, Espinoza P, De la Coussaye J, et al. Inclusion of a rapid test in the current Health Ministry Guidelines with the purpose of improving anti-tetanus prophylaxis prescribed to wounded patients presenting at French Emergency Departments. Med Mal Infect. 2005;35:323–8.
23. Stubbe M, Mortelmans LJ, Desruelles D, et al. Improving tetanus prophylaxis in the emergency department: a prospective, double-blind cost-effectiveness study. Emerg Med J. 2007;24:648–53.
24. Singer AJ, Dagum AB. Current management of acute cutaneous wounds. N Engl J Med. 2008;359:1037–46.
25. Weiss EA, Oldham G, Lin M, et al. Water is a safe and effective alternative to sterile normal saline for wound irrigation prior to suturing: a prospective, double-blind, randomised, controlled clinical trial. BMJ Open. 2013;3: e5001504.
26. Perelman VS, Francis GJ, Rutledge T, et al. Sterile versus nonsterile gloves for repair of uncomplicated lacerations in the emergency department: a randomized controlled trial. Ann Emerg Med. 2004;43:362–70.
27. ACEP. Clinical policy Clinical policy for the initial approach to patients presenting with penetrating extremity trauma. Ann Emerg Med. 1999;33: 612–36.
28. Amirtharajah M, Lattanza L. Open extensor tendon injuries. J Hand Surg [Am]. 2015;40:391–7.
29. Chauhan A, Palmer BA, Merrell GA. Flexor tendon repairs: techniques, eponyms, and evidence. J Hand Surg [Am]. 2014;39:1846–53.
30. Raval P, Khan W, Haddad B, et al. Bite injuries to the hand - review of the literature. Open Orthop J. 2014;8:204–8.
31. Mehling IM, Arsalan-Werner A, Sauerbier M. Evidence-based flexor tendon repair. Clin Plast Surg. 2014;41:513–23.
32. Rrecaj S, Martinaj M, Murtezani A, et al. Physical therapy and splinting after flexor tendon repair in zone II. Med Arch. 2014;68:128–31.
33. Neumeister MW, Amalfi A, Neumeister E. Evidence-based medicine: flexor tendon repair. Plast Reconstr Surg. 2014;133:1222–33.
34. Melamed E, Polatsch D. Partial lacerations of peripheral nerves. J Hand Surg [Am]. 2014;39:1201–3.

19

Analysis of the correlation between blood glucose level and prognosis in patients younger than 18 years of age who had head trauma

Bahadir Danisman[1], Muhittin Serkan Yilmaz[2], Bahattin Isik[1], Cemil Kavalci[3*], Cihat Yel[2], Alper Gorkem Solakoglu[2], Burak Demirci[2], Selim Inan[2] and M Evvah Karakilic[1]

Abstract

Objective: To analyze the correlation between early-term blood glucose level and prognosis in patients with isolated head trauma.

Methods: This study included a total of 100 patients younger than 18 years of age who had isolated head trauma. The admission blood glucose levels of these patients were measured. Age at the time of the incident, sex, mode of occurrence of the trauma, computed tomography findings, and GCSs were recorded. Kruskall Wallis test was used compare of groups. A p value less than 0.05 was considered statistically significant.

Results: The median age of the study population was 7 years and the median GCS was 11. There was a significant negative correlation between blood glucose level and GCS (p < 0.05). A significant correlation in the negative direction was observed between GCS and blood glucose level (r = −0.658, p < 0.05). Seventy-seven percent of the patients were admitted to hospital, while 6% died in ED.

Conclusion: The results of the present study suggest that hyperglycemia at an early stage and a low GCS may be reliable predictors of the severity of head trauma and prognosis. A higher blood glucose level may be an ominous sign that predicts a poor prognosis and an increased risk of death.

Keywords: Head trauma, Blood glucose, GCS

Introduction

Head trauma is common after general body trauma and requires a multidisciplinary approach. It is a severe health problem with long-term rehabilitation of sequel [1]. With an annual mortality rate of about 200/100000, it ranks third among the most common causes of mortality and morbidity in children [2]. The mortality rate of head trauma may goes up to 20-35% [3,4].

Mortality and morbidity of head trauma may be due to the direct injury produced by the trauma itself on the one side, and due to ischemia and hypoxia secondary to head trauma on the other [2]. These effects include traumatic ischemia, infarction, cardiorespiratory dysfunction, secondary hemorrhages, diffuse cerebral edema, and hypoxic ischemia mediated by neuromediators released by body in response to trauma [4]. In addition, it should also be kept in mind that brain injury secondary to head trauma may lead to impaired systemic hemostasis and organ dysfunction.

Blood glucose possesses all properties of an ideal serum marker of systemic injury. It is highly sensitive for cerebral cellular injury secondary to head trauma. Although the pathophysiology of hyperglycemia's neuropathic effect is not entirely clear, it has been reported that it aggravates ischemic acidosis, which in turn worsens brain edema [5,6]. Cochran reported that blood glucose levels more than 300 mg/dl is associated with dead [5].

This study aimed to assess the relationship between early-term blood glucose level and prognosis in patients younger than 18 years of age who were admitted to our emergency department after head trauma.

* Correspondence: cemkavalci@yahoo.com
[3]Emergency Department, Baskent University Faculty of Medicine, Ankara, Turkey
Full list of author information is available at the end of the article

Materials and method

This study was approved by the local ethics committee and performed prospectively at Dışkapı Yıldırım Beyazıt Training and Research Hospital, Department of Emergency Medicine between 01.01.2010-01.01.2011. Written informed consent was obtained from the patient's guardian/parent/next of kin for the publication of this report and any accompanying images. It included 100 patients younger than 18 years of age who presented with isolated head trauma and who met the study inclusion criteria (Table 1).

Age at the time of the incident, sex, Glasgow Coma Scale (GCS) at the time of admission, findings of computed tomography (CT), trauma mechanism, and blood glucose levels were recorded.

The study data were analyzed using the SPSS 13.00 for Windows software package. The descriptive statistics included percentage, number, and median values. Data distribution was tested with the Kolmogorov Smirnov test. Inter-group comparisons were carried out using the Kruskall Wallis test. A p value less than 0.05 was considered statistically significant.

Results

The median age of the study population was 7 [2-16] years, with 67% of the study population being male (Table 2). The most common causes of isolated head trauma were out-of-vehicle traffic accident (37%) and falls (30%). The median GCS level was 11 [3-15] (Table 3). Head trauma was severe in 23 patients, moderate in 29, and mild in 48. CT examination most commonly demonstrated combined findings (52%), with brain edema being the most common isolated finding (25%). Seventeen percent of the cases were discharged after emergency care while 77% of them were hospitalized and 6% died during ED stay (Table 4).

The median blood glucose level was 177 mg/dl in 23 patients with severe head trauma. The median blood glucose levels by trauma severity were summarized on Table 3. Different trauma severities significantly differed with respect to blood glucose levels. A significant negative correlation was detected between GCS and blood glucose level (r = −0.658, p < 0.05).

Table 1 İnclusion/exclusion criteria

İnclusion criteria	Exclusion criteria
1- < 18 year old	1- > 18 year old
2-isolated head trauma	2-Multiple trauma
3- Admitted within 3 hours after trauma	3- Admitted 3 hours after trauma
	4-Admitted exitus patient
	5- Patients with a GCS of 15 and normal CT findings

Table 2 Distribution of patients characteristics according to groups

Variable		Median (Min-Max)/n (%)
Age		7 (2-16)
Sex	Male	67 (67)
	Female	33 (33)
Trauma mechanism	Pedestrian	37 (37)
	Motor vehicle accident	26 (26)
	Falls	30 (30)
	Assault	7 (7)
GCS	Severe head trauma (GCS:3-8)	23 (23)
	Moderate head trauma (GCS:9-13)	29 (29)
	Mild head trauma (GCS:14-15)	48 (48)
CT findings	Brain edema	25 (25)
	Hematoma	14 (14)
	Linear fracture	6 (6)
	Contusion	3 (%3)
	Combined CT findings	52 (%52)
Outcome of patients	Discharge	17 (%17)
	Hospitalization	77 (%77)
	Exitus	6 (%6)

n:total number of the patient (Combined CT findings: Linear fracture and brain edema, linear fracture and epidural hematoma, etc...).
GCS: Glasgow Coma Scale.

Discussion

Head trauma is the most common type of pediatric traumas, and it is considered the leading cause of death between 1–15 years of age [7-10]. The acute stage of severe head trauma is generally characterized by a systemic stress response [10].

Many studies have reported that traffic accidents are the main cause of childhood head traumas [11-13]. Kavalci et al. [14,15] and Durdu et al. [16] reported that the most common trauma mechanism was motor vehicle accident. Our study also found that out-of-vehicle traffic accident was the most common cause of head trauma. Traffic accidents lead to a more destructive process since they apply high energies on the victims.

Murgio et al. reported that 56.4% of the patients had mild head trauma, 38.9% had moderate head trauma, and 4.7% had severe head trauma [17]. Işık et al. reported that 74% of traumas were mild, 22% were

Table 3 The relationship between trauma severity and hyperglycemia

	n	Glucose (Median (min;max))	p
Severe head trauma	23	177 (98-324)	
Moderate head trauma	29	138 (92-244)	p<0.05
Mild head trauma	48	115 (68-180)	

Table 4 The relationship between patient results and hyperglycemia

	N	Glucose (Median (min;max))	p
Discharge	17	103 (68-145)	
Hospitalization	77	118 (86-154)	p<0.05
Exitus	6	233 (148-324)	

moderate, and 4% were severe [8]. A majority of our cases similarly had mild head trauma. However, the rate of severe head trauma in our study was also higher than previous studies. We suggest that this difference may be due to injury by high-energy accidents.

Rovlias et al. reported that patients with head trauma whose blood glucose level was more than 200 mg/dl within 24 hours had worse prognosis [18]. The authors linked this finding to a series of reactions including hyperglycemia following cerebral ischemia [18]. It has also been demonstrated that hyperglycemia in the course of traumatic brain injury adversely affects oxygenation [19]. It has been advocated that, in addition to severity of trauma itself, biochemical and vital parameters should also be taken into account when predicting the severity of head trauma [20]. GCS provides clinicians with very valuable information for predicting head trauma severity. Nevertheless, GCS may also fail in many circumstances. It should be remembered that blood glucose level and vital signs at the acute stage may be good predictors of patient outcomes when GCS is considered insufficient. Furthermore, it looks promising to predict future neurological injury with the help of high blood glucose levels and poor vital signs in patients with normal imaging tests such as CT.

Rovlias et al. [18], in a study with 267 patients with head trauma and a GCS of 3–13, demonstrated that clinical course was worse in patients with a blood glucose level greater than 200 mg/dl. Chiaretti et al. [20] reported that 87.5% of cases with head trauma and a GCS below 8 had a high blood glucose level. Merguerian et al. [21] found a mean blood glucose level of 270 mg/dl in 19 deeply comatose patients with severe head trauma who had a GCS of 3. They also found that all patients with hyperglycemia and a low GCS were lost whereas patients with a low GCS but no hyperglycemia had a mortality rate of 17% on follow-up. Rengachary et al. suggested that blood glucose level elevation was a more potent predictor of clinical worsening than vital signs [22]. Although blood glucose level was closely related to cerebral injury in cases with a GCS of 8 or lower, it was not correlated to the severity of extracranial trauma [23]. Moreover, Babbitt et al. [24] showed that hyperglycemia was related to intracranial injury in younger children. Our study results revealed that the median glucose level was 177 mg/dl in the severe head trauma

group and 233 mg/dl in the patients who died. In addition, there was a negative correlation between blood glucose level and GCS. That is, GCS dropped as blood glucose level increased. Our blood glucose levels have been lower than those reported in previous studies since we drew blood samples within three hours of admission. In agreement with the literature, our study demonstrated a parallel worsening in brain injury with elevating blood glucose level. Hyperglycemia may increase mortality by augmenting brain edema and hypoxia.

Movery et al. reported that blood glucose level increased in proportional to trauma severity. Nevertheless, the authors stated glucose level was not the sole determinant of mortality in clinical practice [25]. Cochran et al. found a significantly higher glucose level in patients with an elevated mortality rate and added that hyperglycemia was closely related to mortality [5]. Similar to Cochran's results, our study demonstrated a significant correlation between mortality and hyperglycemia. This result suggests that hyperglycemia may be an important marker for predicting mortality risk.

Conclusion

In conclusion, the results of this study supports the notion that in patients with head trauma and a low GCS hyperglycemia at an early stage after head trauma may be a reliable marker of cerebral injury and patient prognosis. An elevated blood glucose level may suggest that a patient's prognosis is likely poor and the risk of dying is substantially high.

Competing interests
The authors declare that they have no competing interests.

Authors' contributions
BD, MSY, BI: Article writing, data collection. CK,MEK,CY: Article writing, data collection, statistic analysis. CK: Supervisor of article writing. BD,SI,AGS: Data collection. All authors read and approved the final manuscript.

Author details
[1]Emergency Department, Dıskapi Yıldırım Beyazit Training and Research Hospital, Ankara, Turkey. [2]Emergency Department, Numune Training and Research Hospital, Ankara, Turkey. [3]Emergency Department, Baskent University Faculty of Medicine, Ankara, Turkey.

References
1. Schouten JW, Maas AIR. Epidemiology of traumatic brain injury. In: Bullock MR, Hovda DA, editors. Youmans Neurological Surgery. Volume 4. 6th ed. Philadelphia: Elsevier Saunders; 2011. p. 3270–6.
2. Şahin S, Doğan Ş, Aksoy K. Çocukluk Çağı Kafa Travmaları. Uludağ Ün Tıp Fak Derg. 2002;28:45–51.
3. Işık HS, Bostancı U, Yıldız Ö, Özdemir C, Gökyar A. Retrospective analysis of 954 adult patients with head injury: an epidemiological study. Ulus Travma Acil Cerrahi Derg. 2011;17:46–50.
4. Kihtir T, Kihtir S. Travma tedavi sistemleri. In: Ertekin C, Taviloğlu K, Güloğlu R, Kurtoğlu M, editors. Travma. Ith ed. İstanbul: İstanbul Medikal Yayıncılık; 2005. p. s.65–71.
5. Cochran A, Scaife ER, Hansen KW, Downey EC. Hyperglycemia and outcomes from pediatric traumatic brain injury. J Trauma. 2003;55:1035–8.

6.   Rostami E. Glucose and the injured brain-monitored in the neurointensive care unit. Front Neurol. 2014;5:91.

7.   Geyik AM, Dokur M. Minor head trauma in children. Türk Nöroşir Derg. 2013;23:117–23.

8.   Tuna İC, Akpınar AA, Kozacı N. Demographic analysis of pediatric patients admitted to Emergency Departments with head trauma. JAEM. 2012;11:151–6.

9.   Işık HS, Gökyar A, Yıldız Ö, Bostancı U, Özdemir C. Pediatric head injuries, retrospective analysis of 851 patients: an epidemiological study. Ulus Travma Acil Cerrahi Derg. 2011;17:166–72.

10. Yang SY, Zhang S, Wang ML. Clinical significance of admission hyperglycemia and factors related to it in patients with acute severe head injury. Surg Neurol. 1995;44:373–7.

11. Chinda JY, Abubakar AM, Umaru H, Tahir C, Adamu S, Wabada S. Epidemiology and management of head injury in paediatric age group in North-Eastern Nigeria. Afr J Paediatr Surg. 2013;10:358–61.

12. Cooper A, Barlow B, DiScala C, String D. Mortalty and truncal injury: pediatric perpective. J Pediatric Surg. 1994;29:33–8.

13. Çırak B, Berker M, Özcan OE, Özgen T. An epidemiologic study of head trauma: causes and results of treatment. Ulusal Travma Derg. 1999;5:90–2.

14. Kavalci C, Akdur G, Yemenici S, Sayhan MB. The value of serum BNP for the diagnosis of intracranial injury in head trauma. Tr J Emerg Med. 2012;12:112–6.

15. Kavalci C, Aksel G, Salt O, Yilmaz MS, Demir A, Kavalci G, et al. "Comparison of the Canadian CT head rule and the New Orleans criteria in patients with minor head injury". World J Emerg Surg. 2014;9:31. doi:10.1186/1749-7922-9-31.

16. Durdu T, Kavalci C, Yilmaz MS, Karakilic ME, Arslan ED, Ceyhan ME. Analysis of Trauma Cases Admitted to the Emergency Department. J Clin Anal Med. 2013. doi: 10.4328/JCAM.1279.

17. Murgio A, Andrade FA, Sanchez Munoz MA, Boetto S, Leung KM. International multicenter study of head injury in children. ISHIP group. Childs Nerv Syst. 1999;15:318–21.

18. Rovlias A, Kotsou S. The influence of hyperglycemia on neurological outcome in patients with severe head injury. Neurosurgery. 2000;46:335–42.

19. Young B, Ott L, Dempsey R, Haack D, Tibbs P. Relationship between admission hyperglycemia and neurologic outcome of severely brain-injured patients. Ann Surg. 1989;210:466–72.

20. Chiaretti A, De Benedictis R, Langer A, DiRocco C, Bizzarri C, Iannelli A, et al. Prognostic implications of hyperglycemia in paediatric head injury. Childs Nerv Syst. 1998;14:455–9.

21. Merguerian PA, Perel A, Wald U, Feinsod M, Cotev S. Persistent nonketotic hyperglycemia as a grave prognostic sign in head-injured patients. Crit Care Med. 1981;9:838–40.

22. Rengachary SS, Carey M, Templer J. The sinking bullet. Neurosurg. 1992;30:294–5.

23. Yamashima T, Friede RL. Why do briding veins rupture in to the virtual subdural space? Neurol Neurosurg Psychiatry. 1984;47:121.

24. Babbitt CJ, Halpern R, Liao E, Lai K. Hyperglycemia is associated with intracranial injury in children younger than 3 years of age. Pediatr Emerg Care. 2013;29:279–82.

25. Mowery NT, Gunter OL, Guillamondegui O, Dossett LA, Dortch MJ, Morris Jr JA, et al. Stress insulin resistance is a marker for mortality in traumatic brain injury. J Trauma. 2009;66(1):145–51.

20

Evaluation of clotting factor activities early after severe multiple trauma and their correlation with coagulation tests and clinical data

Manuel Burggraf[1*], Arzu Payas[1], Max Daniel Kauther[1], Carsten Schoeneberg[2] and Sven Lendemans[2]

Abstract

Introduction: Traumatic injuries are amongst the leading causes of death worldwide, frequently as a result of uncontrolled hemorrhage. Critical deficiencies in clotting factors have been noted in trauma-induced coagulopathy. However, the exact underlying conditions that result in devastating coagulopathies remain unclear. The purpose of this study was to elucidate these underlying deficiencies.

Methods: Blood samples were drawn from 45 severely injured trauma patients on their arrival at the resuscitation room, and the activities of all soluble clotting factors and routine coagulation tests were assessed. The Mann–Whitney-U-test was used to assess differences in coagulation activity between the patients and healthy controls. Furthermore, Spearman's rank correlation was used to analyze the blood work.

Results: After severe trauma the levels of serum fibrinogen and calcium were significantly reduced. Furthermore, traumatized patients had a significantly increased International Normalized Ratio (INR) compared to healthy controls. The median activities of all clotting factors were reduced after severe multiple trauma, with the exception of factor VIII, which was increased. Statistically significant differences were observed for factors II (80 vs. 122 %, $P < 0.0001$), V (76 vs. 123 %, $P < 0.0001$), VII (90 vs. 114 %, $P = 0.002$), VIII (200 vs. 108 %, $P < 0.0001$), and X (86 vs. 122 %, $P < 0.0001$). Spearman's correlation indicated a significant negative correlation between INR on arrival with fibrinogen and levels of factors II, V, and VII, whereas Partial Thromboplastin Time was significantly negatively correlated with factor VIII (all $P < 0.0001$).

Conclusions: These findings suggest a general but rather moderate impairment of clotting factor activities following severe multiple trauma. In the concept of a calculated coagulation therapy, this could demand for the use of factor concentrates with higher ratios of clotting factors. Finally, the physiological importance of strongly elevated factor VIII activity remains unclear, but a possible interference with *ex vivo* measurements of Partial Thromboplastin Time has to be considered.

Keywords: Severe multiple trauma, Injury, Coagulation, Coagulopathy, Clotting factor, Coagulation factor, International normalized ratio, Partial thromboplastin time

Introduction

Traumatic injuries account for more than 5 million deaths annually and are among the leading causes of death worldwide [1]. As many as 40 % of all mortalities after severe multiple trauma are related to uncontrolled hemorrhage [2, 3]. Several studies have reported a high incidence of coagulopathy on admission to the emergency department, and in this patient subgroup, mortality is increased by up to 4-fold compared to patients without coagulation abnormalities [4–8]. In fact, hemorrhage is the most common preventable cause of death after severe trauma and might be controlled by early aggressive therapy, either by surgery or correction of coagulopathy [9].

Brohi et al. demonstrated that systemic hypoperfusion in conjunction with tissue damage leads to widespread activation of activated protein C and liberation of tissue

* Correspondence: manuel.burggraf@uk-essen.de
[1]Department for Orthopaedics and Emergency Surgery, University Hospital Essen, University Duisburg-Essen, Hufelandstr. 55, 45147 Essen, Germany
Full list of author information is available at the end of the article

plasminogen activator, potentially causing systemic anticoagulation and hyperfibrinolysis [10, 11]. Hypothermia and acidemia further provoke the development of these clotting disorders [12–14]. Additionally, dilution and consumption of clotting factors may also significantly worsen bleeding disorders in major trauma patients [7]. However, little is known about the actual underlying clotting factor activities after severe injury. Early studies have generally focused on post-transfusional dysfunction at a later phase of the disorder and have described only a small subset of coagulation factors [15–18]. Recent studies from Rizoli et al. and Cohen et al. investigated a broader panel of clotting factors and indeed reported a significant correlation between clotting factor deficiencies and transfusion requirements [19, 20]. However, inclusion criteria aimed at coagulopathic subgroups of patients, either by selecting patients with highly reduced clotting factor activity (<30 %) or those with demonstrated transfusion requirements (at least one unit of red blood cells). It therefore remains unclear to what extent clotting factor deficiencies may generally exist in multiple trauma patients irrespective of the further course.

For this study we investigated the potential derangements of all soluble clotting factor activities early after serious injury and discuss if these changes could be estimated by standard coagulation tests.

Methods
Patients and normal donors
Adult patients were screened for enrollment if they were admitted directly from the scene of an accident to the trauma resuscitation room of our institution (Level 1 academic trauma center in Germany). Only severely injured patients with an Injury Severity Score (ISS) of at least 16 points were included. The study was performed in accordance with the Declaration of Helsinki and approved by the relevant local ethics committee (reference 12-5120-BO). Participants provided written informed consent. Pregnant women and patients known to have congenital coagulopathies or who were on anticoagulant medications were excluded. Ten healthy adult donors served as the control group.

Blood samples
Directly after admission to the resuscitation room, blood samples were drawn from the femoral artery. In addition to routinely collected blood samples, an additional citrate syringe was obtained to assess clotting factor activity. In healthy controls, blood was drawn from a cubital vein. Immediately after collection, blood samples were transferred to the hospital laboratory, and standard coagulation tests for International Normalized Ratio (INR), Partial Thromboplastin Time (PTT), fibrinogen, and calcium were performed. In addition, the activities of clotting factors II, V, VII, VIII, IX, X, XI, XII, and XIII were analyzed. Analysis was performed by comparing samples to standard human plasma assays of clotting factors (SHP, Dade Behring Marburg GmbH, Marburg, Germany). The results were expressed as a percentage of standard activity. If immediate testing of clotting factor activity was not possible, e.g., during off-duty hours, specimens were cryo-stored at −70 °C until the final analysis could be performed the following weekday. Storage of frozen plasma samples is widely accepted and has not been specifically shown to interfere with clotting factor activity [21].

Statistical analysis
Demographic data is reported as mean and standard deviation (SD) when applicable, while results are reported as median values. Differences between demographic data for the study groups were analyzed by t-test (age) or Fisher's exact test (gender). Differences in clotting factor activity among patients and healthy controls were tested using the Mann–Whitney-U-test. Differences in INR, PTT, serum fibrinogen, and calcium among study groups were tested in the same manner. In a second step, Spearman's rank correlation coefficient, rho (ρ), was calculated for traumatized patients by analyzing the results of routine coagulation tests as well as clinical data and clotting factor activity assessments. The 95 % confidence interval (CI) was computed by bootstrapping using a *bias-corrected and accelerated method* based on 1000 bootstrap samples. The correlation was considered negligible for absolute values of ρ between 0.0 and 0.2, weak between 0.21 and 0.4, moderate between 0.41 and 0.7, strong between 0.71 and 0.9, and very strong between 0.91 and 1. A P value smaller than 0.05 (2-tailed) was considered statistically significant for all tests. Data analysis was strictly exploratory. There was no correction for multiple testing. Data were analyzed and graphs were produced using IBM® SPSS® Statistics, Version 20 (Release 20.0.0).

All authors had access to primary clinical data.

Results
Demographic data
A total of 92 patients were enrolled in this study. A total of 45 (49 %) fully met the inclusion criteria for analysis

Table 1 Demographic characteristics of the study population

Characteristics	Patients ($n = 45$)	Healthy controls ($n = 10$)	P
Age; years ± SD	46 ± 19	40 ± 9	0.165
Gender; male (%)	36 (80 %)	7 (70 %)	0.673
ISS; points ± SD	31 ± 9	n/a	n/a
Mechanism; blunt (%)	43 (96 %)	n/a	n/a
Mortality; n (%)	12 (27 %)	n/a	n/a

n/a not applicable

Table 2 Clinical data of the patient group

SBP (prehospital)	SBP (admission)	Lactate	Base excess	Temperature	Hemoglobin	Thrombocytes
124 (±37) mmHg	128 (±25) mmHg	2.4 (±2.0) mmol/l	−3.1 (±4.4) mmol/l	35.7 (±1.1) °C	12.0 (±2.3) g/dl	202 (±55) / nl

Data reported as means (± standard deviation)
SBP systolic blood pressure, *C* celsius

and were included for testing against the healthy controls. Of the enrolled patients, 23 (25 %) were excluded from the study because the final evaluation revealed an ISS below 16, 11 (12 %) were too young, and 6 (6 %) were transferred from other hospitals. Three patients were on anticoagulant medication, and three had no history of trauma. One patient died within minutes of their admission. The baseline characteristics of the study groups are summarized in Table 1. The mean age of patients and healthy controls differed slightly but not significantly (46 years in the patient group and 40 years in the control group, $P = 0.165$). Overall, 80 % of patients and 70 % of healthy controls were male ($P = 0.673$). On average, patients were admitted to our hospital 56 ± 24 min after trauma. Further clinical data is given in Table 2 for the patient group.

Routine tests of coagulation
Figure 1 shows the results of the routine coagulation tests. On admission to the resuscitation room, the median levels of serum fibrinogen in trauma patients and

healthy controls were 230 mg/dL and 296 mg/dL, respectively ($P = 0.031$). Furthermore, traumatized patients had a significantly increased INR compared to the healthy controls (1.10 vs. 0.96, $P < 0.0001$). By contrast, there was no statistically significant difference in PTT between study groups, although there was a tendency toward slightly prolonged clotting time in controls (26.9 vs. 28.8 s, $P = 0.116$). Finally, serum calcium levels were significantly reduced following multiple injury (2.11 [n = 44] vs. 2.30 millimole per liter, $P < 0.0001$).

Influence of trauma on clotting factor activity
The median activities of all clotting factors were reduced after severe multiple trauma, with the exception of factor VIII, which was clearly increased. The results reached statistical significance for factors II (80 vs. 122 %, $P < 0.0001$), V (76 vs. 123 %, $P < 0.0001$), VII (90 vs. 114 %, $P = 0.002$), VIII (200 vs. 108 %, $P < 0.0001$) and X (86 vs. 122 %, $P < 0.0001$). Although not statistically significant, reductions in the median activity of factors IX (91 vs. 110 %, P = 0.141), XI (97 vs. 106 %, $P = 0.270$), XII

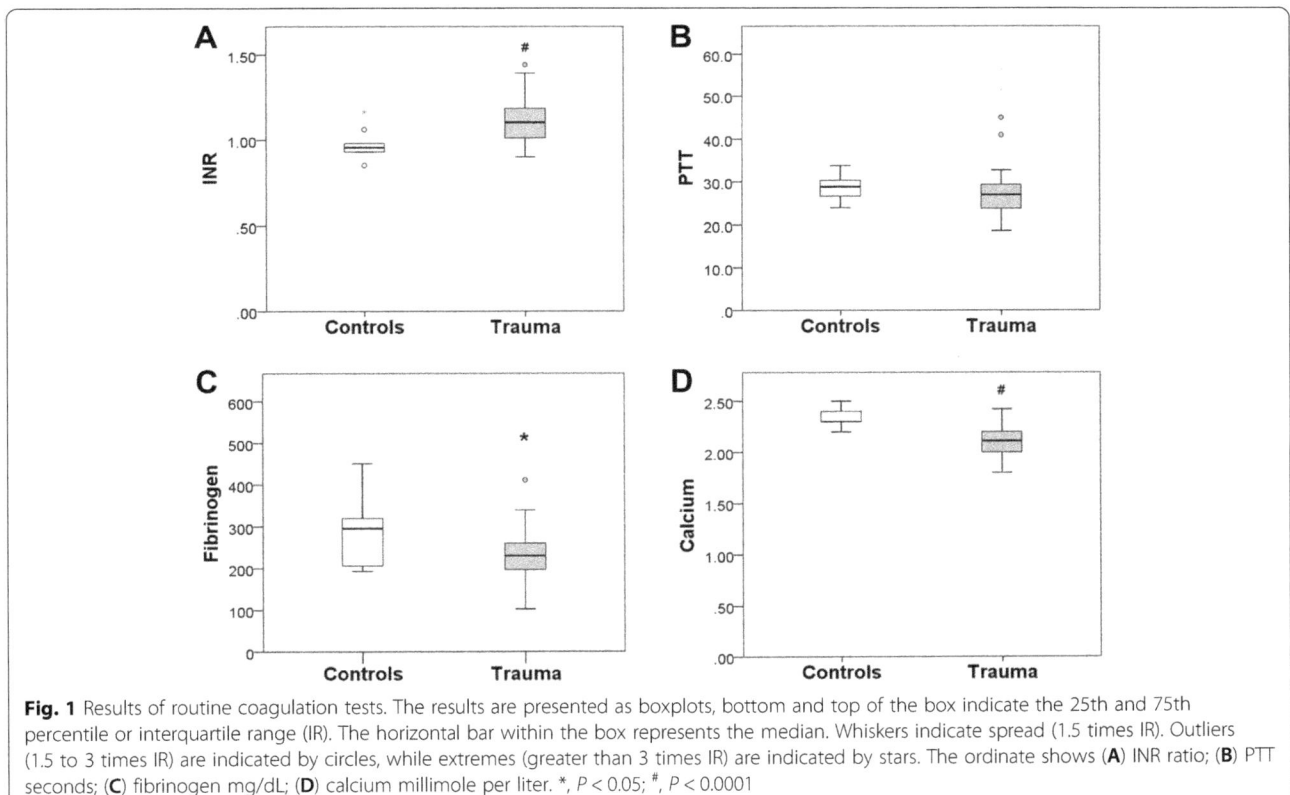

Fig. 1 Results of routine coagulation tests. The results are presented as boxplots, bottom and top of the box indicate the 25th and 75th percentile or interquartile range (IR). The horizontal bar within the box represents the median. Whiskers indicate spread (1.5 times IR). Outliers (1.5 to 3 times IR) are indicated by circles, while extremes (greater than 3 times IR) are indicated by stars. The ordinate shows (**A**) INR ratio; (**B**) PTT seconds; (**C**) fibrinogen mg/dL; (**D**) calcium millimole per liter. *, $P < 0.05$; #, $P < 0.0001$

(89 vs. 99 %, $P = 0.295$) and XIII (84 [n = 44] vs. 102 %, $P = 0.09$) were noted. Interestingly, factor VIII was the only variable, including routine coagulation tests, whose median was beyond the reference range of activity (70 – 150 % for this particular factor) set by the hospital laboratory. The results are presented in Fig. 2.

Correlation of clotting factor activity and tests of coagulation

For the patient group, Spearman's Rank Correlation Coefficient *Rho* (ρ) for routine coagulation tests and clotting factor activity was calculated and is given in Table 3 with associated confidence intervals (CI). A strong (negative) correlation was observed between INR on arrival with serum fibrinogen and factors II, V, and VII ($P < 0.0001$). Correlation with the remaining factors remained moderate ($P < 0.0001–0.005$), with the exception of factor VIII. As shown in Fig. 3, PTT was strongly negatively correlated with factor VIII ($P < 0.0001$).

Thus, PTT was the only variable with a relevant association with elevated factor VIII activity. PTT was also moderately correlated with factors II, V, IX, and XII ($P < 0.0001$). Levels of fibrinogen, also known as clotting factor I, were moderately correlated with levels of other factors, with the exception of factor XII ($P < 0.0001–0.004$), while calcium (factor IV) was barely associated with factors II, V, IX, XI, and XII ($P < 0.01$).

Correlation of clotting factor activity and clinical data

No strong correlation between clotting factor activities and the clinical data of the patients was found. Apart from this, whereas the hemoglobin level at admission showed a moderate correlation with all clotting factors but factor VII ($P < 0.0001–0.05$), the remaining clinical parameters correlated only sparsely and mostly not significant with the various coagulation factors. *Rho* (ρ) for correlation between clinical data and clotting factor activity is given in Table 4 with associated CI.

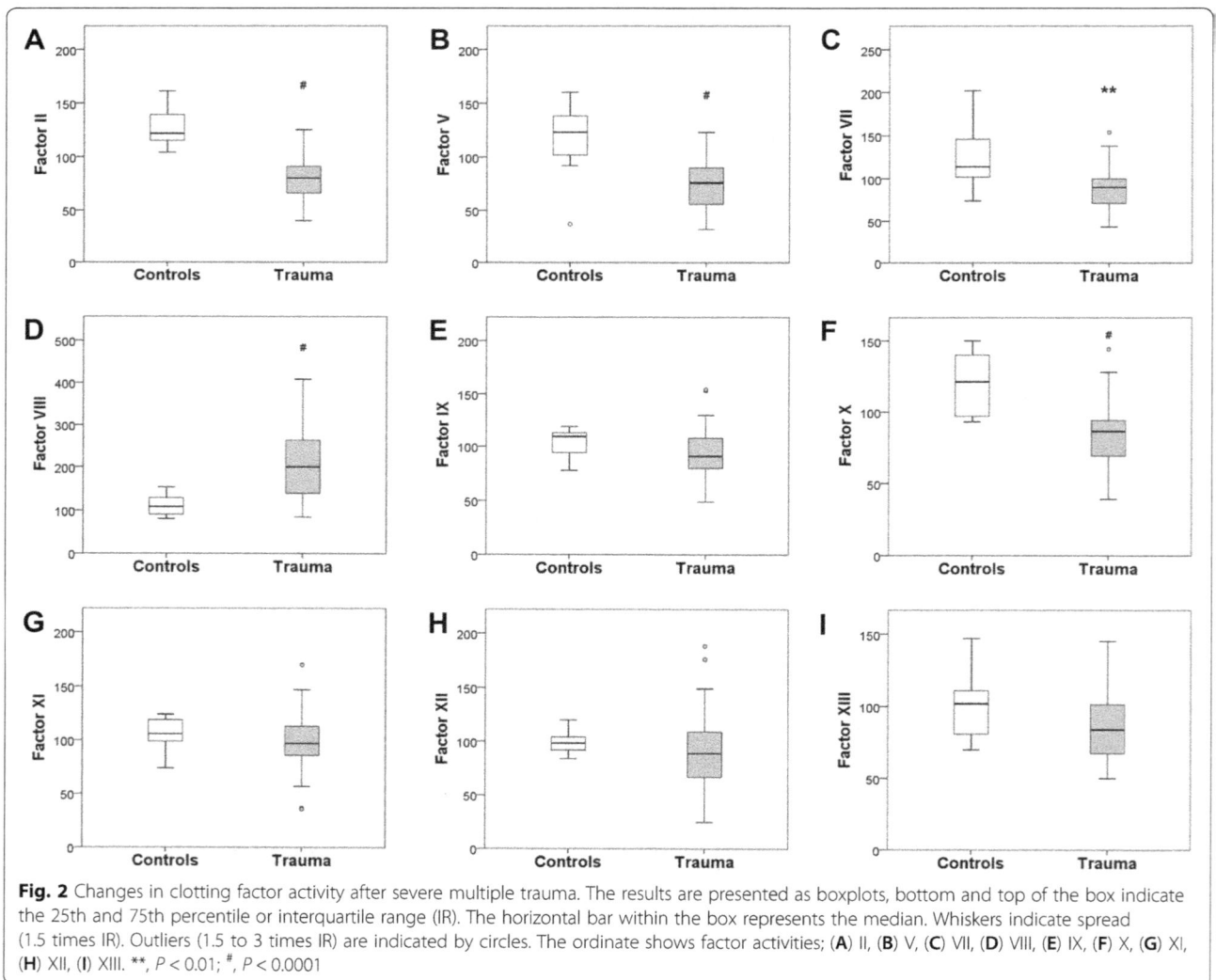

Fig. 2 Changes in clotting factor activity after severe multiple trauma. The results are presented as boxplots, bottom and top of the box indicate the 25th and 75th percentile or interquartile range (IR). The horizontal bar within the box represents the median. Whiskers indicate spread (1.5 times IR). Outliers (1.5 to 3 times IR) are indicated by circles. The ordinate shows factor activities; (**A**) II, (**B**) V, (**C**) VII, (**D**) VIII, (**E**) IX, (**F**) X, (**G**) XI, (**H**) XII, (**I**) XIII. **, $P < 0.01$; #, $P < 0.0001$

Table 3 Correlation between coagulation tests and clotting factor activity in patients

	F	II	Ca	V	VII	VIII	IX	X	XI	XII	XIII
INR	-0.72 (-0.85; -0.45)	-0.74 (-0.86; -0.53)	-0.46 (-0.72; -0.24)	-0.80 (-0.89; -0.58)	-0.75 (-0.88; -0.60)	-0.29 (-0.60; 0.05)	-0.54 (-0.78; -0.38)	-0.57 (-0.79; -0.38)	-0.44 (-0.70; -0.26)	-0.41 (-0.68; -0.18)	-0.42 (-0.63; -0.10)
PTT	-0.49 (-0.68; -0.13)	-0.63 (-0.76; -0.34)	-0.47 (-0.74; -0.20)	-0.65 (-0.79; -0.30)	-0.36 (-0.60; -0.06)	-0.77 (-0.88; -0.63)	-0.63 (-0.83; -0.45)	-0.51 (-0.74; -0.25)	-0.58 (-0.81; -0.41)	-0.58 (-0.79; -0.37)	-0.34 (-0.58; 0.00)
Fibrinogen	/	0.63 (0.36; 0.76)	0.54 (0.35; 0.73)	0.64 (0.39; 0.76)	0.47 (0.17; 0.67)	0.42 (0.13; 0.62)	0.54 (0.34; 0.76)	0.49 (0.22; 0.70)	0.44 (0.20; 0.68)	0.36 (0.11; 0.58)	0.53 (0.23; 0.74)
Calcium	0.54 (0.35; 0.73)	0.46 (0.22; 0.72)	/	0.40 (0.18; 0.66)	0.16 (-0.15; 0.43)	0.37 (0.08; 0.62)	0.50 (0.21; 0.72)	0.40 (0.10; 0.64)	0.46 (0.18; 0.67)	0.46 (0.21; 0.62)	0.38 (0.07; 0.64)

Data reported as Spearman's Rank Correlation Coefficient, Rho (95 % CI)

F fibrinogen, *Ca* calcium

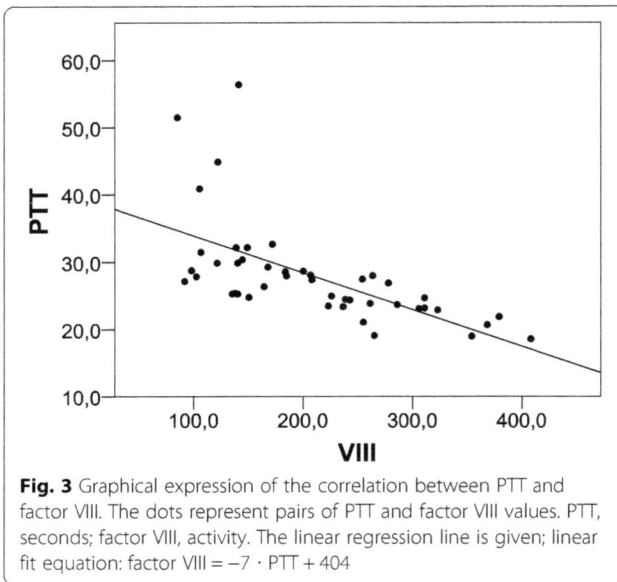

Fig. 3 Graphical expression of the correlation between PTT and factor VIII. The dots represent pairs of PTT and factor VIII values. PTT, seconds; factor VIII, activity. The linear regression line is given; linear fit equation: factor VIII $= -7 \cdot$ PTT $+ 404$

Discussion

The statistical analysis did not reveal statistically significant differences in the baseline demographics of patients and healthy controls. We assume that both groups were comparable and changes in clotting factor activity after severe trauma could be analyzed. A mean ISS of 31 points and an overall mortality of 27 % in patients also implied relevant tissue traumatization. The predominance of blunt injury reflects the medical situation in Germany and has been described previously [7]. However, this might have implications for the generalizability of these findings to different patient populations as they might differ in the incidence of penetrating trauma [22]. Because (isolated) penetrating trauma leads to uncontrolled hemorrhage rather than exorbitant tissue damage and the pathophysiology of the observed changes may depend on the trauma mechanism, divergent findings could be obtainable. One aim of this study was to test for clotting factor impairments as early as possible following trauma to exclude the influence of treatment. In Germany, prehospital emergency physicians are involved in patient care, and thus a potential bias related to individualized patient care prior to admission cannot be fully excluded. Hence, during the enrollment period no general modification of routine prehospital trauma life support was implemented in the study area. In-house protocols for the initial care of polytraumatized patients were also not modified. Furthermore, routine resuscitation room algorithms in our institution provide for blood sampling at the earliest possible time point. In a multidisciplinary strategy, blood is regularly drawn immediately after patient arrival and usually occurs prior to the placement of central venous lines. This strongly reduces the potential

interference of the different tests with relevant fluid resuscitation. Laboratory analysis itself may be affected by the variable degradation timeline of clotting factors. Again, this cannot be fully excluded because several clotting factors showed different half-lives [23]. However, because blood specimens were immediately transported to the laboratory after withdrawal and, if necessary, promptly deep frozen, this is unlikely.

As all primarily admitted patients irrespective of any kind of predefined coagulopathic status were included and results were compared with a reference group, this study differs significantly from the existing ones [19, 20]. The findings of this study demonstrate that, with the exception of factor VIII, clotting factor activities were generally reduced in the early time period following injury. Amongst others, serum levels of fibrinogen and calcium were reduced significantly, a finding that has been described by others [6, 24]. However, our results do not support studies according to which fibrinogen was the earliest and predominantly reduced factor after traumatic blood loss [25, 26]. Consistent with the study of Rizoli et al., we found the activity of factor V the most deficient [19]. This predominance of a factor V deficiency is a strong indicator of an activation of the protein c pathway, which in turn seems to play a key role in the onset of acute traumatic coagulopathy as proposed by Brohi et al. [10, 11, 19]. Hence, the rather low correlation of clinical parameters of tissue hypoperfusion (SBP, lactate, BE) with clotting factor activities is somewhat contrary to the concept of shock induced coagulopathy also supposed by Brohi et al. [10, 11]. In general, the median activities did not fall below the given reference range. This reflects the rather minor rate of only twenty percent of coagulopathic patients according to the inclusion criteria in the study of Rizoli et al. As the authors stated, the threshold of 30 % of activity is somewhat arbitrary and the clinical importance of a less dramatic but simultaneous decline in the activity of multiple clotting factors is unclear. Indeed, in our study the median activities of clotting factors in the normal cohort frequently exceeded the "standard" activity of 100 % and therefore the absolute reduction is even higher. Additionally, those reference ranges were originally established to assess single factor deficiencies and may not be appropriate for trauma patients. Therefore, the imminent reduction in almost all clotting factor activities should not be underestimated as it might act as a potential contributor to trauma-associated coagulopathy. In conclusion, these findings should be considered when treating hemorrhagic patients after severe multiple trauma, as higher ratios of clotting factors might be needed to restore normal coagulation function. Factor concentrates such as prothrombin complex concentrate contain clotting factors in high concentrations and might prove beneficial for treating the deficiencies noted in our study. With respect to the

Table 4 Correlation between clinical data and clotting factor activity in patients

	F	II	Ca	V	VII	VIII	IX	X	XI	XII	XIII
SBP prehospital	0.23 (−0.18; 0.69)	0.20 (−0.19; 0.71)	0.50 (−0.01; 0.80)	0.25 (−0.16; 0.68)	0.03 (−0.50; 0.50)	−0.10 (−0.46; 0.44)	0.16 (−0.27; 0.61)	0.15 (−0.22; 0.68)	0.05 (−0.44; 0.60)	0.11 (−0.23; 0.60)	0.03 (−0.35; 0.61)
SBP admission	0.20 (−0.46; 0.55)	0.31 (−0.19; 0.57)	0.21 (−0.22; 0.64)	0.36 (−0.18; 0.59)	0.11 (−0.45; 0.45)	0.14 (−0.32; 0.48)	−0.01 (−0.41; 0.49)	0.00 (−0.49; 0.42)	0.15 (−0.18; 0.71)	0.08 (−0.17; 0.63)	0.04 (−0.52; 0.49)
Lactate	−0.50 (−0.83; −0.22)	−0.44 (−0.73; 0.11)	−0.43 (−0.79; 0.08)	−0.43 (−0.74; 0.14)	−0.19 (−0.49; 0.42)	−0.19 (−0.66; 0.07)	−0.23 (−0.75; 0.29)	−0.15 (−0.56; 0.38)	−0.12 (−0.64; 0.35)	−0.08 (−0.54; 0.54)	−0.31 (−0.67; 0.08)
Base excess	0.23 (−0.08; 0.73)	0.38 (0.26; 0.77)	0.56 (0.12; 0.88)	0.57 (0.53; 0.86)	0.29 (−0.13; 0.81)	0.01 (−0.25; 0.53)	0.43 (0.46; 0.82)	0.12 (−0.11; 0.63)	0.25 (0.13; 0.76)	0.22 (0.04; 0.73)	−0.05 (−0.31; 0.54)
Temperature	0.18 (−0.25; 0.57)	0.46 (0.02; 0.85)	0.54 (0.08; 0.74)	0.30 (−0.18; 0.78)	0.12 (−0.54; 0.45)	−0.01 (−0.51; 0.41)	0.40 (−0.11; 0.71)	0.29 (−0.32; 0.69)	0.42 (−0.06; 0.79)	0.43 (0.00; 0.90)	0.05 (−0.25; 0.51)
Hemoglobin	0.46 (−0.06; 0.77)	0.52 (0.07; 0.74)	0.60 (0.30; 0.90)	0.45 (0.10; 0.73)	0.32 (−0.36; 0.66)	0.49 (−0.32; 0.53)	0.61 (−0.08; 0.65)	0.58 (−0.13; 0.69)	0.55 (−0.08; 0.71)	0.43 (−0.07; 0.63)	0.54 (−0.01; 0.81)
Thrombocytes	0.49 (−0.02; 0.79)	0.35 (−0.21; 0.68)	0.44 (0.03; 0.76)	0.18 (−0.29; 0.51)	0.17 (−0.34; 0.53)	0.33 (−0.46; 0.39)	0.31 (−0.37; 0.56)	0.36 (−0.26; 0.58)	0.39 (−0.17; 0.71)	0.29 (−0.23; 0.60)	0.40 (0.16; 0.77)

Data reported as Spearman's Rank Correlation Coefficient, Rho (95 % CI)

F fibrinogen, *Ca* calcium, *SBP* systolic blood pressure

increased activity of factor VIII, our results are consistent with the studies of Cohen and Jansen et al. [20, 27]. The latter is based on a subgroup analysis from the work of Rizoli et al. and reported a factor VIII activity level beyond the upper limit of the range in 72 % of all patients. Indeed, elevation of factor VIII activity seems to be the most robust effect of severe multiple trauma in terms of clotting factor activities. A possible explanation is the known role of factor VIII as an acute phase protein [28]. However, because our study design allowed for blood withdrawal quite soon after injury, this might not fully explain the detected levels of factor VIII at such an early time point. Further explanations involve a direct liberation of factor VIII from injured vessels and damaged tissues by unknown mechanisms or, alternatively, active secretion. This might be reasonable, as factor VIII is known to be produced by a wide range of cells [29, 30]. However, the physiological relevance of elevated factor VIII activity after severe trauma remains unclear.

Prothrombin Time (PT) and PTT have major limitations in the diagnosis of trauma induced coagulopathy as they are time-consuming and lack the desirable sensitivity at the critical time of admission. In addition, it is unclear to what extent possible derangements of the underlying coagulation system are reflected by PT and PTT [31]. This has resulted in the emergence of viscoelastic tests (rotational thromboelastometry [ROTEM] or thromboelastography) as a point-of-care diagnostic procedure for detecting acute coagulopathy after trauma [32]. In experimental hypothermia and hemorrhage, ROTEM showed superiority over PT and PTT in predicting coagulation disorders and mortality [33, 34]. In this study, INR (reflecting PT) was significantly elevated whereas differences in PTT were negligible. Indeed, an abnormal PTT is known to occur more infrequently than changes in PT [5]. The strongly elevated factor VIII levels found in this study offer a possible explanation for this phenomenon. As indicated by a strong negative correlation, high plasma levels of factor VIII may "discredit" the measurement of PTT, potentially leading to a reduced (quasi normal) clot formation time ex vivo. In this context, PTT would be useless in an attempt to diagnose traumatic coagulopathy. If viscoelastic tests are not available, INR might be helpful as it highly correlated with reduced levels of fibrinogen and the activities of factors II, V, and VII. This finding is reasonable because INR reflects PT, which was designed to test these factors (formerly called the "extrinsic pathway"). Under these circumstances, INR might be used despite its known limitations to trigger coagulation therapy, e.g., by use of fibrinogen concentrate and PCC. Nevertheless, future studies are desirable to elucidate the potential of viscoelastic tests to predict underlying clotting factor deficiencies in trauma induced coagulopathy.

Conclusions

This prospective study compared clotting factor activities in patients during the early period following severe multiple injury with a normal cohort. With the exception of factor VIII, activities of clotting factors are moderately reduced. This should be considered in the initial treatment after severe multiple trauma. In the concept of a calculated coagulation therapy, this could demand for the use of factor concentrates with higher ratios of clotting factors. Finally, although the physiological importance of elevated factor VIII activity after severe trauma remains unclear, a possible interference with PTT measurement ex vivo has to be considered.

Abbreviations
CI: Confidence interval; INR: International normalized ratio; IR: Interquartile range; ISS: Injury severity score; PT: Prothrombin time; PTT: Partial thromboplastin time; ROTEM: Rotational thromboelastometry; SBP: Systolic blood pressure; SD: Standard deviation; SHP: Standard human plasma.

Competing interests
The authors declare that they have no competing interests.

Authors' contributions
MB conducted the study and drafted the manuscript. AP collected and interpreted data and critically reviewed the manuscript. MDK and CS performed the statistical analysis and made the figures. SL designed and supervised the conduct of the study. All authors contributed substantially to manuscript revision. All authors read and approved the final manuscript.

Acknowledgements
This study was funded by the Department for Orthopaedics and Emergency Surgery, University Hospital Essen, University Duisburg-Essen, Germany.

Author details
[1]Department for Orthopaedics and Emergency Surgery, University Hospital Essen, University Duisburg-Essen, Hufelandstr. 55, 45147 Essen, Germany. [2]Clinic for Accident Surgery and Orthopaedics, Alfried Krupp Hospital Steele, Hellweg 100, 45276 Essen, Germany.

References
1. Herbert HK, Hyder AA, Butchart A, Norton R. Global health: injuries and violence. Infect Dis Clin North Am. 2011;25(3):653–68. doi:10.1016/j.idc.2011.06.004.
2. Sauaia A, Moore FA, Moore EE, Moser KS, Brennan R, Read RA, et al. Epidemiology of trauma deaths: a reassessment. J Trauma. 1995;38(2):185–93.
3. Hoyt DB. A clinical review of bleeding dilemmas in trauma. Semin Hematol. 2004;41(1 Suppl 1):40–3.
4. Brohi K, Singh J, Heron M, Coats T. Acute traumatic coagulopathy. J Trauma. 2003;54(6):1127–30. doi:10.1097/01.TA.0000069184.82147.06.
5. MacLeod JB, Lynn M, McKenney MG, Cohn SM, Murtha M. Early coagulopathy predicts mortality in trauma. J Trauma. 2003;55(1):39–44. doi:10.1097/01.TA.0000075338.21177.EF.
6. Rugeri L, Levrat A, David JS, Delecroix E, Floccard B, Gros A, et al. Diagnosis of early coagulation abnormalities in trauma patients by rotation thrombelastography. J Thromb Haemost. 2007;5(2):289–95. doi:10.1111/j.1538-7836.2007.02319.x.
7. Maegele M, Lefering R, Yucel N, Tjardes T, Rixen D, Paffrath T, et al. Early coagulopathy in multiple injury: an analysis from the German Trauma Registry on 8724 patients. Injury. 2007;38(3):298–304. doi:10.1016/j.injury.2006.10.003.

8. Gonzalez EA, Moore FA, Holcomb JB, Miller CC, Kozar RA, Todd SR, et al. Fresh frozen plasma should be given earlier to patients requiring massive transfusion. J Trauma. 2007;62(1):112–9. doi:10.1097/01.ta.0000250497.08101.8b.

9. Gruen RL, Jurkovich GJ, McIntyre LK, Foy HM, Maier RV. Patterns of errors contributing to trauma mortality: lessons learned from 2,594 deaths. Ann Surg. 2006;244(3):371–80. doi:10.1097/01.sla.0000234655.83517.56.

10. Brohi K, Cohen MJ, Ganter MT, Matthay MA, Mackersie RC, Pittet JF. Acute traumatic coagulopathy: initiated by hypoperfusion: modulated through the protein C pathway? Ann Surg. 2007;245(5):812–8. doi:10.1097/01.sla.0000256862.79374.31.

11. Brohi K, Cohen MJ, Ganter MT, Schultz MJ, Levi M, Mackersie RC, et al. Acute coagulopathy of trauma: hypoperfusion induces systemic anticoagulation and hyperfibrinolysis. J Trauma. 2008;64(5):1211–7. doi:10.1097/TA.0b013e318169cd3c.

12. Wolberg AS, Meng ZH, Monroe 3rd DM, Hoffman M. A systematic evaluation of the effect of temperature on coagulation enzyme activity and platelet function. J Trauma. 2004;56(6):1221–8.

13. Martini WZ, Pusateri AE, Uscilowicz JM, Delgado AV, Holcomb JB. Independent contributions of hypothermia and acidosis to coagulopathy in swine. J Trauma. 2005;58(5):1002–9.

14. Engstrom M, Schott U, Romner B, Reinstrup P. Acidosis impairs the coagulation: A thromboelastographic study. J Trauma. 2006;61(3):624–8. doi:10.1097/01.ta.0000226739.30655.75.

15. Lucas CE, Ledgerwood AM, Mammen EF. Altered coagulation protein content after albumin resuscitation. Ann Surg. 1982;196(2):198–202.

16. Martin DJ, Lucas CE, Ledgerwood AM, Hoschner J, McGonigal MD, Grabow D. Fresh frozen plasma supplement to massive red blood cell transfusion. Ann Surg. 1985;202(4):505–11.

17. Ciavarella D, Reed RL, Counts RB, Baron L, Pavlin E, Heimbach DM, et al. Clotting factor levels and the risk of diffuse microvascular bleeding in the massively transfused patient. Br J Haematol. 1987;67(3):365–8.

18. Harrigan C, Lucas CE, Ledgerwood AM. The effect of hemorrhagic shock on the clotting cascade in injured patients. J Trauma. 1989;29(10):1416–21.

19. Rizoli SB, Scarpelini S, Callum J, Nascimento B, Mann KG, Pinto R, et al. Clotting factor deficiency in early trauma-associated coagulopathy. J Trauma. 2011;71(5 Suppl 1):S427–34. doi:10.1097/TA.0b013e318232e5ab.

20. Cohen MJ, Kutcher M, Redick B, Nelson M, Call M, Knudson MM, et al. Clinical and mechanistic drivers of acute traumatic coagulopathy. J Trauma Acute Care Surg. 2013;75(1 Suppl 1):S40–7. doi:10.1097/TA.0b013e31828fa43d.

21. Woodhams B, Girardot O, Blanco MJ, Colesse G, Gourmelin Y. Stability of coagulation proteins in frozen plasma. Blood Coagul Fibrinolysis. 2001;12(4):229–36.

22. Minei JP, Schmicker RH, Kerby JD, Stiell IG, Schreiber MA, Bulger E, et al. Severe traumatic injury: regional variation in incidence and outcome. Ann Surg. 2010;252(1):149–57. doi:10.1097/SLA.0b013e3181df0401.

23. Zurcher M, Sulzer I, Barizzi G, Lammle B, Alberio L. Stability of coagulation assays performed in plasma from citrated whole blood transported at ambient temperature. Thromb Haemost. 2008;99(2):416–26. doi:10.1160/TH07-07-0448.

24. Vivien B, Langeron O, Morell E, Devilliers C, Carli PA, Coriat P, et al. Early hypocalcemia in severe trauma. Crit Care Med. 2005;33(9):1946–52.

25. Hiippala ST, Myllyla GJ, Vahtera EM. Hemostatic factors and replacement of major blood loss with plasma-poor red cell concentrates. Anesth Analg. 1995;81(2):360–5.

26. Schlimp CJ, Voelckel W, Inaba K, Maegele M, Ponschab M, Schochl H. Estimation of plasma fibrinogen levels based on hemoglobin, base excess and Injury Severity Score upon emergency room admission. Crit Care. 2013;17(4):R137. doi:10.1186/cc12816.

27. Jansen JO, Scarpelini S, Pinto R, Tien HC, Callum J, Rizoli SB. Hypoperfusion in severely injured trauma patients is associated with reduced coagulation factor activity. J Trauma. 2011;71(5 Suppl 1):S435–40. doi:10.1097/TA.0b013e318232e5cb.

28. Begbie M, Notley C, Tinlin S, Sawyer L, Lillicrap D. The Factor VIII acute phase response requires the participation of NFkappaB and C/EBP. Thromb Haemost. 2000;84(2):216–22.

29. Hollestelle MJ, Thinnes T, Crain K, Stiko A, Kruijt JK, van Berkel TJ, et al. Tissue distribution of factor VIII gene expression in vivo–a closer look. Thromb Haemost. 2001;86(3):855–61.

30. Jacquemin M, Neyrinck A, Hermanns MI, Lavend'homme R, Rega F, Saint-Remy JM, et al. FVIII production by human lung microvascular endothelial cells. Blood. 2006;108(2):515–7. doi:10.1182/blood-2005-11-4571.

31. Brohi K, Cohen MJ, Davenport RA. Acute coagulopathy of trauma: mechanism, identification and effect. Curr Opin Crit Care. 2007;13(6):680–5. doi:10.1097/MCC.0b013e3282f1e78f.

32. Theusinger OM, Spahn DR, Ganter MT. Transfusion in trauma: why and how should we change our current practice? Curr Opin Anaesthesiol. 2009;22(2):305–12. doi:10.1097/ACO.0b013e3283212c7c.

33. Kheirabadi BS, Crissey JM, Deguzman R, Holcomb JB. In vivo bleeding time and in vitro thrombelastography measurements are better indicators of dilutional hypothermic coagulopathy than prothrombin time. J Trauma. 2007;62(6):1352–9. doi:10.1097/TA.0b013e318047b805.

34. Martini WZ, Cortez DS, Dubick MA, Park MS, Holcomb JB. Thrombelastography is better than PT, aPTT, and activated clotting time in detecting clinically relevant clotting abnormalities after hypothermia, hemorrhagic shock and resuscitation in pigs. J Trauma. 2008;65(3):535–43. doi:10.1097/TA.0b013e31818379a6.

21

Implementation of a quality improvement project on smoking cessation reduces smoking in a high risk trauma patient population

Jeffry Nahmias*, Andrew Doben, Shiva Poola, Samuel Korntner, Karen Carrens and Ronald Gross

Abstract

Background: Cigarette smoking causes about one of every five deaths in the U.S. each year. In 2013 the prevalence of smoking in our institution's trauma population was 26.7 %, well above the national adult average of 18.1 % according to the CDC website. As a quality improvement project we implemented a multimodality smoking cessation program in a high-risk trauma population.

Methods: All smokers with independent mental capacity admitted to our level I trauma center from 6/1/2014 until 3/31/2015 were counseled by a physician on the benefits of smoking cessation. Those who wished to quit smoking were given further counseling by a pulmonary rehabilitation nurse and offered nicotine replacement therapy (e.g. nicotine patch). A planned 30 day or later follow-up was performed to ascertain the primary endpoint of the total number of patients who quit smoking, with a secondary endpoint of reduction in the frequency of smoking, defined as at least a half pack per day reduction from their pre-intervention state.

Results: During the 9 month study period, 1066 trauma patients were admitted with 241 (22.6 %) identified as smokers. A total of 31 patients with a mean Injury Severity Score (ISS) of 14.2 (range 1–38), mean age of 47.6 (21–71) and mean years of smoking of 27.1 (2–55), wished to stop smoking. Seven of the 31 patients, (22.5 %, 95 % confidence interval [CI] of 10–41 %) achieved self-reported smoking cessation at or beyond 30 days post discharge. An additional eight patients (25.8 %, 95 % CI 12–45 %) reported significant reduction in smoking.

Conclusions: Trauma patients represent a high risk smoking population. The implementation of a smoking cessation program led to a smoking cessation rate of 22.5 % and smoking reduction in 25.8 % of all identified smokers who participated in the program. This is a relatively simple, inexpensive intervention with potentially far reaching and beneficial long-term health implications. A larger, multi-center prospective study appears warranted.
LEVEL OF EVIDENCE: Therapeutic Study, Level V evidence.

Keywords: Trauma preventative care, Smoking, Smoking cessation

* Correspondence: Jeffry.nahmias@baystatehealth.org
Baystate Medical Center, affiliate of Tufts University School of Medicine, 759
Chestnut Street, Springfield, MA 01199, USA

Background

According to the World Health Organization (WHO), in 2012, 21 % of the global population smoked tobacco [1]. Annually, tobacco usage worldwide causes the direct death of over 5 million people with an additional 600,000 people dying from second-hand smoke [2]. In the United States alone, cigarette smoking accounts for one of every five deaths each year [3]. As compared to nonsmokers, the life expectancy of smokers is lowered by 13.2 years for men and 14.5 years for women [4]. Smokers are at an increased risk for chronic obstructive pulmonary disease (COPD) with an absolute risk (AR) of 25 % and lung cancer with an average relative risk (RR) of 15 to 30 [5, 6]. Smoking also increases the likelihood of developing chronic diseases, such as ischemic heart disease (RR = 2.2), cerebrovascular disease (RR = 1.6) and atherosclerotic cardiovascular disease (RR = 1.6) [7]. Smoking is linked to countless malignancies including 40–70 % of bladder cancers and 30 % of pancreatic cancers [8].

Additionally, cigarette smoking poses a financial burden. Assuming a pack of cigarettes costs 7 dollars, smoking one pack a day will cost an individual over $2500 per year. Nationally, from 2001 to 2004, the average financial burden of smoking was approximately $193 billion per year. Of this amount, $96 billion is attributed to health care cost, while the remaining $97 billion is accounted from lost productivity [9].

The Center for Disease Control (CDC) estimates that there are over 42 million adults in the United States who smoke cigarettes [10]. In 2010, the CDC reported that approximately 69 % of smokers were interested in quitting and 52 % of smokers had made a quit attempt in the past year [11]. Multimodal interventions, specifically combined nicotine replacement therapy (NRT) and counseling have demonstrated cessation rates from 20–33 % [12].

A national survey documented an overall decline of cigarette smoking from 21 % in 2005 to 18 % in 2013 [10]. In 2013, only 16.6 % of adults were reported to be smokers in the state of Massachusetts [13]. However at our institution in 2013, the prevalence of smoking among our trauma population was much higher at 27 %. The American College of Surgeons (ACS) has tasked all trauma centers with providing education on alcohol cessation, as studies have shown alcohol to be linked to traumatic injuries. Unlike this stance on alcohol, the ACS has no mandate for smoking cessation counseling. Prior to implementation of this program, our institution had no formalized protocol for smoking cessation. Previous studies have demonstrated that impulsivity is related to heightened nicotine dependence; however the exact relationship is far more complex than a simple causal relationship [14]. The purpose of this study was to implement a multimodality smoking cessation program in a high-risk trauma population. We hypothesized this would lead to smoking cessation in our trauma patient population who previously received no care to address smoking.

Methods

After obtaining Institutional Review Board exemption, all smokers with independent mental capacity were enrolled from June 1, 2014 to March 31st, 2015 at Baystate Medical Center, a level one trauma center. Participants received initial physician counseling regarding smoking cessation. All physician counselors were given a document compiled by the investigators before the start of the intervention. This included detrimental effects of smoking, benefits of smoking cessation, and responses for common reasons that patients refuse to stop smoking. If the patient desired smoking cessation, demographics including: gender, age, injury severity score (ISS), thorax abbreviated injury scale (AIS), and number of years smoking were obtained. They also were given educational pamphlets regarding benefits of smoking cessation and outpatient resources. All patients were offered nicotine replacement therapy (NRT) via a nicotine patch.

If admitted, a pulmonary rehabilitation nurse consultation with further counseling was ordered. Patients agreed to participate in an outpatient survey at 30 days or later. This survey assessed the primary endpoint of smoking cessation as well as the secondary endpoint of significant reduction in smoking defined as at least half a pack per day.

Descriptive statistics (mean and range) for continuous variables and percents for categorical variables were reported for all demographic and clinical variables. Rates of successful smoking cessation and significant smoking reduction and their 95 % confidence intervals were calculated.

Results

During the 9 month study period from June 1st, 2014 until March 31st, 2015, 1066 patients were admitted to Baystate Medical Center, a level one trauma center. Two-hundred forty one patients (22.6 %) were identified as smokers. Only 31 patients (23 male, eight female) wished to pursue smoking cessation. These patients had a mean ISS of 14.2 (range 1–38) and mean thorax AIS of 2.1 (0–5). The participants had a mean age of 47.6 (21–71) and mean years of smoking of 27.1 (2–55). A 100 % survey response was achieved at the 30 day or later designated follow-up. All participants were outpatients at this point with the capability to re-start smoking if desired. Seven of the 31 patients, (22.5 %, 95 % Confidence Interval Confidence Interval [CI] of 10–41 %) achieved smoking cessation at the follow-up. Eight patients (25.8 %, 95 % [CI] of 12–45 %) reported significant reduction in smoking, defined by at least half a pack per day reduction (Table 1). Thirteen of the 24 patients who did not achieve smoking cessation still desired to quit. The most common impediment to smoking cessation of those unable to quit was withdrawal symptoms (20.8 %). The second most common impediment was an inability to procure nicotine replacement therapy as an outpatient (16.7 %). An additional 4.1 % of remaining smokers cited alcohol influence and lack of motivation. On univariate analysis, comparing the subgroups of those who achieved 30 day cessation and those who did not, three variables were statistically significant ($p < .05$): LOS, ISS, and Thorax AIS (Table 2). After controlling for ISS in multiple logistic regression, the difference between the smoking cessation group and non-cessation group in LOS was not statistically significant ($p = 0.19$).

Discussion

Smoking is associated with harmful effects on every organ in the body and is well recognized as the leading cause of preventable illness and death [15]. Smoking adversely affects orthopedic injuries. A recent systematic review was performed by Scolaro et al. included 19 papers (seven prospective, 12 retrospective cohort) examining the effects of smoking on orthopedic trauma. They discovered an adjusted odds ratio of nonunion in smokers of 2.32 and an approximately 6 week longer mean healing time compared to nonsmokers. There was also a trend toward more postoperative wound infections [16].

The link between smoking and pulmonary disease is even more established. The pathophysiology of this process is beyond the scope of this manuscript, but some mechanisms include direct epithelial injury, carcinogen exposure, oxidative stress and mucociliary dysfunction [17]. Smoking is shown to have deleterious effects on respiratory failure in trauma. A retrospective review by Resnick et al. found smokers on average spent five more days of mechanical ventilation compared to nonsmokers [18]. Smoking is also considered one of the main modifiable risk factors for all types of pneumonia, including ventilator-associated pneumonia [19]. Calfee et

Table 1 Description of participants

Participants	31
Male	23
Female	8
Mean age (Range)	47.6 (21–71)
Mean ISS (Range)	14.2 (1–38)
Mean years smoking (Range)	27.1 (2–55)
Stopped smoking at 30 days (percent)	7/31 (23 %)
Significantly decreased smoking (percent)	8/31 (26 %)

Table 2 Demographic and outcomes analysis

Variable	No (Mean/CI)	Yes (Mean/CI)	Significance
Age	46.9(41.6–52.3)	50(33.5–66.5)	0.61
Years smoked	26.3(20.7–32.0)	30(10.0–50.0)	0.58
LOS(CI)	4.3 (2.8–5.8)	7.6 (4.6–10.6)	0.0333
ISS(CI)	11.4 (7.8–15.1)	21.1 (13.5–28.8)	0.0133
Thorax AIS(CI)	1.6 (1.0–2.3)	3.6 (2.7–4.5)	0.0031
Readmit rate	8.30 %	14.30 %	0.639

al found smoking to be a risk factor for acute respiratory distress syndrome (odds ratio 2.28) in patients even with non-pulmonary sepsis [20]. In a prospective observational study conducted by Lucidarme on mechanically ventilated patients, there was a significant difference in morbidity, especially agitation, self-removal of tubes and need for sedatives and restraints when comparing smokers versus nonsmokers [21].

Smoking has also been associated with impaired wound healing. Smoking has deleterious effects on neutrophil responsiveness and migratory and bactericidal function. Smoking also decreases mucosal and subcutaneous blood flow by as much as 40 % in some studies. It additionally causes oxidative stress through creation of reactive oxygen species [22].

In 2006, the American College of Surgeons Committee on Trauma (COT) published their first document on Alcohol Screening and Brief Intervention for Trauma Patients [23]. The need for this document is obvious given that nearly 50 % of trauma admissions have a positive blood alcohol level. In our trauma population we found a significant rate of smoking, 22.6 %. A retrospective chart review by Ferro et al. found an even higher smoking rate of 42.9 % in their trauma population [24]. Hence, like alcohol, this is a common problem in the injured patient.

Smoking cessation creates immediate benefits, which help the injured patient. Within hours of cessation, tissue blood flow and oxygen levels return to normal. At approximately two weeks of abstinence platelet function normalizes. Vitamin C levels and collagen synthesis appear to take approximately 4 weeks to normalize, although some benefit is seen earlier. By 6–8 weeks mucociliary function normalizes and perioperative complications decline. The effects of nicotine replacement therapy is not clear, a systematic review by Sorensen concluded that there is no evidence to suggest that nicotine replacement therapy has a detrimental or beneficial effect on postoperative outcomes or wound healing [22].

In terms of our patient population, there was no difference between those who achieved cessation and those who did not in terms of age, years of smoking, or readmission rate. There was a statistically significant difference in Thorax AIS, ISS, and LOS. Those achieving smoking cessation had a higher thorax AIS. It makes sense that patients with significant pulmonary injuries would be more amenable to cessation as they can easily comprehend the cause and effect relationship. ISS in the smoking cessation group was significantly higher however we do not believe there is a causal relationship. Finally, in terms of LOS being significantly higher for cessation patients, as previously mentioned this difference was no longer statistically significant when we controlled for ISS. Larger studies will be required to better elucidate which patients to focus on for counseling and what potential short term benefits can be achieved with smoking cessation in trauma patients.

The long term benefits of smoking cessation are quite profound. According to the WHO and CDC at one year from cessation the risk of coronary artery disease is half of a smokers and by 5 years the risk of stroke is that of a nonsmoker [1, 2, 4].

The importance of smoking cessation is clear for all patients, but should have the utmost significance for those who are traumatically injured. In our study, we achieved a smoking cessation rate of 22.5 %. The literature contains varied success rates depending on the modalities utilized, patient population and endpoint time, as there is certainly a component of recidivism. A Cochrane review of physician counseling for smoking cessation included 42 trials and found a 1–3 % improvement in cessation with only physician counseling, however, noted a higher rate with more intensive counseling and/or follow-up [25]. A recent randomized trial by Halpern et al. found a 30 day abstinence rate ranging from 10.5 to 22.6 % using financial incentives [26]. Other studies that utilize a multimodality approach, including behavioral therapy, counseling, nicotine replacement and pharmacologic therapy, have reported success rates ranging from 15–68 % [11, 12, 27]. Eisenberg et al. performed a meta-analysis, which included only randomized controlled trials, found an abstinence rate of 16.4 % for nicotine replacement therapy alone, 30.3 % for pharmacologic therapy alone and 35.5 % for combination therapy [28]. Other studies that include nicotine replacement therapy plus behavioral counseling have found abstinence rates ranging from 20–33 % depending on the intensity of counseling [12].

When assessing our financial and fixed resources, our smoking cessation program would need to be easy to implement and cost effective. Thus, the upfront cost of financial incentives was deemed prohibitive. In terms of pharmacologic therapy there are 2 FDA approved options, Varenicline (Chantix) and Buproprion (Zyban). Buproprion therapy is associated with an alarmingly high rate of insomnia (30–50 %), dry mouth (11 %) and other less common side effects such as tremor (3.4 %), rash (2.4 %), and seizures (0.1 %) [29]. Varenicline has two major safety concerns, namely neuropsychiatric and

cardiovascular. The latter led to an FDA advisory in 2011 that there may be increased risk of cardiovascular events in patients with known cardiovascular disease. Other commonly reported side effects include insomnia, nausea, visual disturbances, syncope and moderate to severe skin reactions. Given the relative frequency of adverse medication reactions, we felt it prudent to only use nicotine replacement therapy despite a slightly inferior cessation rate. In the future, we realize that engagement of our primary care physicians to assist with the prescription and maintenance of these medications may be helpful as the most common impediment to quitting was withdrawal symptoms, which may be ameliorated via these medications.

Furthermore, U.S. insurance plans are required to cover tobacco-cessation interventions including behavioral counseling and medications approved by the Food and Drug Administration. This may alleviate our second most common cited impediment to quitting, which was an inability to procure nicotine replacement therapy.

In addition to our rate of cessation we also achieved a 25.8 % reduction in smoking, which we defined by half a pack per day. Multiple studies have shown that even in those not interested in quitting, a reduction in smoking leads to a higher future rate of smoking cessation [30].

Some of the limitations to our study include lack of power, non-randomization, and length of follow-up. In terms of sample size, this was originally designed as a quality improvement project that achieved good results, we hope to continue this process of accrual and potentially expand it to our emergency general surgery patients as well. Since this is not a randomized controlled-blinded trial there are inherent biases such as selection bias as we did not control for potential confounders, including recent attempts to quit, concurrent substance abuse or other factors that may be unrecognized impediments. Additionally, with any interview there is a potential for interviewer bias; an attempt to minimize this was achieved by using a standardized script questionnaire. Finally, there is certainly a known potential for response bias, namely false positives for smoking cessation. Although in the setting of a non-financial gain scenario (i.e. no financial incentive for quitting), this is minimized as much as possible short of confirmatory nicotine testing.

Conclusion

Smoking has significant financial and health ramifications for trauma patients and healthcare as a whole. The implementation of a smoking cessation program led to a smoking cessation rate of 22.5 % and smoking reduction in 25.8 % of all identified smokers who participated in the program. This is a relatively simple and inexpensive intervention with potentially far reaching and beneficial long-term health implications. A multicenter evaluation including trauma and potentially emergency general surgical patients is warranted.

Competing interests
The authors declare that they have no competing interests.

Authors' contributions
JN was responsible for the literature search, study design, data collection, data analysis, data interpretation, writing, and critical revision. SP helped with literature search, interpreting the data, writing the manuscript and revision of the manuscript. SK helped with literature search, interpreting the data, writing the manuscript and revision of the manuscript. AD helped with study design, data interpretation, and revision of the manuscript. KC helped with data collection, study design, and revision of the manuscript. RG helped with study design, data interpretation, and revision of the manuscript. All authors read and approved the final manuscript.

Acknowledgements
We thank Mindy Kim for her assistance in data collection and Jane Sicard for her assistance in statistical analysis.

Funding
This research received no specific grant from any funding agency, commercial or not-for-profit sectors.

References

1. Prevalence of tobacco use. World Health Organization. http://www.who.int/gho/tobacco/use/en/. Accessed 23 Aug 2015.
2. Tobacco. World Health Organization. http://www.who.int/mediacentre/factsheets/fs339/en/. Accessed 23 Aug 2015.
3. U.S. Department of Health and Human Services. The health consequences of smoking—50 years of progress: A report of the surgeon general. Atlanta: U.S. Department of Health and Human Services, Centers for Disease Control and Prevention, National Center for Chronic Disease Prevention and Health Promotion, Office on Smoking and Health; 2014.
4. Centers for Disease Control and Prevention. Annual smoking-attributable mortality, years of potential life lost, and economic costs – United States, 1995–1999. MMWR Morb Mortal Wkly Rep. 2002;51(14):300–3.
5. Sasco AJ, Secretan MB, Straif K. Tobacco smoking and cancer: a brief review of recent epidemiological evidence. Lung Cancer. 2004;45 Suppl 2:S3–9.
6. Løkke A, Lange P, Scharling H, Fabricius P, Vestbo J. Developing COPD: a 25 year follow up study of the general population. Thorax. 2006;61(11):935–9.
7. Jee SH, Suh I, Kim IS, Appel LJ. Smoking and atherosclerotic cardiovascular disease in men with low levels of serum cholesterol: the Korea Medical Insurance Corporation Study. JAMA. 1999;282(22):2149–55.
8. Cancer. World Health Organization. http://www.who.int/tobacco/research/cancer/en/. Accessed 23 Aug 2015.
9. Centers for Disease Control and Prevention. Smoking-attributable mortality, years of potential life lost, and productivity losses — United States, 2000–2004. Morb Mortal Wkly Rep. 2008;57(45):1226–8.
10. Centers for Disease Control and Prevention. Current cigarette smoking among adults–United States, 2005-2013. Morb Mortal Wkly Rep. 2014;63(47):1108–12.
11. Centers for Disease Control and Prevention. Quitting smoking among adults—United States, 2001–2010. Morb Mortal Wkly Rep. 2011;60(44):1513–9.
12. Reus VI, Smith BJ. Multimodal techniques for smoking cessation: a review of their efficacy and utilisation and clinical practice guidelines. Int J Clin Pract. 2008;62(11):1753–68.
13. Centers for Disease Control and Prevention. State Tobacco Activities Tracking and Evaluation System. Interactive Maps: Cigarette Use—Adult Current Smokers—BRFSS. http://www.cdc.gov/tobacco/data_statistics/fact_sheets/adult_data/cig_smoking/. Accessed 23 Aug 2015.
14. Ryan KK, Mackillop J, Carpenter MJ. The relationship between impulsivity, risk-taking propensity and nicotine dependence among older adolescent smokers. Addict Behav. 2013;38(1):1431–4.
15. Danaei G, Ding EL, Mozaffarian D, et al. The preventable causes of death in the United States: comparative risk assessment of dietary, lifestyle, and metabolic risk factors. PLoS Med. 2009;6:e1000058.
16. Scolaro JA, Schenker ML, Yannascoli S, Baldwin K, Mehta S, Ahn J. Cigarette smoking increases complications following fracture: a systematic review. J Bone Joint Surg Am. 2014;96(8):674–81.
17. Centers for Disease Control and Prevention; National Center for Chronic Disease Prevention and Health Promotion; Office on Smoking and Health–United States. How tobacco smoke causes disease: The biology and behavioral basis for smoking attributable disease: A report of the surgeon general. Atlanta: Center for Disease Control and Prevention; 2010.
18. Resnick S, Inaba K, Okoye O, Nosanov L, Grabo D, Benjamin E, Smith J, Demetriades D. Impact of smoking on trauma patients. Ulus Travma Acil Cerrahi Derg. 2014;20(4):248–52.
19. Uckay I, Ahmed QA, Sax H, Pittet D. Ventilator-associated pneumonia as a quality indicator for patient safety? Clin Infect Dis. 2008;46(4):557–63.
20. Calfee CS, Matthay MA, Kangelaris KN, Siew ED, Janz DR, Bernard GR, May AK, Jacob P, Havel C, Benowitz NL, Ware LB. Cigarette smoke exposure and the acute respiratory distress syndrome. Crit Care Med. 2015;43(9):1790–7.
21. Lucidarme O, Seguin A, Daubin C, Ramakers M, Terzi N, Beck P, Charbonneau P, du Cheyron D. Nicotine withdrawal and agitation in ventilated critically ill patients. Crit Care. 2010;14(2):R58.
22. Sorensen LT. Wound healing and infection in surgery: The pathophysiological impact of smoking, smoking cessation, and nicotine replacement therapy. Ann Surg. 2012;255(6):1069–79.
23. Alcohol Screening and Brief Intervention (SBI) for Trauma Patients: COT Quick Guide. https://www.facs.org/~/media/files/quality%20programs/trauma/publications/sbirtguide.ashx. Accessed 23 Aug 2015.
24. Ferro TN, Goslar PW, Romanovsky AA, Petersen SR. Smoking in trauma patients: the effects on the incidence of sepsis, respiratory failure, organ failure, and mortality. J Trauma. 2010;69(2):308–12.
25. Stead LF, Bergson G, Lancaster T. Physician advice for smoking cessation. Cochrane Database Syst Rev. 2008;2:1–77.
26. Halpern SD, French B, Small DS, Saulsgiver K, Harhay MO, Audrain-McGovern J, Loewenstein G, Brennan TA, Asch DA, Volpp KG. Randomized trial of four financial-incentive programs for smoking cessation. N Engl J Med. 2015;372(22):2108–17.
27. Raich A, Martínez-Sánchez JM, Marquilles E, Rubio L, Fu M, Fernández E. Smoking cessation after 12 months with multi-component therapy. Adicciones. 2015;27(1):37–46.
28. Eisenberg MJ, Filion KB, Yavin D, Bélisle P, Mottillo S, Joseph L, Gervais A, O'Loughlin J, Paradis G, Rinfret S, Pilote L. Pharmacotherapies for smoking cessation: a meta-analysis of randomized controlled trials. CMAJ. 2008;179(2):135–44.
29. Corelli RL, Hudmon KS. Medications for smoking cessation. West J Med. 2002;176(2):131–5.
30. Carpenter MJ. Both smoking reduction with nicotine replacement therapy and motivational advice increase future cessation among smokers unmotivated to quit. J Consult Clin Psychol. 2004;72(3):371–81.

22

Casualties of peace: an analysis of casualties admitted to the intensive care unit during the negotiation of the comprehensive Colombian process of peace

Carlos A. Ordoñez[1,2], Ramiro Manzano-Nunez[1,3], Maria Paula Naranjo[1,3], Esteban Foianini[6*] [ID], Cecibel Cevallos[2], Maria Alejandra Londoño[4], Alvaro I. Sanchez Ortiz[1,3], Alberto F. García[1,2] and Ernest E. Moore[5]

Abstract

Background: After 52 years of war in 2012, the Colombian government began the negotiation of a process of peace, and by November 2012, a truce was agreed. We sought to analyze casualties who were admitted to the intensive care unit (ICU) before and during the period of the negotiation of the comprehensive Colombian process of peace.

Methods: Retrospective study of hostile casualties admitted to the ICU at a Level I trauma center from January 2011 to December 2016. Patients were subsequently divided into two groups: those seen before the declaration of the process of peace truce (November 2012) and those after (November 2012–December 2016). Patients were compared with respect to time periods.

Results: Four hundred forty-eight male patients were admitted to the emergency room. Of these, 94 required ICU care. Sixty-five casualties presented before the truce and 29 during the negotiation period. Median injury severity score was significantly higher before the truce. Furthermore, the odds of presenting with severe trauma (ISS > 15) were significantly higher before the truce (OR, 5.4; (95% CI, 2.0–14.2); $p < 0.01$). There was a gradual decrease in the admissions to the ICU, and the performance of medical and operative procedures during the period observed.

Conclusion: We describe a series of war casualties that required ICU care in a period of peace negotiation. Despite our limitations, our study presents a decline in the occurrence, severity, and consequences of war injuries probably as a result in part of the negotiation of the process of peace. The hysteresis of these results should only be interpreted for their implications in the understanding of the peace-health relationship and must not be overinterpreted and used for any political end.

Keywords: Wounds and injuries, Military personnel, Peace, Casualties, Trauma, Critical care, Critical care outcomes

* Correspondence: ruralcirugiatrauma@gmail.com; efoianini@hotmail.com
[6]Department of Surgery, Clinica Foianini, Santacruz de la Sierra, Bolivia
Full list of author information is available at the end of the article

Background

After decades of a civil war that caused thousands of military and civilian victims [1, 2] in 2012, the Colombian Government started a process of peace with the left-wing guerrillas "Fuerzas Armadas Revolucionarias de Colombia" (FARC). The process of peace aimed to put a definitive end to the rural violence that plagued the country for more than a half century. To this end, both parties (government and guerillas) agreed to a truce that started in November 2012 [3].

Collective violence in the form of war is responsible for illness and death [4, 5]. It has been estimated that 191 million people died as a result of armed conflict during the twentieth century [4]. Among the many adverse effects of armed conflict, war-fighters carry a higher risk of suffering the immediate and deadly impact of war and military operations as they can be killed or injured on the battlefield [6]. Despite the catastrophic consequences of war on the health of populations, the majority of healthcare research in this field has been focused on analyzing the epidemiology of combat injuries on the battlefield during ongoing war periods [7–10]. However, there are no contemporary descriptions of hostile casualties during times of peace negotiation and implementation.

We hypothesized that the negotiation of the Colombian process of peace reduced the number of severe injuries and their consequences. As intensive care unit (ICU) admissions can provide an indirect measure of severe injuries, we sought to analyze casualties who were admitted to the ICU before and during the period of the negotiation of the comprehensive Colombian process of peace.

Methods

Study design

Following our hypothesis, a retrospective study was carried out to analyze casualties who were admitted to the ICU before and during the period of the negotiation of the comprehensive Colombian process of peace. According to the process of peace timeline, we set up two study periods: the first period was the one before the declaration of the truce [3] (January 2011–November 2012) and the second was the one after the truce (November 2012–December 2016: the negotiation period).

Data source

For this retrospective observational study, we used data from the prospective Trauma Registry of the Panamerican Trauma Society. A description of this registry is found elsewhere [11, 12]. Data was complemented with information from medical charts. We reviewed data of hostile casualties admitted to the intensive care unit from 2011 to 2016 at La Fundación Valle del Lili (FVL)

University Hospital, in Cali, Colombia. The FVL Institutional Review Board approved the study protocol.

FVL is a level I trauma center with 510 beds, 80 in adult intensive care units (ICUs), of which ten are reserved for trauma patients. It serves as a referral facility for both civilian and military trauma from the southwest region of the country. The FVL referral area for military trauma covers the southwest region of Colombia (131,301 km^2), which corresponds to the departments of Nariño, Cauca, Valle del Cauca, and the southern part of Chocó. FVL is the only level I trauma center of the southwest region of the country with a partnership agreement with the Colombian Army for the care of the soldiers wounded in combat.

Historically, the FVL referral area (Southwest Region) has been the most affected by violence between guerrilla groups and military forces [13, 14].

Patients

An initial screening of the Trauma Registry and FVL medical charts identified all soldiers admitted to the emergency room from January 2011 to December 2016. We were able to identify all soldiers because FVL electronic medical records contain data on the insurance company of each patient, and soldiers are the only ones that are covered by the "Dirección de Sanidad Militar" Colombian Army insurance. Furthermore, all hostile casualties are classified as "soldier wounded in combat" at the moment of arrival to the emergency room.

We included hostile casualties. Soldiers who were injured severely enough to be admitted to the intensive care unit were included. Soldiers who arrived at the ER but were not injured in action were excluded. A warfighter was classified as a hostile casualty if he was a victim of terrorist activity or became a casualty in action [15]. Soldiers wounded in combat (hostile casualties) were managed following institutional protocols by the same group of surgeons during the period observed.

We recorded data on demographics, trauma, and clinical characteristics, the severity of the injury, resuscitation and operative strategies, organ dysfunction, activation of the trauma transfusion protocol, and mortality.

We calculated organ dysfunction as defined by Vincent et al. [16] (SOFA Score). Patients who needed the activation of the trauma transfusion protocol were those who (1) died early from hemorrhage, (2) patients who, within 24 h of admission received ≥ 3 U PRBCs within 1 h, (3) patients who received massive transfusion (MT) (MT > 10 U in 24 h), and (3) patients with a hemorrhage that required plasma and platelet transfusion. Patients suffering severe trauma were those who had an Injury Severity Score (ISS) greater than 15.

Statistical analysis

Descriptions of all patients were performed using relative and absolute frequencies for qualitative variables. Continuous variables were summarized by reporting medians and inter-quartile ranges. Variables of interest were compared between groups (group before the truce vs. group after the truce) using the Wilcoxon-Mann-Whitney U Test for continuous variables and the Fisher exact test for categorical variables. We considered multivariate regression analysis to asses for differences in severe trauma occurrence (ISS > 15) between periods. All analyses were conducted using Stata statistical software. A $p < 0.05$ was considered significant.

Results

During the 6 years observed, 448 soldiers wounded in action were admitted to the emergency room. Figure 1 provides an overview of the variations in the number of hostile casualties admitted to the ER for the years 2011 to 2016. There was a gradual decrease in the number of warfighters admitted to the ER since the beginning of the truce. Moreover, the numbers of blast and gunshot rifle injuries also declined over this period. In 2012, 142 soldiers wounded in combat were admitted to the ER. This number decreased to 84, 63, 32, and 6 ER admissions in 2013, 2014, 2015, and 2016, respectively.

Of all casualties admitted to the ER during the period observed, 94 required ICU care. Sixty-five presented before the negotiation of the process of peace period and 29 during the negotiation period.

All patients were male, and half were less than 25 years old. Soldiers were victims of blast (52%) and gunshot rifle injuries (48%) in almost equal proportions. Twenty-five of those with blast injuries suffered land mine

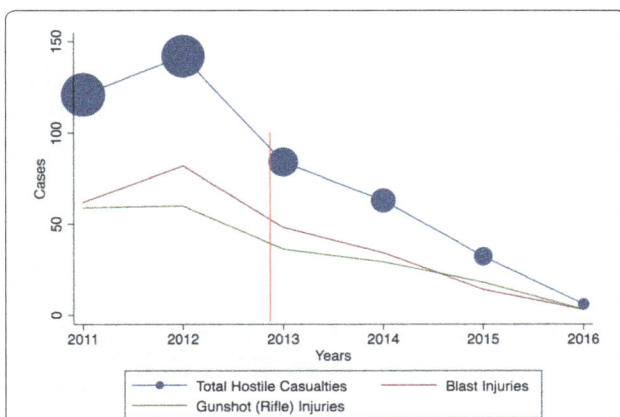

Fig. 1 Variations in hostile casualties' admissions and trauma mechanisms 2011–2016. (Description: shows the variations in hostile casualties admissions to the ER and trauma mechanisms during the period observed. Blue circles: graphic representation of the proportion of ICU admissions each year)

injuries. On admission, half of the patients had a shock index greater than 0.9 and one-third (31%) presented with hypotension (SBP < 90 mmHg). Soldiers suffered predominantly severe traumatic injuries. The median (IQR) Injury Severity Score was 20 (14–29), with 70% of patients scoring more than 15.

Differences in demographics, initial clinical variables, and injury severity by periods are presented in Table 1. There were no statistically significant differences between groups with respect to age, vital signs, mode of transportation to the ER, and mechanism of trauma. Injury Severity Scores were significantly higher in patients who presented before the truce than in patients who presented after [ISS, median (IQR): 25 (16-30) vs 14 (10-22); $p < 0.01$]. The proportion of patients presenting with an ISS greater than 15 was significantly higher before the truce ($p < 0.01$).

As shown in Table 2, no significant differences were found between periods with respect to resuscitation strategies, operative interventions, multi-organ failure, and mortality. However, fewer patients required surgery, damage control laparotomy (DCL), and the activation of the trauma transfusion protocol in the negotiation period after the truce. Moreover, fewer amputations and ostomies (intestinal diversions) were performed during the period of peace negotiation. Furthermore, the occurrence of severe trauma and serious injuries gradually decreased in the period of peace negotiation (Table 3).

As shown in Fig. 2, there was a considerable reduction in the performance of procedures related to trauma care during the period observed. In 2012, 33 patients were admitted to ICU, ten required damage control laparotomy, and 12 underwent the application of the trauma transfusion protocol. These numbers decreased to three DCL, three Trauma Transfusion Protocol (TTP) activations, and nine ICU admissions in 2014, then dropped to zero DCL, zero TTP activations, and one ICU admission in 2016.

Finally, the odds of suffering severe trauma were higher in patients who presented before the truce than in patients who presented after the negotiation period (unadjusted OR = 5.4; (95% CI, 2.0–14.2); $p < 0.01$). Although we considered multivariate regression analysis to assess for differences in severe trauma occurrence between periods, the only significant difference that we found in univariate analysis was for injury severity, and thus, we decided to present the unadjusted odds ratio for severe trauma occurrence.

Discussion

To our knowledge, this is the first known analysis of warfighters requiring ICU care during a period of peace negotiation. We found that casualties presenting before the negotiation period were more likely to suffer severe trauma. Moreover, we describe a gradual decrease in the

Table 1 Demographics, initial clinical variables, and injury severity with respect to periods

	Before the negotiation period ($n = 65$)	During the negotiation period ($n = 29$)	p
Age	25 (21–30)	26 (24–29)	0.41
SBP	110 (82–134)	116 (84–131)	0.98
Shock Index	0.90(0.67–1.3)	0.92(0.67–1.2)	0.99
HR	102 (84–120)	110 (88–120)	0.58
Tachycardia*, n	38	21	0.25
Hypotension**, n	22	8	0.63
Mode of transport			
Helicopter, n	53	25	0.76
Ambulance, n	12	4	0.76
Trauma mechanism			
Gunshot rifle, n	30	15	0.66
Blast injuries, n	35	14	0.66
Landmine injuries, n	16	9	0.61
Trauma severity			
ISS, median (IQR)	25 (16–30)	14 (10–22)	< 0.01
ISS > 15, n (%)	53 (81.5)	13 (44.8)	< 0.01

SBP systolic blood pressure, HR heart rate, ISS Injury Severity Score
*Heart rate > 90 bpm; **systolic blood pressure < 90 mmHg

Table 2 Resuscitation and operative strategies, multi-organ failure, and mortality with respect to periods

	Before the negotiation period ($n = 65$)	During the negotiation period ($n = 29$)	p
PRBCs *	2 (0–4)	2 (0–3)	0.27
Crystalloids *	5050 (3350–7650)	4400 (3350–6400)	0.35
Required activation of the TTP	28	10	0.49
Required surgery, n	61	26	0.67
DCL, n	14	7	0.79
Ostomies, n	10	1	0.16
Amputations, n	13	5	1
SOFA score *	3 (1–7)	3 (1–7)	0.97
Organ dysfunction			
Renal dysfunction, n	9	9	0.08
Hemodynamic dysfunction, n	14	8	0.6
Coagulopathy, n	41	20	0.8
Respiratory dysfunction, n	48	17	0.13
Organ failure			
Cardiovascular failure, n	13	8	0.5
Coagulation failure, n	6	2	1
Respiratory failure, n	16	7	1
Mortality, n	1	0	0.9

PRBCs packed red blood cells, TTP Trauma Transfusion Protocol, DCL damage control laparotomy
*Median (IQR)

Table 3 Injuries, ostomies, and amputations per year

Year	2011 (n = 32)	2012 (n = 33)	2013 (n = 13)	2014 (n = 9)	2015 (n = 6)	2016 (n = 1)
Severe trauma (ISS > 15), n	28	25	9	0	3	1
Serious extremity Injuries*, n	19	11	7	1	1	0
Serious chest Injuries*, n	5	8	1	3	0	0
Serious abdominal Injuries*, n	7	17	2	2	1	0
Ostomies, n	3	7	1	0	0	0
Amputations, n	9	4	4	0	1	0

ISS Injury Severity Score
*Serious injuries: AIS ≥ 3

admission of hostile casualties to the ICU, the performance of damage control resuscitation and surgical procedures, and the consequences related to military trauma during the period observed. This number started to decline from 2013 onwards.

A total of 448 hostile casualties were registered of which 20% were injured severely enough to require ICU admission. Previous descriptions of critical care provision in austere war environments reported higher volumes of patients admitted to the ICU in shorter time periods [17, 18]. The first description of contemporary ICU data from the Operation Iraqi Freedom [18] reported the 1-month experience in the care of 47 critically ill patients. Our series report a 6-year experience in the care of 94 war fighters injured in combat. Although the volume of patients admitted to the ICU in our series seems to be smaller, this is likely to be a consequence of the characteristics of the armed conflict. Colombian conflict was below conventional war and above the routine peaceful competition between the state and independent groups. In this conflict, military operations were deployed to confront

subversion (FARC) and high-velocity weaponry or high-order explosives were regularly used.

War has a deadly impact on human health [4]. Many people, but especially soldiers can suffer the direct consequences of war. The existing literature on war injuries is extensive and consistently describes increasing numbers of warfighters suffering war injuries [6–10]. For example, the Colombian armed forces reported that for the years 2005–2010 the number of soldiers wounded in combat increased and this was accompanied by an increase in the number of service members suffering severe trauma [19, 20]. In contrast, this study shows a gradual decrease in the admission warfighters to the ICU, the procedures related to trauma care, and the surgical interventions performed (damage control surgery, ostomies, and amputations). Furthermore, the number of patients suffering severe trauma (ISS > 15) and/or serious injuries (AIS ≥ 3) gradually decreased during the period observed, and thus, we present a pattern that has not previously been described.

In the context of collective violence in the form of war, the severity of injuries suffered by warfighters could be seen as a measure of the intensity of the war. Therefore, the reduction in the proportion of warfighters suffering severe injuries could be a proxy indicator for the positive impact of peace negotiation on war casualties. Regarding the latter, the current study found that there was a significant difference in average Injury Severity Scores between periods. Moreover, the odds of presenting with severe trauma were higher before the negotiation period. The reason why the proportion of warfighters suffering severe trauma was significantly lower during the negotiation period seems to be clear. The truce established in November 2012 was an agreement between the Colombian government and the FARC to stop hostile actions. During this truce, the efforts made by the leaders of both parties and their commitment to preventing the conflict from resuming, although not directly, inferred in reducing the number of injuries and associated consequences that we saw. On the other hand, the reason why average injury severity scores differed between periods is unclear. It could be

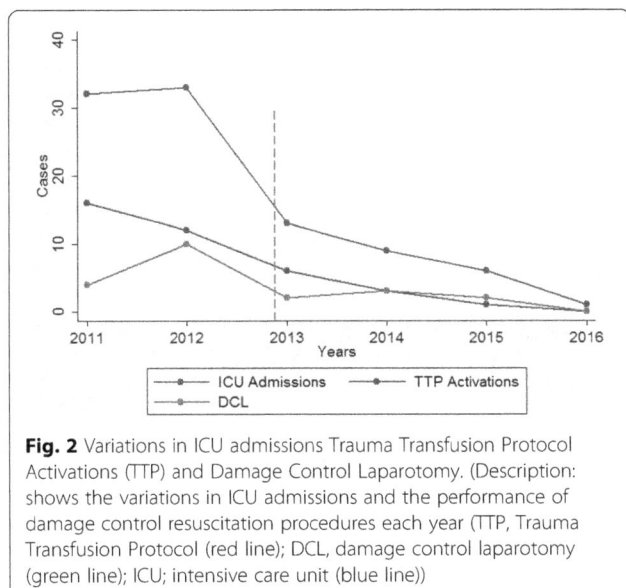

Fig. 2 Variations in ICU admissions Trauma Transfusion Protocol Activations (TTP) and Damage Control Laparotomy. (Description: shows the variations in ICU admissions and the performance of damage control resuscitation procedures each year (TTP, Trauma Transfusion Protocol (red line); DCL, damage control laparotomy (green line); ICU; intensive care unit (blue line))

that during the negotiation period, hostile actions were performed with less lethal weapons not involving classical high-velocity weaponry or high-order explosives, and thus, the nature of anatomical damage in soldiers' victims of hostile acts in the late period could differ from that of warfighters in the time before the truce.

The number of casualties admitted to the ICU decreased gradually during the period observed, and this was accompanied by a reduction in the activations of the trauma transfusion protocol and the number of damage control surgeries performed (Fig. 2). Damage control resuscitation (DCR) is a structured intervention that includes early blood product transfusion, early hemorrhage control by damage control surgery, and restoration of physiologic stability [21, 22]. These interventions could have a great impact on resource utilization as patients managed following principles of DCR may require a longer intensive care unit and hospital stay and, thus, higher medical resources and costs. Traditionally, combat troops have required specialized medical resources for the resuscitation and the management of combat related injuries. As war increases its intensity, there is a proportional increase in the need for the deployment of more advanced medical capabilities to increases the odds of survival of the wounded in combat [23]. Therefore, war is not only a social catastrophe but also an economic one, and thus, our findings could go beyond the immediate reduction in the number of soldiers suffering trauma and requiring advanced trauma care and could have significant policy implications. It could be that in the future period of peace, advanced medical capabilities for the care of the wounded in combat will no longer be required and these resources could be used in civilian populations.

In the study that we present, the situation after (negotiation period) may differ in respects other than the exposure to peacebuilding if compared to the situation before (war period). For example, indications for laparotomy or resuscitation strategies such as transfusion protocols may vary over time [24, 25], and these variations could affect procedures rates and patient outcomes. Therefore, one can argue that the evolution and improvements in trauma care may be responsible in part for the differences observed. However, all included patients were treated by the same group of well-trained trauma surgeons following institutional protocols. Furthermore, during the study period, no significant improvements in the principles of trauma surgery and trauma care were developed, and thus, we believe that no other factors different from the process of peace could plausibly have caused any observed change in outcomes. Therefore, it is very probable that the period of peace negotiation was responsible in part for the pattern observed, and thus, our description, although limited, is an advance in the understanding of the beneficial effects of peace in the health of populations [26, 27].

Finally, although the Colombian armed conflict only delivered suffering and destruction, we must acknowledge how civilian trauma was positively affected by the experience of the war. Our hospital is located in the largest city of southwest Colombia and was initially conceived as a large non-profit, high-complexity center dedicated to the people of the southwest region of Colombia. However, as war increased its intensity, our center became a mixed military-civilian center, and we had to provide surgical critical care to the wounded in combat. We learned how to perform simple surgical maneuvers to optimize times during damage control surgery [28–30] and thus be able to control contamination and stop the bleeding on time. Therefore, it is likely possible that competencies acquired from warfighters were translated to daily practice and played a key role in improving outcomes of injured patients in the civilian sector.

Limitations

Although our hospital is the only referral level I trauma center for military casualties in the southwest region of Colombia, we can only have access to casualties admitted to the emergency department. Moreover, we had no data of casualties from other areas of the country and those who died before reaching a medical facility; all of which may have introduced significant selection and information bias. However, other reports also have shown a reduction in the number emergency department admissions of soldiers wounded in combat in different regions of the country probably as a result of the period of peace negotiation [31, 32]. For example, commenting on the effects of the process of peace on military casualties, the director of the Central Military Hospital argues [33]: *"I see very positive changes. Saving one life is already a very big win, but we went from having about 400-500 amputees [a year] to, this year, having much fewer cases. Over the course of the year (2017), we have had about 19 injured".*

Further selection bias could be introduced as we only included soldiers admitted to the ICU. However, we wanted to have a description and analysis of a homogeneous population suffering severe trauma. Therefore, we decided to include soldiers wounded enough to require ICU care as this could be an indirect measure of severe trauma. Finally, the methodology used does not provide substantial evidence about the positive effect of peace negotiation on war casualties. However, our results are of importance for advancing the knowledge of peace-health relationship [26, 27] and for achieving the universal desire for peace.

Despite these results, questions remain, and future studies should investigate the long-term outcomes of severely wounded warfighters in the post-conflict period. Also, additional explorations of the effect of peace on civilian trauma should be undertaken. Finally, further multicentric designs such as time series analysis will need to be conducted to support our initial observations.

Conclusion

We describe a series of war casualties who required ICU care in a period of peace negotiation. Despite our limitations, our study presents a decline in the occurrence, severity, and consequences of war injuries probably as a result in part of the negotiation of the process of peace. The hysteresis of these results should only be interpreted for their implications in the understanding of the peace-health relationship and must not be overinterpreted and used for any political end.

Acknowledgements
The authors would like to thank the FVL Clinical Research Center for their constant support.

Funding
No funding. This article received no specific grant from any funding agency in the public, commercial, or non-for-profit sectors.

Authors' contributions
CAO, RMN, MPN, EF, CC, MAL, AIS, AFG, and EEM contributed equally to this work. CAO and AFG designed the research. CAO, RMN, MPN, EF, CC, MAL, AIS, AFG, and EEM performed the research, analyzed the data, and wrote the paper. All authors made important intellectual contributions to the manuscript, and all authors approved the final version before submission. CAO supervised all the process.

Competing interest
The authors declare that they have no competing interests.

Author details
[1]Division of Trauma and Acute Care Surgery, Fundación Valle del Lili, Cali, Colombia. [2]Department of Surgery, Universidad del Valle, Cali, Colombia. [3]Clinical Research Center, Fundación Valle del Lili, Cali, Colombia. [4]School of Medicine, Universidad ICESI, Cali, Colombia. [5]Department of Surgery, Trauma Research Center, University of Colorado, Denver, CO, USA. [6]Department of Surgery, Clinica Foianini, Santacruz de la Sierra, Bolivia.

References
1. RNI. Registro Único de Víctimas (Colombian Victims Registry) [Internet]. Available from: http://rni.unidadvictimas.gov.co/RUV Accessed 11 Jan 2017.
2. Rubiano AM, Sánchez Ál, Guyette F, Puyana JC. Trauma care training for National Police Nurses in Colombia. Prehosp Emerg Care. 2010;14:124–30. Available from: http://www.ncbi.nlm.nih.gov/pmc/articles/PMC3413284/
3. BBC. Colombia: FARC declares unilateral truce at landmark talks [Internet]. BBC news. 2012 [cited 2017 Jan 11]. Available from: http://www.bbc.com/news/world-latin-america-20399152. Accessed 11 Jan 2017.
4. Sidel VW, Levy BS. The health impact of war. Int J Inj Control Saf Promot. 2008;15:189–95.
5. Haagsma JA, Graetz N, Bolliger I, Naghavi M, Higashi H, Mullany EC, et al. The global burden of injury: incidence, mortality, disability-adjusted life years and time trends from the Global Burden of Disease study 2013. Inj Prev. 2015;22:3–18. Available from: http://injuryprevention.bmj.com/content/early/2015/10/20/injuryprev-2015-041616
6. Gawande A. Casualties of War—military care for the wounded from Iraq and Afghanistan. N Engl J Med. 2004;351:2471–5.
7. Eastridge BJ, Mabry RL, Seguin P, Cantrell J, Tops T, Uribe P, et al. Death on the battlefield (2001–2011): Implications for the future of combat casualty care. J Trauma Acute Care Surg. 2012;73. Available from: http://journals.lww.com/jtrauma/Fulltext/2012/12005/Death_on_the_battlefield__2001_2011___.10.aspx
8. Belmont PJJ, Goodman GP, Zacchilli M, Posner M, Evans C, Owens BD. Incidence and Epidemiology of Combat Injuries Sustained During "The Surge" Portion of Operation Iraqi Freedom by a U.S. Army Brigade Combat Team. J Trauma Acute Care Surg. 2010;68. Available from: http://journals.lww.com/jtrauma/Fulltext/2010/01000/Incidence_and_Epidemiology_of_Combat_Injuries.35.aspx
9. Kelly JF, Ritenour AE, McLaughlin DF, Bagg KA, Apodaca AN, Mallak CT, et al. Injury Severity and Causes of Death From Operation Iraqi Freedom and Operation Enduring Freedom: 2003–2004 Versus 2006. J Trauma Acute Care Surg. 2008;64. Available from: http://journals.lww.com/jtrauma/Fulltext/2008/02001/Injury_Severity_and_Causes_of_Death_From_Operation.6.aspx
10. Antebi B, Benov A, Mann-Salinas EA, Le TD, Cancio LC, Wenke JC, et al. Analysis of injury patterns and roles of care in US and Israel militaries during recent conflicts: two are better than one. J Trauma Acute Care Surg. 2016;81:S87–94.
11. Ordoñez CA, Morales M, Rojas-Mirquez JC, Bonilla-Escobar FJ, Badiel M, Miñán Arana F, et al. Trauma Registry of the Pan American Society of Trauma: one year of experience in two referral centers in the Colombian southwestern. Colomb Médica. 2016;47(3)
12. Ramachandran A, Ranjit A, Zogg CK, Herrera-Escobar JP, Appelson JR, Pino LF, et al. Comparison of epidemiology of the injuries and outcomes in two first-level trauma centers in Colombia using the Pan-American Trauma Registry System. World J Surg. 2017:1–7.
13. Bergquist CW, Peñaranda R, Sánchez G. G. Violence in Colombia, 1990-2000 : waging war and negotiating peace. Lanham, MD: Rowman & Littlefield; 2001.
14. Glade J. Drug, guerrilla violence is crippling Colombia's southwestern Cauca department. Colomb Reports. 2011. Available from: https://colombiareports.com/drug-guerrilla-violence-is-crippling-cauca/. Accessed 11 Jan 2017.
15. United States Department of Defense. Department of Defense Dictionary of Military and Associated Terms. US Dep Def Jt Publ. 2015. Available from: http://www.dtic.mil/doctrine/new_pubs/jp1_02.pdf. Accessed 11 Jan 2017.
16. Vincent JL, Moreno R, Takala J, Willatts S, De Mendonça A, Bruining H, et al. The SOFA (Sepsis-related Organ Failure Assessment) score to describe organ dysfunction/failure. Intensive Care Med. 1996;22:707–10.
17. Lundy JB, Swift CB, McFarland CC, Mahoney LCP, Perkins RM, Holcomb JB. A descriptive analysis of patients admitted to the intensive care unit of the 10th combat support hospital deployed in Ibn Sina, Baghdad, Iraq, from October 19, 2005, to October 19, 2006. J Intensive Care Med. 2010;25:156–62. Available from: http://journals.sagepub.com/doi/abs/10.1177/0885066609359588?journalCode=jica
18. Lockey DJ, Nordmann GR, Field JM, Clough D, Henning JDR. The deployment of an intensive care facility with a military field hospital to the 2003 conflict in Iraq. Resuscitation. 2017;62:261–5. Available from: https://doi.org/10.1016/j.resuscitation.2004.06.003
19. Camargo J, Pérez LE, Franco C, Rodríguez E, Sánchez W. "Plan pantera", trauma militar en Colombia. Rev Colomb Cir. 2014;29:293-304. Available from: http://www.scielo.org.co/pdf/rcci/v29n4/v29n4a5.pdf
20. Arias C, Villamil E, Gutierrez J, Morales H, Sanchez W. Trauma vascular periférico de guerra en Colombia: análisis epidemiológico de ocho años. Rev Colomb Cirugía. 2012;2:26.
21. Mizobata Y. Damage control resuscitation: a practical approach for severely hemorrhagic patients and its effects on trauma surgery. J Intensive Care. 2017;5:-4. Available from: https://doi.org/10.1186/s40560-016-0197-5
22. Holcomb JB. Damage Control Resuscitation. J Trauma Acute Care Surg. 2007;62(6 Suppl):S36-7. Available from: http://journals.lww.com/jtrauma/Fulltext/2007/06001/Damage_Control_Resuscitation.29.aspx
23. Patel TH, Wenner KA, Price SA, Weber MA, Leveridge A, McAtee SJ. A U.S. Army Forward Surgical Team's Experience in Operation Iraqi Freedom. J Trauma Acute Care Surg. 2004;57. Available from: http://journals.lww.com/jtrauma/Fulltext/2004/08000/A_U_S__Army_Forward_Surgical_Team_s_Experience_in.1.aspx
24. ME K, LZ K, Narayan R, AI E. A paradigm shift in trauma resuscitation: evaluation of evolving massive transfusion practices. JAMA Surg. 2013;148:834–40.
25. Brinck T, Handolin L, Lefering R. The effect of evolving fluid resuscitation on

the outcome of severely injured patients: an 8-year experience at a tertiary trauma center. Scand J Surg. 2015;105:109–16.

26. Joshi M. Comprehensive peace agreement implementation and reduction in neonatal, infant and under-5 mortality rates in post-armed conflict states, 1989–2012. BMC Int Health Hum Rights. 2015;15:27. Available from: https://doi.org/10.1186/s12914-015-0066-7

27. Gaffar AM, Mahfouz MS. Peace impact on health: population access to iodized salt in south Sudan in post-conflict period. Croat Med J. 2011;52: 178–82. Available from: https://www.ncbi.nlm.nih.gov/pmc/articles/PMC3083250/

28. Ordoñez CA, Pino LF, Badiel M, Sánchez AI, Loaiza J, Ballestas L, et al. Safety of performing a delayed anastomosis during damage control laparotomy in patients with destructive colon injuries. J Trauma. 2011;71:1512–8. Available from: http://www.ncbi.nlm.nih.gov/pmc/articles/PMC3413258/

29. Garcia A, Martinez J, Rodriguez J, Millan M, Valderrama G, Ordoñez C, et al. Damage control techniques in the management of severe lung trauma. J Trauma Acute Care Surg. 2015;78:45–51.

30. Ordoñez CA, Parra MW, Salamea JC, Puyana JC, Millán M, Badiel M, et al. A comprehensive five-step surgical management approach to penetrating liver injuries that require complex repair. J Trauma Acute Care Surg. 2013;75:207–11.

31. CERAC. Assessing the merits of an imperfect peace: the FARC's unilateral ceasefire in 2013-14. Blog CERAC. 2014. Available from: http://blog.cerac.org.co/assessing-the-merits-of-an-imperfect-peace-the-farcs-unilateral-ceasefire-in-2013-14. Accessed 11 Jan 2017.

32. "Hace 51 años no se presentaba una reducción tan grande del conflicto armado": Cerac. El Espectador [Internet]. 2016; Available from: https://www.elespectador.com/noticias/politica/hace-51-anos-no-se-presentaba-una-reduccion-tan-grande-articulo-611701. Accessed 11 Jan 2017.

33. Daniels JP. Frontline: caring for soldiers after the peace deal in Colombia. Lancet. 2017;390:1939.

23

WSES classification and guidelines for liver trauma

Federico Coccolini[1*], Fausto Catena[2], Ernest E. Moore[3], Rao Ivatury[4], Walter Biffl[5], Andrew Peitzman[6], Raul Coimbra[7], Sandro Rizoli[8], Yoram Kluger[9], Fikri M. Abu-Zidan[10], Marco Ceresoli[1], Giulia Montori[1], Massimo Sartelli[11], Dieter Weber[12], Gustavo Fraga[13], Noel Naidoo[14], Frederick A. Moore[15], Nicola Zanini[16] and Luca Ansaloni[1]

Abstract

The severity of liver injuries has been universally classified according to the American Association for the Surgery of Trauma (AAST) grading scale. In determining the optimal treatment strategy, however, the haemodynamic status and associated injuries should be considered. Thus the management of liver trauma is ultimately based on the anatomy of the injury and the physiology of the patient. This paper presents the World Society of Emergency Surgery (WSES) classification of liver trauma and the management Guidelines.

Keywords: Liver trauma, Minor, Moderate, Severe, Classification, Guidelines, Surgery, Hemorrage, Operative management, Non-operative management

Background

The severity of liver injuries is universally classified according to the American Association for the Surgery of Trauma (AAST) grading scale (Table 1) [1]. The majority of patients admitted for liver injuries have grade I, II or III and are successfully treated with nonoperative management (NOM). In contrast, almost two-thirds of grade IV or V injuries require laparotomy (operative management, OM) [2]. However in many cases there is no correlation between AAST grade and patient physiologic status. Moreover the management of liver trauma has markedly changed through the last three decades with a significant improvement in outcomes, especially in blunt trauma, due to improvements in diagnostic and therapeutic tools [3–5]. In determining the optimal treatment strategy, the AAST classification should be supplemented by hemodynamic status and associated injuries. The anatomical description of liver lesions is fundamental in the management algorithm but not definitive. In fact, in clinical practice the decision whether patients need to be managed operatively or undergo NOM is based mainly on the clinical conditions and the associated injuries, and less on the AAST liver injury grade. Moreover, in some situations patients conditions lead to an emergent transfer to the operating room (OR) without the opportunity to define the grade of liver lesions before the surgical exploration; thus confirming the primary importance of the patient's overall clinical condition. Utimately, the management of trauma requires an assessment of the anatomical injury and its physiologic effects.

This paper aims to present the World Society of Emergency Surgery (WSES) classification of liver trauma and the treatment Guidelines, following the WSES position paper emerged from the Second WSES World Congress [6].

As stated in the position paper, WSES includes surgeons from around the globe. This Classification and Guidelines statement aims to direct the management of liver trauma, acknowledging that there are acceptable alternative management options. In reality, not all trauma surgeons work in the same conditions and have the same facilities and technologies available [6].

Methods

The discussion of the present guidelines started in 2011 during the WSES World Congress in Bergamo (Italy). From that first discussion, through the Delphi process came the published position paper [6]. A group of experts in the field coordinated by a central coordinator

* Correspondence: federico.coccolini@gmail.com
[1]General Emergency and Trauma Surgery Department, Papa Giovanni XXIII Hospital, Piazza OMS 1, 24127 Bergamo, Italy
Full list of author information is available at the end of the article

Table 1 AAST Liver Trauma Classification

Grade	Injury type	Injury description
I	Haematoma	Subcapsular <10 % surface
	Laceration	Capsular tear <1 cm parenchymal depth
II	Haematoma	Subcapsular 10–50 % surface area; intraprenchymal, <10 cm diameter
	Laceration	1–3 cm parenchymal depth, <10 cm in length
III	Haematoma	Subcapsular >50 % surface area or expanding, ruptured subcapsular or parenchymal haematoma. Intraprenchymal haematoma >10 cm
	Laceration	>3 cm parenchymal depth
IV	Laceration	Parenchymal disruption 25–75 % of hepatic lobe
	Vascular	Juxtavenous hepatic injuries i.e. retrohepatic vena cava/centrl major hepatic veins
VI	Vascular	Hepatic avulsion

Advance one grade for multiple injuries up to grade III
AAST liver injury scale (1994 revision)

was contacted to express their evidence-based opinion on several issues about the liver trauma management differentiated into blunt and penetrating trauma and evaluating the conservative and operative management for both.

The central coordinator assembled the different answers derived from the first round and drafted the first version that was subsequently revised by each member of the expert group separately in the second round. The definitive version about which the agreement was reached consisted in the position paper published in 2013 [6].

In July 2013 the position paper was discussed during the WSES World Congress in Jerusalem (Israel) and then a subsequent round of consultation among a group of experts evaluated the associated WSES classification and the new evidence based improvements. Once reached the agreement between the first experts group, another round among a larger experts group lead to the present form of the WSES classification and guidelines of liver trauma to which all the experts agreed. Levels of evidence have been evaluated in agreement with the Oxford guidelines.

WSES classification

The WSES position paper suggested dividing hepatic traumatic lesions into minor (grade I, II), moderate (grade III) and major/severe (grade IV, V, VI) [6]. This classification has not previously been clearly defined by the literature. Frequently low-grade AAST lesions (i.e. grade I-III) are considered as minor or moderate and treated with NOM [7, 8]. However some patients with high-grade lesions (i.e. grade IV-V laceration with parenchymal disruption involving more than 75 % of the hepatic lobe or more than 3 Couinaud segments within a single lobe) may be hemodynamically stable and

successfully treated nonoperatively [2]. On the other hand, "minor" lesions associated with hemodynamic instability often must be treated with OM. This demonstrates that the classification of liver injuries into minor and major must consider not only the anatomic AAST classification but more importantly, the hemodynamic status and the associated injuries.

The Advanced Trauma Life Support (ATLS) definition considers as "unstable" the patient with: blood pressure <90 mmHg and heart rate >120 bpm, with evidence of skin vasoconstriction (cool, clammy, decreased capillary refill), altered level of consciousness and/or shortness of breath [9].

The WSES Classification divides Hepatic Injuries into three classes:

- Minor (WSES grade I).
- Moderate (WSES grade II).
- Severe (WSES grade III and IV).

The classification considers either the AAST classification either the hemodynamic status and the associated lesions (Table 2).

Minor hepatic injuries:

- *WSES grade I* includes AAST grade I-II hemodynamically stable either blunt or penetrating lesions.

Moderate hepatic injuries:

- *WSES grade II* includes AAST grade III hemodynamically stable either blunt or penetrating lesions.

Severe hepatic injuries:

- *WSES grade III* includes AAST grade IV-VI hemodynamically stable either blunt or penetrating lesions.
- *WSES grade IV* includes AAST grade I-VI hemodynamically unstable either blunt or penetrating lesions.

Basing on the present classification WSES indicates a management algorithm explained in Fig. 1.

Recommendations for non operative management (NOM) in blunt liver trauma (BLT)

Blunt trauma patients with hemodynamic stability and absence of other internal injuries requiring surgery, should undergo an initial attempt of NOM irrespective of injury grade (GoR 2 A).

Table 2 WSES Liver Trauma Classification

	WSES grade	Blunt/Penetrating (Stab/Guns)	AAST	Haemodynamic	CT-scan	First-line Treatment
MINOR	WSES grade I	B/P SW/GSW	I-II	Stable		
MODERATE	WSES grade II	B/P SW/GSW	III	Stable	Yes + Local Exploration in SW#	NOM* + Serial Clinical/Laboratory/ Radiological Evaluation
SEVERE	WSES grade III	B/P SW/GSW	IV-V	Stable		
	WSES grade IV	B/P SW/GSW	I-VI	Unstable	No	OM

(*SW* Stab Wound, *GSW* Gun Shot Wound; OM: Operative Management; NOM: Non Operative Management; *NOM should only be attempted in centers capable of a precise diagnosis of the severity of liver injuries and capable of intensive management (close clinical observation and haemodynamic monitoring in a high dependency/intensive care environment, including serial clinical examination and laboratory assay, with immediate access to diagnostics, interventional radiology and surgery and immediately available access to blood and blood products; # wound exploration near the inferior costal margin should be avoided if not strictly necessary because of the high risk to damage the intercostal vessels)

NOM is contraindicated in the setting of hemodynamic instability or peritonitis (GoR 2 A).

NOM of moderate or severe liver injuries should be considered only in an environment that provides capability for patient intensive monitoring, angiography, an immediately available OR and immediate access to blood and blood product (GoR 2 A).

In patients being considered for NOM, CT-scan with intravenous contrast should be performed to define the anatomic liver injury and identify associated injuries (GoR 2 A).

Angiography with embolization may be considered the first-line intervention in patients with hemodynamic stability and arterial blush on CT-scan (GoR 2 B).

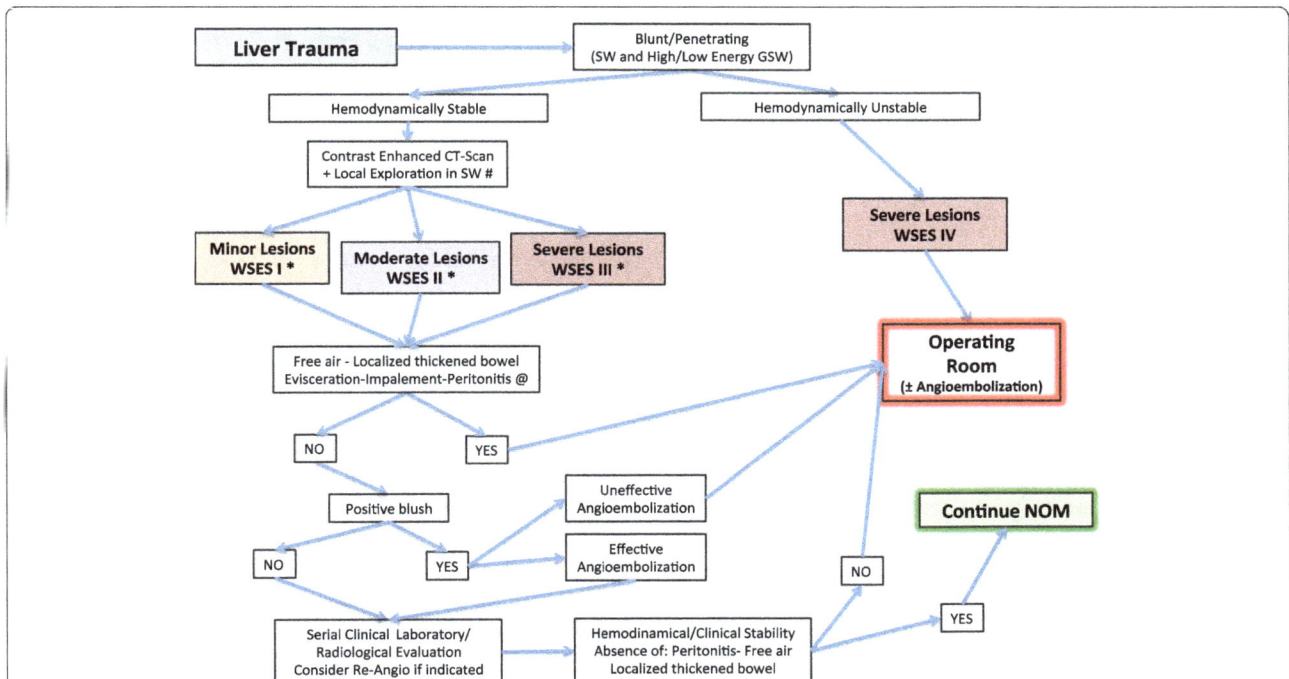

Fig. 1 Liver Trauma Management Algorithm. (*SW* Stab Wound, *GSW* Gun Shot Wound; *NOM should only be attempted in centers capable of a precise diagnosis of the severity of liver injuries and capable of intensive management (close clinical observation and haemodynamic monitoring in a high dependency/intensive care environment, including serial clinical examination and laboratory assay, with immediate access to diagnostics, interventional radiology and surgery and immediately available access to blood and blood products; # wound exploration near the inferior costal margin should be avoided if not strictly necessary because of the high risk to damage the intercostal vessels; @ extremely selected patients hemodynamically stable with evisceration and/or impalement and/or diffuse peritonitis with the certainty of an exclusive and isolated abdominal lesion could be considered as candidate to be directly taken to the operating room without contrast enanched CT-scan)

In hemodynamically stable blunt trauma patients without other associated injuries requiring OM, NOM is considered the standard of care [10–12]. In case of hemodynamic instability or peritonitis NOM is contraindicated [7, 11, 13].

The requirements to attempt NOM of moderate and severe injuries are the capability to make a diagnosis of the severity of liver injuries, and to provide intensive management (continuous clinical monitoring, serial hemoglobin monitoring, and around-the-clock availability of CT-scan, angiography, OR, and blood and blood products) [14–19]. No evidence exists at present to define the optimal monitoring type and duration.

In patients with ongoing resuscitative needs, the angioembolization is considered as an "extension" of resuscitation. However with the aim to reduce the need for transfusions and surgery, angioembolization can be applied safely but generally only in selected centers [13, 20, 21]. If required it can be safely repeated. Positive results associated with its early use have been published [22, 23].

In blunt hepatic trauma, particularly after high-grade injury, complications occur in 12–14 % of patients [13, 24]. Diagnostic tools for complications after NOM include: clinical examination, blood tests, ultrasound and CT-scan. Although routine follow-up with CT-scan is not necessary, [2, 13, 24] in the presence of abnormal inflammatory response, abdominal pain, fever, jaundice or drop of hemoglobin level, CT-scan is recommended [13]. Bleeding, abdominal compartment syndrome, infections (abscesses and other infections), biliary complications (bile leak, hemobilia, biloma, biliary peritonitis, biliary fistula) and liver necrosis are the most frequent complications associated with NOM [14, 24]. Ultrasound is useful in the assessment of bile leak/biloma in grade IV-V injuries, especially with a central laceration.

Re-bleeding or secondary hemorrhage are frequent (as in the rupture of a subcapsular hematoma or a pseudo-aneurysm) [13, 24]. In the majority of cases (69 %), "late" bleeding can be treated non-operatively [13, 24]. Post-traumatic hepatic artery pseudo-aneurysms are rare and they can usually be managed with selective embolization [6, 25].

Biliary complications can occur in 30 % of cases. Endoscopic retrograde cholangio-pancreatography (ERCP) and eventual stenting, percutaneous drainage and surgical intervention (open or laparoscopic) are all effective ways to manage biliary complications [13]. In presence of intrahepatic bilio-venous fistula (frequent associated with bilemia) ERCP represents an effective tool [26].

CT-scan or ultrasound-guided drainage are both effective in managing peri-hepatic abscesses (incidence 0–7 %) [13, 22, 24]. In presence of necrosis and devascularization of hepatic segments surgical management would be indicated [6, 24]. Hemobilia is uncommon and frequently associated with pseudo-aneurysm [2, 6, 24]. In hemodynamically stable and non-septic patients embolization is safe and

could be considered as the first approach; otherwise surgical management is mandatory [6, 24].

Lastly, the liver compartment syndrome is rare and has been described in some case reports as a consequence of large sub-capsular hematomas. Decompression by percutaneous drainage or by laparoscopy has been described [24, 27].

No standard follow-up and monitoring protocol exist to evaluate patients with NOM liver injuries [6]. Serial clinical evaluation and hemoglobin measurement are considered the pillars in evaluating patients undergone to NOM [10]. Abdominal ultrasound could help in managing non-operatively managed liver trauma patients.

Recommendations for NOM in penetrating liver trauma (PLT)

NOM in penetrating liver trauma could be considered only in case of hemodynamic stability and absence of: peritonitis, significant free air, localized thickened bowel wall, evisceration, impalement (GoR 2 A).

NOM in penetrating liver trauma should be considered only in an environment that provides capability for patient intensive monitoring, angiography, an immediately available OR and immediate access to blood and blood product (GoR 2 A).

CT-scan with intravenous contrast should be always performed to identify penetrating liver injuries suitable for NOM (GoR 2 A).

Serial clinical evaluations (physical exams and laboratory testing) must be performed to detect a change in clinical status during NOM (GoR 2 A).

Angioembolisation is to be considered in case of arterial bleeding in a hemodynamic stable patient without other indication for OM (GoR 2 A).

Severe head and spinal cord injuries should be considered as relative indications for OM, given the inability to reliably evaluate the clinical status (GoR 2A).

The most recent published trials demonstrate a high success rate for NOM in 50 % of stab wounds (SW) in the anterior abdomen and in about 85 % in the posterior abdomen [6, 28]. The same concept has also been applied to gunshot wounds (GSWs) [29, 30]. However, a distinction should be made between low and high-energy penetrating trauma in deciding either for OM or NOM. In case of low energy, both SW and GSW, NOM can be safely applied. High energy GSW and other ballistic injuries are less amenable to NOM because of the high-energy transfer, and in 90 % of cases an OM is required [6, 31, 32]. Of note, a 25 % non-therapeutic laparotomy rate is reported in abdominal GSWs [31]. This confirms that in selective cases NOM could be pursued either in GSWs.

Clinical trials report a high success rate of NOM in penetrating liver injuries (69 to 100 %) [29, 30, 32–37]. Absolute requirements for NOM are: hemodynamic stability, absence of peritonitis, and an evaluable abdomen [6]. Evisceration and impalement are other indications for OM [30, 32, 34]. Current guidelines suggest that hemodynamically stable patients presenting with evisceration and/or impalement and/or diffuse peritonitis should be considered candidates to be directly taken to the OR without CT-scan [30]. These findings are particularly important in cases of gunshot injuries. Other suggested predictive criteria of NOM failure in abdominal GSWs according to Navsaria et al. are: associated head and spinal cord injuries (that preclude regular clinical examination) and significant reduction in hemoglobin requiring more than 2–4 units of blood transfusion in 24 h [6, 29].

In SWs the role of CT scan has been questioned [28, 34]. Local wound exploration (LWE) is considered accurate in determining the depth of penetration; sometimes in little wounds it would be necessary to enlarge a little the incision [6, 30]. However, wound exploration near the inferior costal margin should be avoided if not strictly necessary because of the high risk to damage the intercostal vessels. Emergency laparotomy has been reported to be necessary even in some cases with negative CT-scan [34]. CT-scan may be necessary in obese patients and when the wound tract is long, tangential and difficult to determine the trajectory [6, 34].

In NOM of GSWs the CT-scan can help in determining the trajectory. However not all authors consider it mandatory [29, 31]. Velmahos et al. reported a CT-scan specificity of 96 % and a sensitivity of 90.5 % for GSWs requiring laparotomy [38]. The gold standard to decide for OM or NOM remains the serial clinical examination [6, 31].

NOM is contraindicated in case of CT-scan detection of free intra- or retro-peritoneal air, free intra-peritoneal fluid in the absence of solid organ injury, localized bowel wall thickening, bullet tract close to hollow viscus with surrounding hematoma [33] and in high energy penetrating trauma. In NOM strict clinical and hemoglobin evaluation should be done (every 4–6 h for at least 48 h); once stabilized the patient could be transferred to the ward [28, 29, 34].

There is considerable variation in local CT-scan imaging practices, and no uniform standard exists. Variations are dependent on imaging hardware, radiation exposure, contrast dose, and image sequences, among other factors. For example, image acquisition may occur in a triphasic fashion (non-contrast, arterial, and portal venous phases), or as a single phase following a split bolus contrast injection, providing a mixed arterial and portal venous phase. These variables have not been standardized across centers, or in the literature, and require expert radiologist consideration and manipulation for optimal diagnostic yield, and are dependent on the study indication.

Even in penetrating liver trauma, the angioembolization is considered as an "extension" of resuscitation in those patients presenting with ongoing resuscitative needs. However angioembolization can be applied safely only in selected centers [13, 20, 21]. If required it can be safely repeated.

The main reluctance of surgeons to employ NOM in penetrating trauma is related to the fear of missing other abdominal lesions, especially hollow viscus perforation [6, 33]. Published data clearly showed that in patients without peritonitis on admission, no increase in mortality rates with missed hollow viscus perforation has been reported [39]. On the other hand, non-therapeutic laparotomy has been demonstrated to increase the complication rate [39]. Nevertheless OM in penetrating liver injuries has a higher liver-related complication rate (50–52 %) than in blunt ones [6, 33].

Concomitant severe head injuries

The otimal management of concomitant severe head and liver injuries is debated. In patients with severe head injuries hypotension may be deleterious, and OM could be suggested as safer [24, 36]. Recently, a large cohort of 1106 non-operatively managed low-energy gunshot liver injuries, has been published by Navsaria et al. [36]. The presence of concomitant liver and severe head injuries has been considered one of the main exclusion criteria to NOM. Authors stated that: "Hemodynamically stable patients with unreliable clinical examinations (head and/ or high spinal cord injury) must also undergo an urgent exploratory laparotomy". Another paper analyzing 63 patients by Navsaria et al. suggested as predictive criteria for NOM failure in abdominal low-energy GSWs is the association with head and spinal cord injuries precluding meaningful clinical examination [29].

Follow-up after successful NOM

Clear and definitive direction for post-injury follow-up and normal activity resumption in those patients who experienced NOM haven't been published yet. General recommendations are to resume usual activity after 3–4 months in patients with an uncomplicated hospital course. This derives from the observation that the majority of liver lesions heal in almost 4 months [10, 24]. If the CT-scan follow-up (in grade III-V lesions) has shown significant healing normal activity can be resumed even after 1 month [24].

Patients should to be counseled not to remain alone for long periods and to return to the hospital immediately if they experience increasing abdominal pain, light-headedness, nausea or vomiting [6, 10].

Recommendations for operative management (OM) in liver trauma (blunt and penetrating)

Patients should undergo OM in liver trauma (blunt and penetrating) in case of hemodynamic instability, concomitant internal organs injury requiring surgery, evisceration, impalement (GoR 2 A).

Primary surgical intention should be to control the hemorrhage, to control bile leak and to institute an intensive resuscitation as soon as possible (GoR 2 B).

Major hepatic resections should be avoided at first, and considered subsequently (delayed fashion) only in case of large devitalized liver portions and in centers with the necessary expertise (GoR 3 B).

Angioembolisation is a useful tool in case of persistent arterial bleeding (GoR 2 A).

As exsanguination represents the leading cause of death in liver injuries OM decision mainly depends on hemodynamic status and associated injuries [6].

In those cases where no major bleeding are present at the laparotomy, the bleeding may be controlled by compression alone or with electrocautery, bipolar devices, argon beam coagulation, topical hemostatic agents, or omental packing [6, 8, 24, 40, 41].

In presence of major haemorrhage more aggressive procedures can be necessary. These include first of all hepatic manual compression and hepatic packing, ligation of vessels in the wound, hepatic debridement, balloon tamponade, shunting procedures, or hepatic vascular isolation. It is important to provide concomitant intraoperative intensive resuscitation aiming to reverse the lethal triad [6, 8, 41].

Temporary abdominal closure can be safely considered in all those patients when the risk of developing abdominal compartment syndrome is high and when a second look after patient's hemodynamic stabilization is needed [8, 40, 41].

Anatomic hepatic resection can be considered as a surgical option [2, 42, 43]. In unstable patients and during damage control surgery a non-anatomic resection is safer and easier [6, 8, 24, 44]. For staged liver resection, either anatomic either non-anatomic ones can be safely made with stapling device in experienced hands [44].

If despite the fundamental initial maneuvers (hepatic packing, Pringle maneuver) the bleeding persists and

evident lesion to a hepatic artery is found, an attempt to control it should be made. If repair is not possible a selective hepatic artery ligation can be considered as a viable option. In case of right or common hepatic artery ligation, cholecystectomy should be performed to avoid gallbladder necrosis [44, 45]. Post-operative angioembolization is a viable option, when possible, allowing hemorrhage control while reducing the complications [6, 8, 24, 46]. After artery ligation, in fact, the risk of hepatic necrosis, biloma and abscesses increases [6].

Portal vein injuries should be repaired primarily. The portal vein ligation should be avoided because liver necrosis or massive bowel edema may occur. Liver Packing and a second look or liver resection are preferable to portal ligation [6, 44].

In those cases where Pringle maneuver or arterial control fails, and the bleeding persists from behind the liver, a retro-hepatic caval or hepatic vein injury could be present [6, 46]. Three therapeutic options exist: 1) tamponade with hepatic packing, 2) direct repair (with or without vascular isolation), and 3) lobar resection [7]. Liver packing is the most successful method of managing severe venous injuries [6, 24, 47–49]. Direct venous repair is problematic in non-experienced hands, with a high mortality rate [6, 24].

When hepatic vascular exclusion is necessary, different types of shunting procedures have been described, most of them anecdotally. The veno-veno bypass (femoral vein to axillary or jugular vein by pass) or the use of fenestrated stent grafts are the most frequent type of shunt used by surgeons familiar with their use [8, 24, 44, 50]. The atrio-caval shunt bypasses the retro-hepatic cava blood through the right atrium using a chest tube put into the inferior cava vein. Mortality rates in such a complicated situations are high [8]. Liver exclusion is generally poorly tolerated in the unstable patient with major blood loss [6].

In the emergency, in cases of liver avulsion or total crush injury, when a total hepatic resection must be done, hepatic transplantation has been described [44].

The exact role of post-operative angio-embolization is still not well defined [51–55]. Two principal indications have been proposed: 1) after primary operative hemostasis in stable or stabilized patients, with an evidence at contrast enhanced CT-scan of active bleeding, and 2) as adjunctive hemostatic control in patients with uncontrolled suspected arterial bleeding despite emergency laparotomy [6, 56].

Conclusions

The management of trauma poses in definitive the attention in treating also the physiology and decision can be more effective when both anatomy of injury and its physiological effects are combined.

Abbreviations
AAST: American Association for Surgery for Trauma; ATLS: Advanced Trauma Life Support; BLT: Blunt liver trauma; DCS: Damage Control Surgery; ERCP: Endoscopic retrograde cholangio-pancreatography; GSW: Gunshot wound; NOM: Non-Operative Management; OM: Operative Management; OR: Operating Room; SW: Stab wounds; WSES: World Society of Emergency Surgery

Acknowledgements
None.

Funding
None.

Authors' contributions
FC, FaCa, EM, RI, WB, AP, RC, SR, YK, FM AZ, MC, GM, MS, DW, GF, NN, FAM, NZ, LA, manuscript conception and draft critically revised the manuscript and contribute with important scientific knowledge giving the final approval.

Competing interest
The authors declare that they have no competing interests.

Author details
[1]General Emergency and Trauma Surgery Department, Papa Giovanni XXIII Hospital, Piazza OMS 1, 24127 Bergamo, Italy. [2]Emergency and Trauma Surgery, Parma Maggiore Hospital, Parma, Italy. [3]Trauma Surgery, Denver Health, Denver, CO, USA. [4]Virginia Commonwealth University, Richmond, VA, USA. [5]Acute Care Surgery, The Queen's Medical Center, Honolulu, HI, USA. [6]Department of Surgery, Trauma and Surgical Services, University of Pittsburgh School of Medicine, Pittsburgh, USA. [7]Department of Surgery, UC San Diego Health System, San Diego, USA. [8]Trauma & Acute Care Service, St Michael's Hospital, Toronto, ON, Canada. [9]Division of General Surgery Rambam Health Care Campus, Haifa, Israel. [10]Department of Surgery, College of Medicine and Health Sciences, UAE University, Al-Ain, United Arab Emirates. [11]Department of Surgery, Macerata Hospital, Macerata, Italy. [12]Department of General Surgery, Royal Perth Hospital, Perth, Australia. [13]Faculdade de Ciências Médicas (FCM)-Unicamp, Campinas, SP, Brazil. [14]Department of Surgery, University of KwaZulu-Natal, Durban, South Africa. [15]Department of Surgery, University of Florida, Gainesville, FL, USA. [16]General Surgery Department, Infermi Hospital, Rimini, Italy.

References
1. Moore EE, Cogbill TH, Jurkovich GJ, Shackford SR, Malangoni MA, Champion HR. Organ injury scaling: spleen and liver (1994 revision). J Trauma. 1995;38: 323–4.
2. Piper G, Peitzman AB. Current management of hepatic trauma. Surg Clin N Am. 2010;90:775–85.
3. Bouras AF, Truant S, Pruvot FR. Management of blunt hepatic trauma. J Visc Surg. 2010;147(6):e351–8.
4. Badger SA, Barclay R, Campbell P, Mole DJ, Diamond T. Management of liver trauma. World J Surg. 2009;33:2522–37.
5. Peitzman AB, Richardson JD. Surgical treatment of injuries to the solid abdominal organs: a 50-years perspective from the Journal of Trauma. J Trauma. 2010;69:1011–21.
6. Coccolini F, Montori G, Catena F, Di Saverio S, Biffl W, Moore EE, Peitzman AB, Rizoli S, Tugnoli G, Sartelli M, Manfredi R, Ansaloni L. Liver trauma: WSES position paper. World J Emerg Surg. 2015;10:39.
7. Croce MA, Fabian TC, Menke PG, Waddle-Smith L, Minard G, Kudsk KA, Patton Jr JH, Schurr MJ, Pritchard FE. Nonoperative management of blunt hepatic trauma is the treatment of choice for hemodynamically stable patients. Results of a prospective trial. Ann Surg. 1995;221(6):744–53.
8. Kozar RA, Feliciano VD, Moore EE, Moore FA, Cocanour CS, West MA, Davis JW, McIntyre Jr RC. Western trauma association/critical decision in trauma: operative management of blunt hepatic trauma. J Trauma. 2011;71(1):1–5.
9. American College of Surgeons. Advanced trauma life support for doctors (ATLS) student manual. 8th ed. 2008.
10. Parks NA, Davis JW, Forman D, Lemaster D. Observation for Nonoperative management of blunt liver injuries: how long is long enough? J Trauma. 2011;70(3):626–9.
11. Hommes M, Navsaria PH, Schipper IB, Krige JE, Kahn D, Nicol AJ. Management of blunt liver trauma in 134 severely injured patients. Injury. 2015;46(5):837–42.
12. Boese CK, Hackl M, Müller LP, Ruchholtz S, Frink M, Lechler P. Nonoperative management of blunt hepatic trauma: a systematic review. J Trauma Acute Care Surg. 2015;79(4):654–60.
13. Kozar RA, Moore FA, Moore EE, West M, Cocanour CS, Davis J, Biffl WL, McIntyre Jr RC. Western trauma association critical decisions in trauma: nonoperative management of adult blunt hepatic trauma. J Trauma. 2009;67:1144–9.
14. Stassen NA, Bhullar I, Cheng JD, Crandall M, Friese R, Guillamondegui O, Jawa R, Maung A, Rohs Jr TJ, Sangosanya A, Schuster K, Seamon M, Tchorz KM, Zarzuar BL, Kerwin A, Eastern Association for the Surgery of Trauma. Non operative management of blunt hepatic injury: an Eastern association for the surgery of trauma practice management guideline. J Trauma Acute Care Surgery. 2012;73(5 Suppl 4):S288–93.
15. Velmahos GC, Toutouzas KG, Radin R, Chan L, Demetriades D. Nonoperative treatment of blunt injury to solid abdominal organs. Arch Surg. 2003;138:844.
16. Yanar H, Ertekin C, Taviloglu K, Kabay B, Bakkaloglu H, Guloglu R. Nonoperative treatment of multiple intra-abdominal solid organ injury after blunt abdominal trauma. J Trauma. 2008;64(4):943–8.
17. Fang JF, Wong YC, Lin BC, Hsu YP, Chen MF. The CT risk factors for the need of operative treatment on initially stable patients after blunt hepatic trauma. J Trauma. 2006;61:547–53.
18. Fang JF, Chen RJ, Wong YC, Lin BC, Hsu YB, Kao JL, Kao YC. Pooling of contrast material on computed tomography mandates aggressive management of blunt hepatic injury. Am J Surg. 1998;176:315–9.
19. Poletti AP, Mirvis SE, Shanmuganathan K, Takada T, Killeen KL, Perlmutter D, Hahn J, Mermillod B. Blunt abdominal trauma patients: can organ injury be excluded without performing computer tomography? J Trauma. 2004;57:1072–81.
20. Wahl WL, Ahrns KS, Brandt MM, Franklin GA, Taheri PA. The need for early angiographic embolization in blunt hepatic injuries. J Trauma. 2002;52: 1097–101.
21. Mohr AM, Lavery RF, Barone A, Bahramipour P, Magnotti LJ, Osband AJ, Sifri Z, Livingston DH. Angioembolization for liver injuries: low mortality, high morbidity. J Trauma. 2003;55(5):1077–81.
22. Stein DM, Scalea TM. Nonoperative management of spleen and liver injuries. J Int Care Med. 2006;21:296.
23. Letoublon C, Amariutei A, Taton N, Lacaze L, Abba J, Risse O, Arvieux C. Management of blunt hepatic trauma. J Visc Surg. 2016;153(4 Suppl):33–43.
24. Fabian TC, Bee TK. Ch.32 Liver and biliary tract. In: Feliciano DV, Mattox KL, Moore EE, editors. Trauma. 7th ed. United States of America: The McGraw-Hill Companies, Inc; 2008. p. 851–70.
25. Marcheix B, Dambrin C, Cron C, Sledzianowski JF, Aguirre J, Suc B, Cerene A, Rousseau H. Transhepatic percutaneous embolisation of a post-traumatic pseudoaneurysm of hepatic artery. Ann Chir. 2004;129(10):603–6.
26. Harrell DJ, Vitale GC, Larson GM. Selective role for endoscopic retrograde cholangiopancreatography in abdominal trauma. Surg Endosc. 1998;12(5):400–4.
27. Letoublon C, Chen Y, Arvieux C, Voirin D, Morra I, Broux C, Risse O. Delayed celiotomy or laparoscopy as part of the nonoperative management of blunt hepatic trauma. World J Surg. 2008;32:1189–93.
28. Biffl WL, Kaups KL, Cothren CC, Brasel KJ, Dicker RA, Bullard MK, Haan JM, Jurkovich GJ, Harrison P, Moore FO, Schreiber M, Knudson MM, Moore EE. Management of patients with anterior abdominal stab wounds: a Western Trauma Association multicenter trial. J Trauma. 2009;66(5):1294–301.
29. Navsaria PH, Nicol AJ, Krige JE, Edu S. Selective nonoperative management of liver gunshot injuries. Ann Surg. 2009;249(4):653.
30. Biffl WL, Leppaniemi A. Management Guidelines for Penetrating Abdominal Trauma. World J Surg. 2015;39(6):1373–80.
31. Lamb CM, Garner JP. Selective non-operative management of civilian gunshot wounds to the abdomen: a systematic review of the evidence. Injury. 2014;45(4):659–66.

32. Biffl WL, Moore EE. Management guidelines for penetrating abdominal trauma. Curr Opin Crit Care. 2010;16(6):609–17.

33. Demetriades D, Hadjizacharia P, Constantinou C, Brown C, Inaba K, Rhee P, Salim A. Selective nonoperative management of penetrating abdominal solid organ injuries. Ann Surg. 2006;244(4):620–8.

34. Biffl WL, Kaups LK, Pham TN, Rowell SE, Jurkovich GJ, Burlew CC, Elterman J, Moore EE. Validating the western trauma association algorithm managing patients with anterior abdominal stable wounds: a western trauma association multi center trial. J Trauma. 2011;71(6):1494–502.

35. Demetriades D, Rabinowitz B. Indications for operation in abdominal stab wounds. A prospective study of 651 patients. Ann Surg. 1987;205(2):129–32.

36. Navsaria PH, Nicol AJ, Edu S, Gandhi R, Ball CG. Selective nonoperative management in 1106 patients with abdominal gunshot wounds: conclusions on safety, efficacy, and the role of selective CT imaging in a prospective single-center study. Ann Surg. 2015;261(4):760–4.

37. Omoshoro-Jones JA, Nicol AJ, Navsaria PH, Zellweger R, Krige JE, Kahn DH. Selective non-operative management of liver gunshot injuries. Br J Surg. 2005;92(7):890–5.

38. Velmahos GC, Constantinou C, Tillou A, Brown CV, Salim A, Demetriades D. Abdominal computed tomographic scan for patients with gunshot wounds to the abdomen selected for non-operative management. J Trauma. 2005; 59(5):1155–60.

39. Demetriades D, Velmahos G. Indication for and technique of Laparotomy. In: Moore, Feliciano, Mattox, editors. Trauma. 6th ed. New York: McGrraw-Hill; 2006.

40. Letoublon C, Reche F, Abba J, Arvieux C. Damage control laparotomy. J Visc Surg. 2011;148(5):e366–70.

41. Letoublon C, Arvieux C. Traumatisme fermés du foie, Principes de technique et de tactique chirurgicales. EMC. Techniques chirurgicales – Appareil digestif, 40–785. 2003. p. 20.

42. Strong RW, Lynch SV, Wall DR, Liu CL. Anatomic resection for severe liver trauma. Surgery. 1998;123:251–7.

43. Polanco P, Stuart L, Pineda J, Puyana JC, Ochoa JB, Alarcon L, Harbrecht BG, Geller D, Peitzman AB. Hepatic resection in the management of complex injury to the liver. J Trauma. 2008;65(6):1264–9.

44. Peitzman AB, Marsh JW. Advanced operative techniques in management of complex liver injury. J Trauma Acute Care Surg. 2012;73(3):765–70.

45. Richardson JD, Franklin GA, Lukan JK, Carrillo EH, Spain DA, Miller FB, Wilson MA, Polk Jr HC, Flint LM. Evolution in the management of hepatic trauma: a 25-year perspective. Ann Surg. 2000;232(3):324–30.

46. Frenklin GA, Casos SR. Current advances in the surgical approach to abdominal trauma. Injury. 2006;37:1143–56.

47. Beal SL. Fatal hepatic hemorrhage: an unresolved problem in the management of complex liver injuries. J Trauma. 1990;30:163.

48. Fabian TC, Croce MA, Stanford GG, Payne LW, Mangiante EC, Voeller GR, Kudsk KA. Factors affecting morbidity following hepatic trauma. A prospective analysis od 482 injuries. Ann Surg. 1991;213:540.

49. Cue JI, Cryer HG, Miller FB, Richardson JD, Polk Jr HC. Packing and planned re-exploration for hepatic and retroperitoneal hemorrhage: critical refinements of a useful technique. J Trauma. 1990;30(8):1007.

50. Biffl WL, Moore EE, Franciose RJ. Venovenous bypass and hepatic vascular isolation as adjuncts in the repair of destructive wounds to the retrohepatic inferior vena cava. J Trauma. 1998;45:400–3.

51. Misselbeck TS, Teicher E, Cipolle MD, Pasquale MD, Shah KT, Dangleben DA, Badellino MM. Hepatic angioembolization in trauma patients:indications and complications. J Trauma. 2009;67:769–73.

52. Johnson JW, Gracias VH, Gupta R, Guillamondegui O, Reilly PM, Shapiro MB, Kauder DR, Schwab CW. Hepatic angiography in patients undergoing damage control laparotomy. J Trauma. 2002;52:1102–6.

53. Asensio JA, Petrone P, García-Núñez L, Kimbrell B, Kuncir E. Multidisciplinary approach for the management of complex hepatic injuries AAST-OIS grades IV-V: a prospective study. Scand J Surg. 2007;96(3):214–20.

54. Dabbs DN, Stein DM, Scalea TM. Major hepatic necrosis: a common complication after angioembolization for treatement of high grade injuries. J Trauma. 2009;66:621–7.

55. Mohr AM, Lavery RF, Barone A, Bahramipour P, Magnotti LJ, Osband AJ, Sifri Z, Livingston DH. Angiographic embolization for liver injuries: low mortality, high morbidity. J Trauma. 2003;55(6):1077–81.

56. Letoublon C, Morra I, Chen Y, Monnin V, Voirin D, Arvieux C. Hepatic arterial embolization in the management of blunt hepatic trauma: indications and complications. J Trauma. 2011;70(5):1032–6.

24

Massive hemothorax due to inferior phrenic artery injury after blunt trauma

Makoto Aoki[1,2*], Kei Shibuya[2], Minoru Kaneko[1], Ayana Koizumi[2], Masato Murata[1], Jun Nakajima[1], Shuichi Hagiwara[1], Masahiko Kanbe[1], Yoshinori Koyama[2], Yoshito Tsushima[2] and Kiyohiro Oshima[1]

Abstract

Injury to the inferior phrenic artery after blunt trauma is an extremely rare event, and it may occur under unanticipated conditions. This case report describes an injury to the left inferior phrenic artery caused by blunt trauma, which was complicated by massive hemothorax, and treated with transcatheter arterial embolization (TAE).

An 81 year-old female hit by a car while walking at the traffic intersection was transferred to the emergency department, computed tomography scanning revealed active extravasations of the contrast medium within the retrocrural space and from branches of the internal iliac artery. The patient underwent repeated angiography, and active extravasation of contrast medium was observed between the retrocrural space and the right pleural space originating from the left inferior phrenic artery. The injured left inferior phrenic artery was successfully embolized with N-butyl cyanoacrylate, resulting in stabilization of the patient's clinical condition.

Inferior phrenic artery injury should be recognized as a rare phenomenon and causative factor for hemothorax. TAE represents a safe and effective treatment for this complication and obviates the need for a thoracotomy.

Keywords: Inferior phrenic artery, Blunt trauma, Transcatheter arterial embolization, N-butyl cyanoacrylate

Background

Injury to the inferior phrenic artery after blunt trauma is an extremely rare event, and it may occur under un-anticipated conditions. In the present case, blunt trauma led to left inferior phrenic artery injury associated with massive hemothorax, which was treated with TAE alone. To the author's knowledge, this is the first report of massive hemothorax due to inferior phrenic artery injury treated definitively by TAE. Furthermore, previous cases of inferior phrenic artery injury after blunt trauma are reviewed.

Review
Case presentation

Following a collision with a car while walking at the traffic intersection, an 81 year-old female was transferred to the emergency department by helicopter. The patient had medication for hypertension and wasn't on

* Correspondence: aokimakoto@gunma-u.ac.jp
[1]Department of Emergency Medicine, Gunma University Graduate School of Medicine, Maebashi, Gunma, Japan
[2]Department of Diagnostic and Interventional Radiology, Gunma University Graduate School of Medicine, Maebashi, Gunma, Japan

antiplatelet or anticoagulant medications. On hospital arrival (50 min after injury) the patient was alert, with a systolic/diastolic blood pressure (SBP/DBP) of 126/86 mmHg, a heart rate of 110 beats/min. Physical examination revealed tenderness in the pelvic region and contusion in the left knee joint. Initial laboratory studies revealed the following values; hemoglobin, 12.0 g/dl; white blood cell (WBC) count, 11,500/µl; platelet count, 16.9×10^4/µl; creatinine (Cr), 0.45 mg/dl; prothrombin time international ratio, 1.00; activated partial thromboplastin time, 26.5 s; Arterial blood gas analysis measured on arrival revealed the following values; pH, 7.430; PCO_2, 30.6 mmHg; PO_2, 69.0 mmHg; HCO_3^-, 21.8 mmol/l; base excess, −3.6 mmol/l; lactate, 2.4 mmol/l.

Computed tomography (CT) scanning with contrast medium (80 min after injury) demonstrated that active extravasations were detected in the retrocrural space (Fig. 1a) and from branches of the internal iliac artery (Fig. 1b) with fractures to the pubic and ischial bones. In addition, No other injuries were observed in the abdominal solid organs, and obvious lung injury, rib fracture and diaphragm rupture were not found. In primary

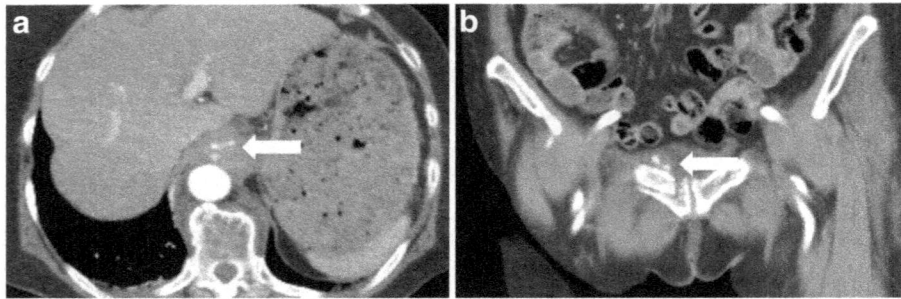

Fig. 1 a Enhanced CT revealed contrast material extravasation within the retrocrural space on arterial phase (arrow). **b** Enhanced CT revealed contrast material extravasation above the pubic bone fractures on arterial phase (arrow)

management intravenous lines were secured and a rapid infusion with normal saline was started, however, approximately 60 min after arrival, the patient's vital signs became unstable (98/58 mmHg and 111 beats/min for SBP/DBP and heart rate, respectively). Immediately blood transfusion was started. To control the continuous bleeding from the pelvic fractures, angiography was performed. The right and left iliac arteries were cannulated with a 5-Fr cobra catheter (Medikit Co. Ltd., Tokyo, Japan). Digital subtraction angiography (DSA) of the internal iliac artery did not demonstrate obvious bleeding from both the internal and the external iliac artery, however, the patient situation was impending and embolization of the bilateral internal iliac arteries was empirically performed with gelatin sponge particles (Serescue; Nippon Kayaku Co. Ltd., Tokyo, Japan) based on the CT scans performed at arrival. CT scans performed during angiography demonstrated that the hematoma extended into the retrocrural space. Injury of the aorta and aortic branches was suspected. Each branch of aorta, comprising the left gastric artery, the celiac artery (including the left inferior phrenic artery) and superior mesenteric artery, was cannulated with a 5-Fr shepherd's hook catheter (Terumo Clinical Supply Co. Ltd., Gifu, Japan) and a 5-Fr Michelson catheter (Medikit Co. Ltd., Tokyo, Japan). However, obvious extravasation was not confirmed. The patient recovered from shock and was transferred to the intensive care unit (ICU), but shock occurred again at 3 h post-ICU admission. Enhanced CT scans were performed again and revealed the hematoma extending from within the retrocrural space to the right pleural space, and extravasation within the retrocrural space (Fig. 2). Therefore, angiography was immediately repeated. The left inferior phrenic artery was cannulated with a 5-Fr Michelson catheter, and DSA of the left inferior phrenic artery showed extravasation (Fig. 3a). NBCA was mixed with iodized oil (Lipiodol; Andre Guerbet, Aulnay-sous-Bois, France) at a ratio of 1:3, and the

mixture was injected. Post-embolization angiography was performed to confirm the absence of extravasation, and completion of TAE (Fig. 3b). Massive hemothorax in the right pleural space was demonstrated on post-embolization chest CT. A thoracostomy tube was inserted, and approximately 1000 ml of bloody fluid was collected. After TAE, the increase of hemothorax was not confirmed. The patient needed 14 units of red blood cells and 8 units of fresh frozen plasma within 24 h from injury. The post-treatment course was uneventful and clinical symptoms revealing a diaphragmatic injury were not seen. The patient was enrolled in orthopediac department for the operation of left knee joint on the 17th day and transferred to another hospital for rehabilitation without complications on the 39th day.

Discussion

This was an unusual case of hemothorax because it was not accompanied by damage to the thoracic and abdominal organs. Only one case was previously reported in

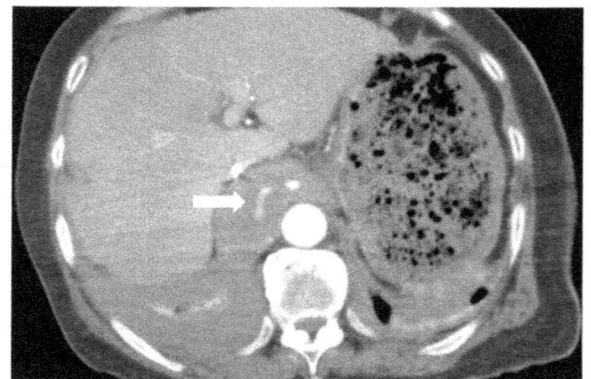

Fig. 2 Enhanced CT showed the extension of the hematoma from within the retrocrural space to the right pleural space, and the extravasation of the retrocrural space (arrow)

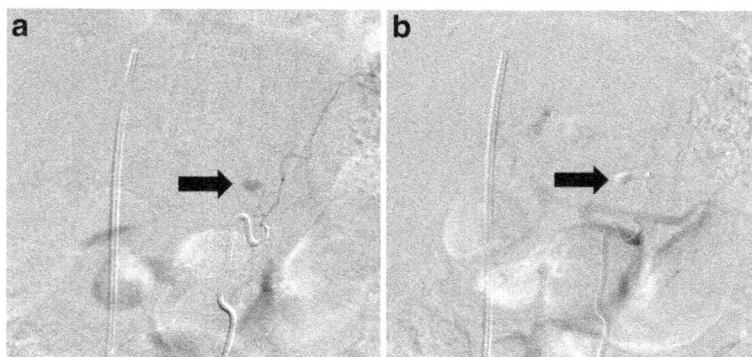

Fig. 3 a Digital subtraction angiography of the left inferior phrenic artery angiography demonstrated contrast material extravasation (arrow). **b** After transcatheter arterial embolization, N-Butyl Cyanoacrylate (NBCA) and Lipiodol were detected (arrow)

which hemothorax was caused by inferior phrenic artery injury, without multiple organ injury [1], however, this is the first report of an injured left inferior phrenic artery injury resulting in contralateral right hemothorax. Data from the present case suggest that damage to the left inferior phrenic artery injury led to a hemorrhage in mediastinum, which subsequently ruptured into the right pleural region.

The inferior phrenic artery originates between the middle of the second lumbar vertebrae and the twelfth thoracic vertebrae [2]. The right and left inferior phrenic arteries arise from the ascending (anterior), descending (posterior), superior suprarenal, and middle suprarenal branches. The ascending branch of the left inferior phrenic artery divides into the esophageal and accessory splenic branches [3]. According to various branches of the inferior phrenic artery, the injury of inferior phrenic artery has the potential to cause multiple clinical conditions. To date only four cases of inferior phrenic artery injury (excluding this report) have been reported, and each case was related to a different condition (Table 1) [1, 4–6]. TAE was selected as the treatment in four of the five reported cases, but different embolic materials were used. In the present case, TAE was performed for hemostasis, and NBCA was selected as the embolic material because the patient exhibited coagulopathy induced by severe trauma, with vital signs indicating shock. NBCA is considered to be the most appropriate

embolic material for cases with hemorrhagic diathesis because it does not depend on the coagulation process for its therapeutic effect [7]. In contrast to Ogawa et al., we succeeded in complete treatment by TAE with NBCA [1]. This is the first report concerning an inferior phrenic artery injury complicated with massive hemothorax, and treated only by TAE using NBCA.

Lee et al. described a patient with inferior phrenic artery injury accompanied by diaphragmatic injury, and laparotomy was selected [6]. Laparotomy is the best choice for single stage restoration. The present case was definitively treated by TAE and not accompanied by diaphragmatic injury, however, the combination of laparoscopy and thoracoscopy could be safe management and more useful for detecting the diaphragmatic injury [8].

In the other four cases, there were no concomitant injuries and complications. TAE may circumvent the need for thoracotomy or laparotomy, if the arterial injury is not associated with diaphragmatic rupture and stomach herniation into the left hemithorax [6]. TAE is commonly considered the most reliable and feasible therapeutic alternative to thoracotomy for control of intrathoracic arterial hemorrhages [9, 10] and is useful alternative treatment for a thoracotomy, which could be fatal in this 80+ year old patient. The authors propose that TAE represents the optimal strategy for management of inferior phrenic artery injury without diaphragmatic injury, and advances in microcatheter designs and

Table 1 The characteristics of the reported cases of inferior phrenic artery injury due to blunt trauma

Author	N	Clinical presentation	Diaphragmatic injury	Subsequent Treatment	Embolic material of TAE
Blaise	1	Pericardial tamponade	None	TAE	Polyvinyl alcohol particles
Mizobata	2	Intraperitoneal hemorrhage and Subcapsular hematoma	None	TAE	NS
Lee	1	Intrapetironeal hemorrhage	Grade V	Laparotomy	
Ogawa	1	Hemothorax	None	TAE and thoracotomy	Coil embolization
Aoki (present)	1	Hemothorax	None	TAE	NBCA

N number of patients, *TAE* transcatheter arterial embolization, *NS* not shown, *NBCA* N-butyl cyanoacrylate

embolic agents have contributed to the safety and effectiveness of TAE.

Conclusions

In the summary we described the case of the left inferior phrenic artery injury who suffered blunt trauma. The findings suggest that hemothorax may be induced by inferior phrenic artery injury and this is very rare phenomenon. TAE can be a safe and effective treatment for the inferior phrenic artery bleeding and obviates the need for a thoracotomy.

Consent statement

Written informed consent was obtained from the patient for publication of this Case report and any accompanying images. A copy of the written consent is available for review by the Editor-in-Chief of this journal.

Competing interests
The authors declare that they have no competing interests.

Authors' contributions
All authors read and approved the final manuscript.

Acknowledgements
There is no one to acknowledge except for the co-authors listed.

References

1. Ogawa F, Naito M, Iyoda A, Satoh Y. Report of a rare case: occult hemothorax due to blunt trauma without obvious injury to other organs. J Cardiothorac Surg. 2013;8:205.
2. Pick JM, Anson BJ. The inferior phrenic artery: origin and suprarenal branches. Anat Rec. 1940;78:413–27.
3. Loukas M, Hullett J, Wagner T. Clinical anatomy of the inferior phrenic artery. Clin Anat. 2005;18(5):357–65.
4. Jones BV, Vu D. Diagnosis of posttraumatic pericardial tamponade by plain film and computed tomography and control of bleeding by embolotherapy of the left inferior phrenic artery. Cardiovasc Intervent Radiol. 1993;16(3):183–5.
5. Mizobata Y, Yokota J, Yajima Y, Sakashita K. Two cases of blunt hepatic injury with active bleeding from the right inferior phrenic artery. J Trauma. 2000;48(6):1153–5.
6. Lee JW, Kim S, Kim CW, Kim KH, Jeon TY. Massive hemoperitoneum due to ruptured inferior phrenic artery pseudoaneurysm after blunt trauma. Emerg Radiol. 2006;13(3):147–9.
7. Yonemitsu T, Kawai N, Sato M, Tanihata H, Takasaka I, Nakai M, et al. Evaluation of transcatheter arterial embolization with gelatin sponge particles, microcoils, and n-butyl cyanoacrylate for acute arterial bleeding in a coagulopathic condition. J Vasc Interv Radiol. 2009;20(9):1176–87.
8. Ochsner MG, Rozycki GS, Lucente F, Wherry DC, Champion HR. Prospective evaluation of thoracoscopy for diagnosing diaphragmatic injury in thoracoabdominal trauma: a preliminary report. J Trauma. 1993;34(5):704–9.
9. Carrillo EHHB, Senler SO, Dykes JR, Maniscalco SP, Richardson JD. Embolization therapy as an alternative to thoracotomy in vascular injuries of the chest wall. Am Surg. 1998;64:7.
10. Chemelli AP, Thauerer M, Wiedermann F, Strasak A, Klocker J, Chemelli-Steingruber IE. Transcatheter arterial embolization for the management of iatrogenic and blunt traumatic intercostal artery injuries. J Vasc Surg. 2009;49(6):1505–13.

25

Pelvic trauma: WSES classification and guidelines

Federico Coccolini[1*], Philip F. Stahel[2], Giulia Montori[1], Walter Biffl[3], Tal M Horer[4], Fausto Catena[5], Yoram Kluger[6], Ernest E. Moore[7], Andrew B. Peitzman[8], Rao Ivatury[9], Raul Coimbra[10], Gustavo Pereira Fraga[11], Bruno Pereira[11], Sandro Rizoli[12], Andrew Kirkpatrick[13], Ari Leppaniemi[14], Roberto Manfredi[1], Stefano Magnone[1], Osvaldo Chiara[15], Leonardo Solaini[1], Marco Ceresoli[1], Niccolò Allievi[1], Catherine Arvieux[16], George Velmahos[17], Zsolt Balogh[18], Noel Naidoo[19], Dieter Weber[20], Fikri Abu-Zidan[21], Massimo Sartelli[22] and Luca Ansaloni[1]

Abstract

Complex pelvic injuries are among the most dangerous and deadly trauma related lesions. Different classification systems exist, some are based on the mechanism of injury, some on anatomic patterns and some are focusing on the resulting instability requiring operative fixation. The optimal treatment strategy, however, should keep into consideration the hemodynamic status, the anatomic impairment of pelvic ring function and the associated injuries. The management of pelvic trauma patients aims definitively to restore the homeostasis and the normal physiopathology associated to the mechanical stability of the pelvic ring. Thus the management of pelvic trauma must be multidisciplinary and should be ultimately based on the physiology of the patient and the anatomy of the injury. This paper presents the World Society of Emergency Surgery (WSES) classification of pelvic trauma and the management Guidelines.

Keywords: Pelvic, Trauma, Management, Guidelines, Mechanic, Injury, Angiography, REBOA, ABO, Preperitoneal pelvic packing, External fixation, Internal fixation, X-ray, Pelvic ring fractures

Background

Pelvic trauma (PT) is one of the most complex management in trauma care and occurs in 3% of skeletal injuries [1–4]. Patients with pelvic fractures are usually young and they have a high overall injury severity score (ISS) (25 to 48 ISS) [3]. Mortality rates remain high, particularly in patients with hemodynamic instability, due to the rapid exsanguination, the difficulty to achieve hemostasis and the associated injuries [1, 2, 4, 5]. For these reasons, a multidisciplinary approach is crucial to manage the resuscitation, to control the bleeding and to manage bones injuries particularly in the first hours from trauma. PT patients should have an integrated management between trauma surgeons, orthopedic surgeons, interventional radiologists, anesthesiologists, ICU doctors and urologists 24/7 [6, 7].

At present no comprehensive guidelines have been published about these issues. No correlation has been demonstrated to exist between type of pelvic ring anatomical lesions and patient physiologic status. Moreover the management of pelvic trauma has markedly changed throughout the last decades with a significant improvement in outcomes, due to improvements in diagnostic and therapeutic tools. In determining the optimal treatment strategy, the anatomical lesions classification should be supplemented by hemodynamic status and associated injuries. The anatomical description of pelvic ring lesions is fundamental in the management algorithm but not definitive. In fact, in clinical practice the first decisions are based mainly on the clinical conditions and the associated injuries, and less on the pelvic ring lesions. Ultimately, the management of trauma requires an assessment of the anatomical injury and its physiologic effects.

This paper aims to present the World Society of Emergency Surgery (WSES) classification of pelvic trauma and the treatment Guidelines.

* Correspondence: federico.coccolini@gmail.com
[1]General, Emergency and Trauma Surgery, Papa Giovanni XXIII Hospital, P.zza OMS 1, 24128 Bergamo, Italy
Full list of author information is available at the end of the article

WSES includes surgeons from whole world. This Classification and Guidelines statements aim to direct the management of pelvic trauma, acknowledging that there are acceptable alternative management options. In reality, as already considered for other position papers and guidelines, not all trauma surgeons work in the same conditions and have the same facilities and technologies available [8].

Notes on the use of the guidelines

The Guidelines are evidence-based, with the grade of recommendation also based on the evidence. The Guidelines present the diagnostic and therapeutic methods for optimal management of pelvic trauma. The practice Guidelines promulgated in this work do not represent a standard of practice. They are suggested plans of care, based on best available evidence and the consensus of experts, but they do not exclude other approaches as being within the standard of practice. For example, they should not be used to compel adherence to a given method of medical management, which method should be finally determined after taking account of the conditions at the relevant medical institution (staff levels, experience, equipment, etc.) and the characteristics of the individual patient. However, responsibility for the results of treatment rests with those who are directly engaged therein, and not with the consensus group.

Methods

Eight specific questions were addressed regarding the management of PT assessing the main problems related to the hemodynamic and the mechanical status:

- 1 Which are the main diagnostic tools necessary prior to proceed in hemodynamically unstable PT?
- 2 Which is the role of pelvic binder in hemodynamically unstable pelvic fracture?
- 3 Which is the role of Resuscitative Endovascular Balloon Occlusion of the Aorta (REBOA) in hemodynamically unstable pelvic trauma?
- 4 Which patients with hemodynamically unstable PT warrant preperitoneal pelvic packing?
- 5 Which patients with hemodynamically unstable pelvic ring injuries require external pelvic fixation?
- 6 Which patients with hemodynamically unstable PT warrant angioembolization?
- 7 What are the indications for definitive surgical fixation of pelvic ring injuries?
- 8 What is the ideal time-window to proceed with definitive internal pelvic fixation?

A computerized search was done by the bibliographer in different databanks (MEDLINE, SCOPUS, EMBASE)

citations were included for the period between January 1980 to December 2015 using the primary search strategy: pelvis, pelvic, injuries, trauma, resuscitation, sacral, bone screws, fractures, external fixation, internal fixation, anterior e posterior fixation, hemodynamic instability/stability, packing, pubic symphisis, angioembolization, pelvic binder/binding, aortic, balloon, occlusion, resuscitative, definitive, stabilization combined with AND/OR. No search restrictions were imposed. The dates were selected to allow comprehensive published abstracts of clinical trials, consensus conference, comparative studies, congresses, guidelines, government publication, multicenter studies, systematic reviews, meta-analysis, large case series, original articles, randomized controlled trials. Case reports and small cases series were excluded. No randomized controlled trials were found. Narrative review articles were also analyzed to determine other possible studies. Literature selection is reported in the flow chart (Fig. 1). The Level of Evidence (LE) was evaluated using the GRADE system [9] (Table 1).

The discussion of the present guidelines has been realized through the Delphi process. A group of experts in the field coordinated by a central coordinator was contacted separately to express their evidence-based opinion on the different questions about the hemodynamically and mechanically unstable pelvic trauma management. Pelvic trauma patterns were differentiated into hemodynamically and mechanically stable and unstable ones. Conservative and operative management for all combinations of these conditions were evaluated. The central coordinator assembled the different answers derived from the first round and drafted the first version that was subsequently revised by each member of an enlarged expert group separately. The central coordinator addressed the definitive amendments, corrections and concerns. The definitive version about which the agreement was reached consisted in the published guidelines.

Mechanisms of injuries

Principal mechanisms of injuries that cause a pelvic ring fracture are due to a high energy impact as fall from height, sports, road traffic collision (pedestrian, motorcyclist, motor vehicle, cyclist), person stuck by vehicles [1, 5]. Ten to fifteen percent of patients with pelvic fractures arrive to the ED in shock and one third of them will die reaching a mortality rate in the more recent reports of 32% [10]. The causes of dying are represented in the major part by uncontrolled bleeding and by patient's physiologic exhaustion.

Anatomy of pelvis and pelvic injuries

Pelvic ring is a close compartment of bones containing urogenital organs, rectum, vessels and nerves. Bleeding from pelvic fractures can occur from veins (80%) and

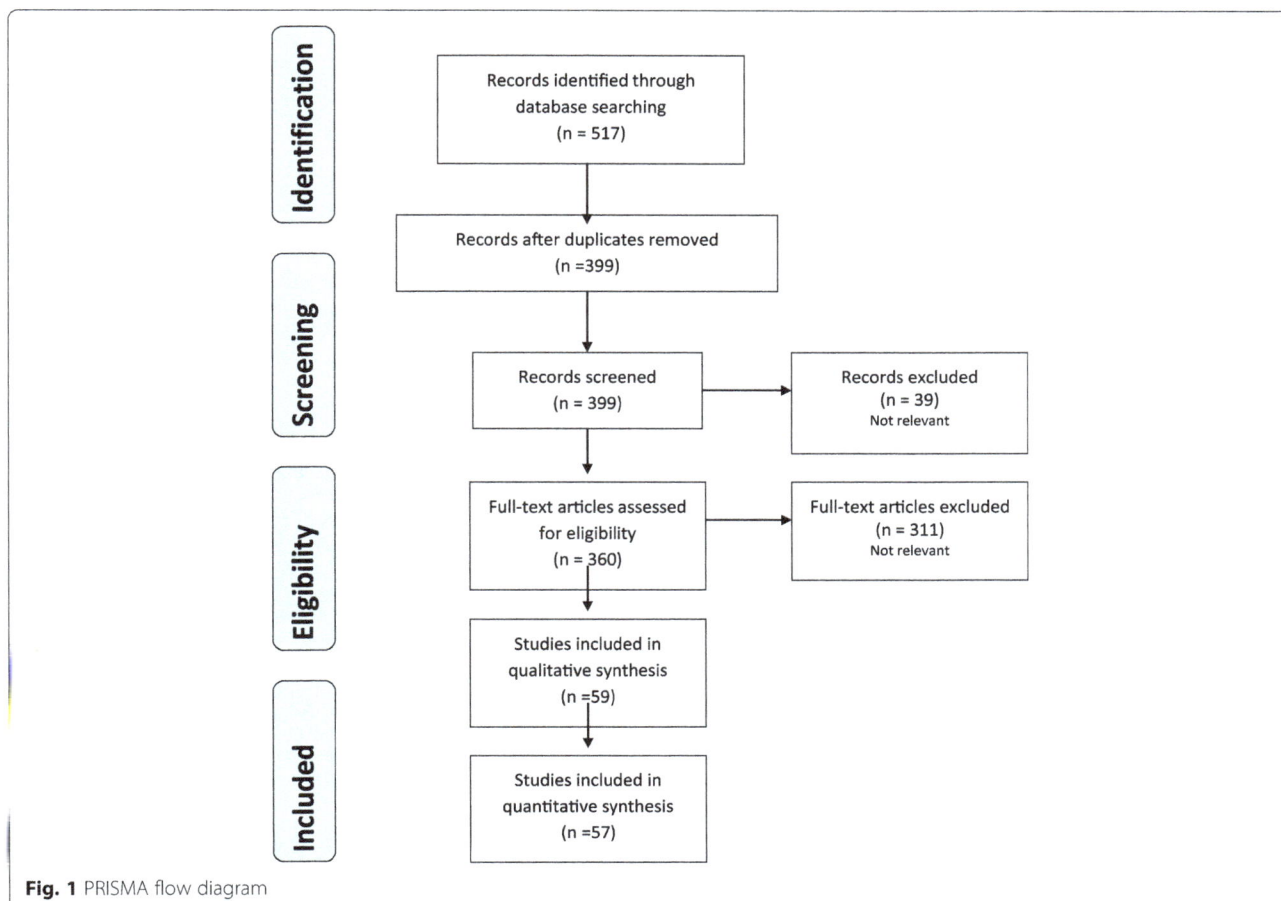

Fig. 1 PRISMA flow diagram

from arteries (20%) [7, 11]. Principal veins injured are presacral plexus and prevescical veins, and the principals arteries are anterior branches of the internal iliac artery, the pudendal and the obturator artery anteriorly, and superior gluteal artery and lateral sacral artery posteriorly [7, 11]. Others sources of bleeding include bones fractures [1]. Among the different fracture patterns affecting the pelvic ring each has a different bleeding probability. No definitive association between fracture pattern and bleeding exist but some pattern as APC III are associated to a greater transfusion rate according to some studies [12]. Part of the bleeding is from the bones as clearly showed since 1973. The necessity to fix the bones fractures by repositioning them has been explained by Huittimen et al. [13]. In cases of high-grade injuries, thoraco-abdominal associated injuries can occur in 80%, and others local lesions such as bladder, urethra (1.6-25% of cases), vagina, nerves, sphincters and rectum (18–64%), soft tissues injuries (up to 72%). These injuries should be strongly suspected particularly in patients with perineal hematoma or large soft tissue disruption [1, 3, 14]. These patients need an integrate management with other specialists. Some procedures like

supra-pubic catheterization of bladder, colostomy with local debridement and drainage, and antibiotic prevention are important to avoid aggravating urethral injuries or to avoid fecal contamination in case of a digestive tract involvement [1]. Although these conditions must be respected and kept in mind the first aim remains the hemodynamic and pelvic ring stabilization.

Physiopathology of the injuries

The lesions at the level of the pelvic ring can create instability of the ring itself and a consequent increase in the internal volume. This increase in volume, particular in open book lesions, associated to the soft tissue and vascular disruption, facilitate the increasing hemorrhage in the retroperitoneal space by reducing the tamponing effect (pelvic ring can contain up to a few liters of blood) and can cause an alteration in hemodynamic status [7, 15]. In the management of severely injured and bleeding patients a cornerstone is represented by the early evaluation and correction of the trauma induced coagulopathy. Resuscitation associated to physiologic impairment and to suddenly activation and deactivation of several procoagulant and anticoagulant factors contributes to the insurgence of this

Table 1 GRADE system to evaluate the level of evidence and recommendation

Grade of recommendation	Clarity of risk/benefit	Quality of supporting evidence	Implications
1A			
Strong recommendation, high-quality evidence	Benefits clearly outweigh risk and burdens, or vice versa	RCTs without important limitations or overwhelming evidence from observational studies	Strong recommendation, applies to most patients in most circumstances without reservation
1B			
Strong recommendation, moderate-quality evidence	Benefits clearly outweigh risk and burdens, or vice versa	RCTs with important limitations (inconsistent results, methodological flaws, indirect analyses or imprecise conclusions) or exceptionally strong evidence from observational studies	Strong recommendation, applies to most patients in most circumstances without reservation
1C			
Strong recommendation, low-quality or very low-quality evidence	Benefits clearly outweigh risk and burdens, or vice versa	Observational studies or case series	Strong recommendation but subject to change when higher quality evidence becomes available
2A			
Weak recommendation, high-quality evidence	Benefits closely balanced with risks and burden	RCTs without important limitations or overwhelming evidence from observational studies	Weak recommendation, best action may differ depending on the patient, treatment circumstances, or social values
2B			
Weak recommendation, moderate-quality evidence	Benefits closely balanced with risks and burden	RCTs with important limitations (inconsistent results, methodological flaws, indirect or imprecise) or exceptionally strong evidence from observational studies	Weak recommendation, best action may differ depending on the patient, treatment circumstances, or social values
2C			
Weak recommendation, Low-quality or very low-quality evidence	Uncertainty in the estimates of benefits, risks, and burden; benefits, risk, and burden may be closely balanced	Observational studies or case series	Very weak recommendation; alternative treatments may be equally reasonable and merit consideration

frequently deadly condition. The massive transfusion protocol application is fundamental in managing bleeding patients. As clearly demonstrated by the literature blood products, coagulation factors and drugs administration has to be guided by a tailored approach through advanced evaluation of the patient's coaugulative asset [16–22]. Some authors consider a normal hemodynamic status when the patient does not require fluids or blood to maintain blood pressure, without signs of hypoperfusion; hemodynamic stability as a counterpart is the condition in which the patient achieve a constant or an amelioration of blood pressure after fluids with a blood pressure >90 mmHg and heart rate <100 bpm [23]; hemodynamic instability is the condition in which the patient has an admission systolic blood pressure <90 mmHg, or > 90 mmHg but requiring bolus infusions/transfusions and/or vasopressor drugs and/or admission base deficit (BD) >6 mmol/l and/or shock index > 1 [24, 25] and/or transfusion requirement of at least 4–6 Units of packed red blood cells within the first 24 hours [5, 16, 26]. The Advanced Trauma Life Support (ATLS) definition considers as "unstable" the patient with: blood pressure < 90 mmHg and

heart rate > 120 bpm, with evidence of skin vasoconstriction (cool, clammy, decreased capillary refill), altered level of consciousness and/or shortness of breath [26]. The present classification and guideline utilize the ATLS definition. Some authors suggested that the sacroiliac joint disruption, female gender, duration of hypotension, an hematocrit of 30% or less, pulse rate of 130 or greater, displaced obturator ring fracture, a pubic symphysis diastasis can be considered good predictors of major pelvic bleeding [2, 15, 27]. However unfortunately the extent of bleeding is not always related with the type of lesions and there is a poor correlation between the grade of the radiological lesions and the need for emergent hemostasis [7, 15, 28].

WSES Classification

The anatomical description of pelvic ring lesions is not definitive in the management of pelvic injuries. The classification of pelvic trauma into minor, moderate and severe considers the pelvic ring injuries anatomic classification (Antero-Posterior Compression APC; Lateral Compression LC; Vertical Shear VS; CM: Combined Mechanisms) and more importantly, the hemodynamic status. As already stated the ATLS definition considers as "unstable" the patient with: blood pressure < 90 mmHg and heart rate > 120 bpm, with evidence of skin vasoconstriction (cool, clammy, decreased capillary refill), altered level of consciousness and/or shortness of breath [26].

The WSES Classification divides Pelvic ring Injuries into three classes:

- *Minor* (WSES grade I) comprising hemodynamically and mechanically stable lesions
- *Moderate* (WSES grade II, III) comprising hemodynamically stable and mechanically unstable lesions
- *Severe* (WSES grade IV) comprising hemodynamically unstable lesions independently from mechanical status.

The classification (Table 2) considers the Young-Burgees classification (Fig. 2), the hemodynamic status and the associated lesions.

Minor pelvic injuries:

- *WSES grade I (should be formatted in bold and cursive as the other grade of classification)* includes APC I, LC I hemodynamically stable pelvic ring injuries.

Moderate pelvic injuries:

- *WSES grade II* includes APC II – III and LC II - III hemodynamically stable pelvic ring injuries.
- *WSES grade III* includes VS and CM hemodynamically stable pelvic ring injuries.

Severe pelvic injuries:

- *WSES grade IV* includes any hemodynamically unstable pelvic ring injuries.

Basing on the present classification WSES indicates a management algorithm explained in Fig. 3.

Principles and cornerstones of the management
The management of pelvic trauma as for all the other politraumatized patients needs to pose in definitive the attention in treating also the physiology; decisions can be more effective when combining evaluation of anatomy, mechanical consequences of injury and their physiological effects. During daily clinical practice the first decisions are based mainly on the clinical conditions and the associated injuries, and less on the pelvic ring lesions. The management of trauma in fact aims firstly to restore the altered physiology. The main aims of proper PT management are bleeding control and stabilization of the hemodynamic status, restoring of the eventual coagulation disorders and the mechanical integrity and stability of the pelvic ring, and preventing complications (septic, urogenital, intestinal, vascular, sexual functions, walking) (×9); then to definitively stabilize the pelvis.

Recommendations for diagnostic tools use in Pelvic Trauma

- *- The time between arrival in the Emergency Department and definitive bleeding control should be minimized to improve outcomes of patients with hemodynamically unstable pelvic fractures [Grade 2A].*
- *- Serum lactate and base deficit represent sensitive diagnostic markers to estimate the extent of traumatic-haemorrhagic shock, and to monitor response to resuscitation [Grade 1B].*
- *- The use of Pelvic X-ray and E-FAST in the Emergency Department is recommended in hemodynamic and mechanic unstable patients with pelvic trauma*

Table 2 WSES pelvic injuries classification (*: patients hemodynamically stable and mechanically unstable with no other lesions requiring treatment and with a negative CT-scan, can proceed directly to definitive mechanical stabilization. LC: Lateral Compression, APC: Antero-posterior Compression, VS: Vertical Shear, CM: Combined Mechanism, NOM: Non-Operative Management, OM: Operative Management, REBOA: Resuscitative Endo-Aortic Balloon)

	WSES grade	Young-Burgees classification	Haemodynamic	Mechanic	CT-scan	First-line Treatment
MINOR	WSES grade I	APC I – LC I	Stable	Stable	Yes	NOM
MODERATE	WSES grade II	LC II/III - APC II/III	Stable	Unstable	Yes	Pelvic Binder in the field ± Angioembolization (if blush at CT-scan) OM – Anterior External Fixation *
	WSES grade III	VS - CM	Stable	Unstable	Yes	Pelvic Binder in the field ± Angioembolization (if blush at CT-scan) OM - C-Clamp *
SEVERE	WSES grade IV	Any	Unstable	Any	No	Pelvic Binder in the field Preperitoneal Pelvic Packing ± Mechanical fixation (see over) ± REBOA ± Angioembolization

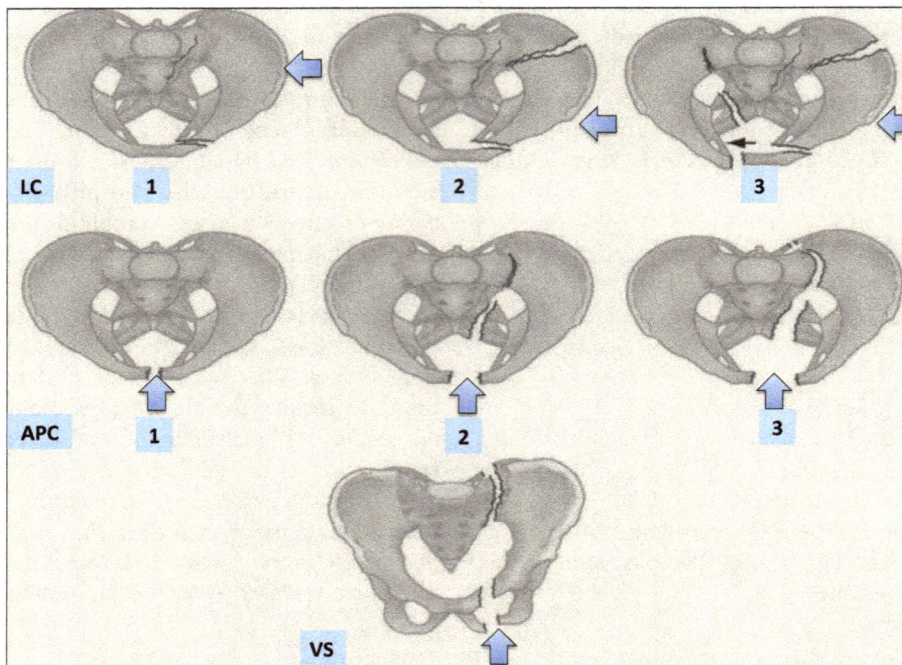

Fig. 2 Young and Burgees classification for skeletal pelvic lesions

and allows to identify the injuries that require an early pelvic stabilization, an early angiography, and a rapid reductive maneuver, as well as laparotomy [Grade 1B].

— *- Patients with pelvic trauma associated to hemodynamic normality or stability should undergo further diagnostic workup with multi phasic CT-scan with intravenous contrast to exclude pelvic hemorrhage [Grade 1B].*

— *- CT-scan with 3-Dimensional bones reconstructions reduces the tissue damage during invasive procedures, the risk of neurological disorders after surgical fixation, operative time, and irradiation and the required expertise [Grade 1B].*

— *- Retrograde urethrogram or/and urethrocystogram with contrast CT-scan is recommended in presence of local perineal clinical hematoma and pelvic disruption at Pelvic X-ray [Grade 1B].*

— *- Perineal and a rectal digital examination are mandatory in case of high suspicious of rectal injuries [Grade 1B].*

— *- In case of a positive rectal examination, proctoscopy is recommended [Grade 1C].*

Diagnostic workup strategies in the emergency room must be standardized and streamlined in order to avoid an unnecessary delay to definitive bleeding control, the time between trauma and operating room has been shown to inversely correlate with survival in patients with traumatic pelvic hemorrhage [29].

Sensitive **laboratory markers** of acute traumatic hemorrhage include serum lactate and base deficit by arterial blood gas analysis [29]. In contrast, hemoglobin level and hematocrit do not represent sensitive early markers of the extent of traumatic hemorrhagic shock [29]. As coagulopathic patients with traumatic hemorrhagic shock form unstable pelvic ring injuries have a significantly increased post-injury mortality [16], the presence of coagulopathy should be determined early by "point-of-care" bedside testing using Thromboelastography (TEG) or Rotational Thromboelastometry (ROTEM), which allow targeted resuscitation with blood products and improved post-injury survival rates [17, 19–22]. At first, the evaluation of a PT should be based on the mechanism of injury (particularly in case of high-energy impact, more frequent in blunt trauma) and physical examination to search a pelvic ring deformity or instability, a pelvic or perineal hematoma, or a rectal/urethral bleeding [1]. Lelly maneuver can be useful in evaluating the pelvic ring stability but it should be done cautiously because it can sometime increase the bleeding by dislocating bones margin. In case of hemodynamic instability, particularly in blunt trauma, chest and pelvic x-rays and extended focused assessment for sonographic evaluation of trauma patients (E-FAST) are performed according to ATLS protocols. Chest X-rays and E-FAST are performed to exclude others sours of hemorrhage in the thorax and in the abdomen [1, 7, 30, 31]. The Eastern Association for the Surgery of Trauma guidelines [2]

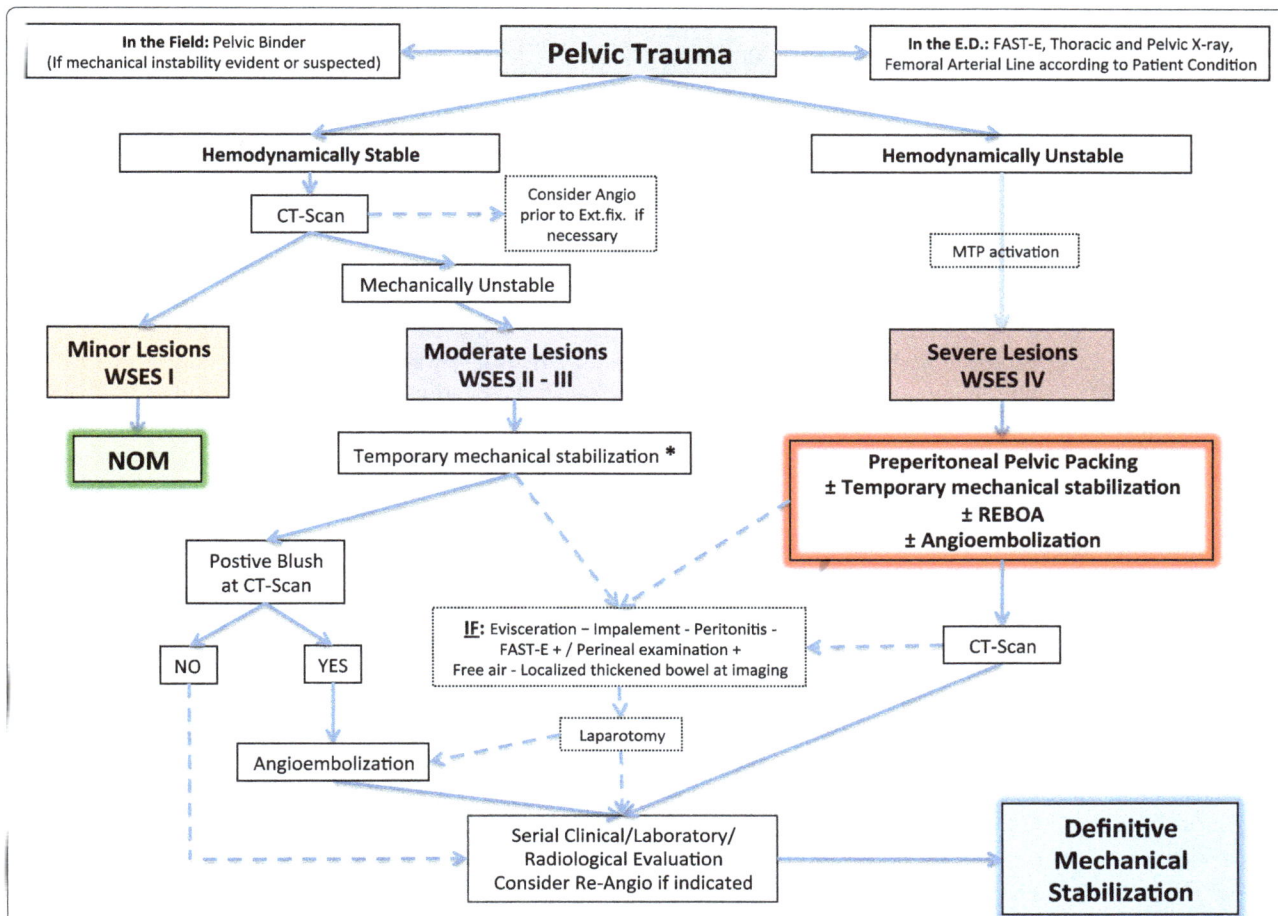

Fig. 3 Pelvic Trauma management algorithm (*: patients hemodynamically stable and mechanically unstable with no other lesions requiring treatment and with a negative CT-scan, can proceed directly to definitive mechanical stabilization. MTP: Massive Transfusion Protocol, FAST-E: Eco-FAST Extended, ED: Emergency Department, CT: Computed Tomography, NOM: Non Operative Management, HEMODYNAMIC STABILITY is the condition in which the patient achieve a constant or an amelioration of blood pressure after fluids with a blood pressure >90 mmHg and heart rate <100 bpm; HEMODYNAMIC INSTABILITY is the condition in which the patient has an admission systolic blood pressure <90 mmHg, or > 90 mmHg but requiring bolus infusions/transfusions and/or vasopressor drugs, or admission base deficit (BD) >6 mmol/l, or shock index > 1, or transfusion requirement of at least 4–6 Units of packed red blood cells within the first 24 h)

reported that E-FAST is not enough sensitive to exclude a pelvic bleeding, however it could be considered adequate to exclude the need for a laparotomy in unstable patients.

Pelvic X-ray (PXR) in hemodynamically unstable patients helps in identifying life-threatening pelvic ring injuries [18, 32, 33]. It is important but its execution must not delay in proceeding with life-saving maneuvers. Sensitivity and sensibility rates are low (50–68% and 98% respectively) and the false negative rates are high (32%) [23, 34]. For these reason some authors suggested to abandon PXR in case of stable patients [11, 23, 34]. The principal injuries related with hemodynamic instability are sacral fractures, open-book injuries and vertical-shear injuries (APC II-III, LC II-III and VS) [34]. To clearly define injury pattern, it is fundamental to achieve

early pelvic stabilization and to early plan for the subsequent diagnostic-therapeutic approach. Moreover PXR is important to evaluate the hip dislocation in order to provide a prompt reductive maneuver [34]. However PXR alone does not predict mortality, hemorrhage or need for angiography [2]. In hemodynamically normal patients with nor pelvic instability nor hip dislocation nor positive physical examination scheduled for CT-scan PXR could be omitted [11].

At the end of primary evaluation a radiological workup is performed. In case of hemodynamic normality or stability *Computed Tomography (CT)* is the gold standard with a sensitivity and specificity for bones fractures of 100% [1, 23, 34]. The main two factors that are important to plan a correct decision-making process and to steer the angiography are the presence at CT of intravenous contrast extravasation and the pelvic hematoma size [2, 35]. CT has an accuracy of 98% for identifying patients with blush, however an absence of blush in contrast CT does not always exclude an active pelvic bleeding [2, 28]. In presence of a pelvic hematoma ≥500 cm3 an arterial injury should be strongly suspected even in absence of a visible contrast blush [2]. CT is useful also to evaluate any injuries of other organs, retroperitoneum, and bones but also to better decide the subsequent surgical management [34]. A recent study supports the use of a multidetector CT with a three phases protocol (arterial, portal and delayed phase) with a subsequent digital subtraction angiography (DSA) in case of suspect of arterial hemorrhage so as to better evaluate bleeding or hematoma [35]. This protocol could significantly reduce the rate of subsequent interventions due to others hemorrhagic foci [35].

CT with 3-Dimensional bone reconstruction is helpful reducing tissue damage during invasive procedure, reducing the subjective expertise required from clinical staff and improving patient recovery times [36]. Chen and coll. reported successful rates of screw positioning in 93.8% of cases after 3D CT reconstruction, particularly in patients with sacral fractures and ilio-sacral joint dislocations [36]. This approach permits to also reduce the neurological disorders after surgical fixation, operative times, and irradiation.

In 7-25% of pelvic ring fractures lower urinary tract and urethra are damaged. However the diagnosis of urethral injuries remains difficult at the initial evaluation and about 23% of them are missed [14]. Clinical signs suggesting a urethral injury are perineal/scrotal hematoma, blood from the urethral meatus, the presence of a high-riding or non-palpable prostate at rectal exploration, the presence of an unstable pelvic fracture. The insertion of a transurethral catheter without other previous investigations in patients with a pelvic injury could be associated with severe complications: either acute like complete transection of the urethra, or chronic like stricture formation, impotence and urinary incontinence [14]. For this reason ATLS guidelines, the World Health Organization and some authors [14] suggested a *retrograde urethrogram (RUG)* prior the urethral catheterization. RUGs is recommended when local clinical signs or a disruption in the PXR are found, particularly in the presence of higher degree of soft tissue disruption, bone displacement, or multiple fractures [14]. In case a positive of RUG or when high suspicion of urethral injury are present, a suprapubic catheter with delayed cystogram is recommended [14]. Magnetic resonance images seem promising to detect type of injuries and could be a useful tool in combination with RUGs or in alternative but only in stable patients [14]. However the sequence between RUG and *urethrocystogram with*

contrast CT is controversial [2]. Performing a RUG before CT could increase the rate of indeterminate and false-negative CT-scans [2]. For this reason when hemodynamic status permits in case of suspected urethral injuries the late contrast CT-scan with a urologic study is recommended [2].

The high incidence of ano-rectal lesions (18–64%) requires careful study of the ano-rectal region. At first a *perineal and a rectal digital examination* to detect blood, rectal wall weakness and non-palpable prostate should be done. In case of positive rectal examination a *rigid proctoscopy* should be strongly considered [3].

Tile Classification and Young and Burgess Classification (Fig. 2) are the most commonly used classifications for pelvic ring injuries. These classifications are based on the direction of forces causing fracture and the associated instability of pelvis with four injury patterns: lateral compression, antero-posterior compression (external rotation), vertical shear, combined mechanism [12]. The Young and Burgess classification is more beneficial for specialists, as a counterpart the second seems to be more easily remembered and applied.

Role of pelvic binder in hemodynamically unstable pelvic fractures

— *- The application of non-invasive external pelvic compression is recommended as an early strategy to stabilize the pelvic ring and decrease the amount of pelvic haemorrhage in the early resuscitation phase. [Grade 1A]*
— *- Pelvic binders are superior to sheet wrapping in the effectiveness of pelvic haemorrhage control [Grade 1C].*
— *- Non-invasive external pelvic compression devices should be removed as soon as physiologically justifiable, and replaced by external pelvic fixation, or definitive pelvic stabilization, if indicated [Grade 1B].*
— *- Pelvic binders should be positioned cautiously in pregnant women and elderly patients [Grade 2A].*
— *- In a patient with pelvic binder whenever it's possible, an early transfer from the spine board reduces significantly the skin pressure lesions [Grade 1A].*

Pelvic binder (PB) could be a "home-made" (as a bedsheet) or commercial binder (as T-POD® (Bio Cybernetics Inter-national, La Verne, CA, USA), SAM-Sling® (SAM Medical Products, Newport, OR, USA), Pelvi Binder® (Pelvic Binder Inc., Dallas, TX, USA)). Nowadays, according to ATLS guidelines PB should be used before mechanical fixation when there are signs of a pelvic ring fracture [26]. The PB right position should be around the great trochanter and the symphysis pubis to apply a pressure to reduce pelvic fracture and to adduct lower limbs in order to decrease the pelvic internal volume. Commercial pelvic binders are more effective in control pelvic bleeding than the "home-made" ones [36]. However in low resources setting or in lacking of commercial devices, "home-made" pelvic binder con be effectively and safely used.

PB is a cost-effective and a non-invasive tool that could be used by physicians and volunteers during the maneuvers aiming to stabilize a trauma patient, particularly in the immediate resuscitative period and the pre-hospital setting [1, 28, 37]. Sometimes PB can be used as bridge to definitive mechanical stabilization in those patients hemodynamically stable and mechanically unstable with no other lesions requiring treatment and with a negative CT-scan; those patients in many cases can proceed directly to definitive mechanical stabilization. Biomechanical studies on cadaver showed an effective pelvic volume reduction with an improved hemorrhage control [38–41]. These data are confirmed in vivo [42–44]. The Eastern Association for Surgery for Trauma's pelvic trauma guidelines reporting data from the large retrospective study of Croce et al. recommended the use of PB to reduce a pelvic unstable ring [2, 42]. The use of PB alone doesn't seem to reduce mortality [2, 42]. Authors reported a decrease in used units of blood from 17.1 to 4.9 ($p = 0.0001$) in the first 24 h, and from 18.6 to 6 after 48 h in patients treated with external fixation and PB, respectively [42]. However, comparing PB with external pelvic fixation in patients with sacroiliac fractures, Krieg et al. found a higher transfusion needs in the first 24 and 48 h in patients who underwent external fixation [43].

Some complications could occur if the binder is not removed rapidly and if it's over-tightened: PB should not be kept for more than 24–48 h. Skin necrosis and pressure ulcerations could be increased by PB continuous application of a pressure above 9.3 kPa for more than 2–3 h [40]. As the long-term effects of pelvic binder remain unclear at present, including the potential risk of soft tissue complications from prolonged compression [45], the general recommendation is to remove pelvic binders as soon as physiologically justifiable [26], and to consider replacing binders by external pelvic fixation.

In elderly patients, even a minor trauma could cause major pelvic fractures or bleedings due to the bones fragility and the decrease in function of regulation systems as the vasospasm [46]. Lateral compression fracture pattern is more frequent, and fractures are usually not displaced. For this reason angiography seems to have more hemostatic effect than PB [44].

Even in pregnant women, the pelvis can be closed with internal rotation of the legs and PB positioning [47].

Role of REBOA in hemodynamic unstable pelvic ring injuries

- - *Resuscitative thoracotomy with aortic cross-clamping represents an acute measure of temporary bleeding control for unresponsive patients "in extremis" with exsanguinating traumatic hemorrhage. [Grade 1A]*
- - *REBOA technique may provide a valid innovative alternative to aortic cross-clamping [Grade 2B].*
- - *In hemodynamic unstable patients with suspected pelvic bleeding (systolic blood pressure <90 mmHg or non-responders to direct blood products transfusion), REBOA in zone III should be considered as a bridge to definitive treatment [Grade 2B].*
- - *In major trauma patients with suspected pelvic trauma, arterial vascular access via femoral artery (e.g. 5Fr) introducer might be considered as the first step for eventually REBOA placement [Grade 2C].*
- - *Partial-REBOA or/and intermittent-REBOA should be considered to decrease occlusion time and ischemic insult [Grade 2C].*

Resuscitative Endovascular Balloon Occlusion of the Aorta (REBOA) has emerged in recent years as alternative to emergent Resuscitative thoracotomy (RT) in hemodynamic unstable trauma patients [48–51]. The usage of REBOA and other Endo-Vascular hybrid Trauma Management (EVTM) methods is increasing worldwide in general trauma care including pelvic bleeding and now a part of the clinical praxis and guidelines in major trauma centers [6, 48–50, 52–58]. Several retrospective publications on REBOA in trauma care came lately from Japan, where REBOA has been practiced widely in the last 10–15 years but there are only few series concentrating on pelvic bleeding and REBOA [53, 57, 59, 60]. The method itself though, as a bleeding control method, has been used widely in endovascular surgery under the name Aortic Balloon Occlusion (ABO) [61–64]. REBOA is described as a "bridge to surgery" method and in pelvic bleeding as an alternative for RT with following open surgery or embolization (or both) for definitive bleeding control. REBOA can be placed in Zone I (supra-celiac or descending aorta) or Zone III (infra-renal) but preferably not in zone II (pararenal) due to risk of visceral organ ischemia. It's been speculated that Zone III REBOA be optimal for pelvic bleeding as the ischemic insult on visceral organs is prevented and long occlusion time (4–6 h) is possible [48, 49, 52]. Trauma patients though, might have multiple injuries and unclear source of bleeding upon arrival, which makes it challenging to decide if Zone III REBOA is suitable for hemodynamic stabilization. In the majority of reported series, REBOA was placed in zone I first and then redeployed in Zone III. REBOA seems to elevate the systolic blood pressure in bleeding patients while preserving carotid and coronary flow and this data is confirmed in animal studies though there is no clear evidence of mortality benefit in the reported literature [49, 65–68]. One must consider though that the reported usage of REBOA is a mixture of different bleeding mechanism and localizations as there is not enough data of isolated pelvic bleedings reported [57, 59]. New information from the AORTA, ABOTrauma Registry and DIRECT IABO studies show preliminary beneficial results in trauma patients and some evidence that zone III REBOA as well as partial-REBOA and intermittent-REBOA might have positive effect on survival rates [54]. Zone III REBOA seems to have some benefits as time gain for surgical strategic consideration by temporary hemodynamic stabilization. It also allows time for fluid replacement as well as preparation of bleeding control procedures (surgery/angiography or hybrid procedures) [49, 52, 54, 69]. REBOA is highly dependent on a functional femoral artery access and its early establishment might be of considerable value [52, 70]. REBOA for pelvic bleeding in hemodynamic unstable patients has the advantage of being a minimal invasive procedure with less metabolic and surgical burden on the trauma patient but this is only based on expert opinion and animal experiments rather than firm data [66, 68, 71–74]. Its usage is though increasing dramatically worldwide, especially in the USA despite lack of high quality evidence and prospective trials and RCT data are needed. Two important factors to consider when using REBOA in pelvic bleeding are:

- the vascular access for REBOA, because of a functional femoral artery access must be gained first and it's still remained to be answered who should do it and at what stage and localization should it be done. As a main rule only qualified experienced people should do this; as a counterpart however any surgeon who also does ICU or vascular should be facile at these. Lastly it must be kept in mind that having an arterial line bring some additional issues to manage: on one hand when placed it needs to be connected to ulterior lines (i.e. fluids, cable, etc.) on the other hand it also provides the most accurate blood pressure readings.

- the estimated source of bleeding is crucial for determination of REBOA zone placement. For pelvic bleeding, zone III is postulated to be preferred [48, 49, 52].

Moreover there are some major limitations to REBOA. As mentioned, REBOA is only a temporary solution and a definitive bleeding control must follow. One of the major problems of REBOA is the ischemia-reperfusion organ injury followed by multiple organ failure that might be prevented by short REBOA time, intermittent REBOA (iREBOA), Zone

III REBOA and new methods as partial REBOA (pREBOA) described lately [67, 75, 76].

The insertion of REBOA is not free from risks. During maneuvers inside emergency room in a hemodynamically unstable patient, it can be time-consuming to obtain percutaneous, or US guided, or surgically exposed femoral access. Vascular injuries can be present in severe pelvic injuries or otherwise produced particularly in elderly with calcific vessels and, nowadays, most trauma surgeons reserve REBOA only in patients in extremis, with multiple sites of bleeding, as a bridge to more definitive damage control surgical techniques.

Finally, a new evolving concept is the EvndoVascular hybrid Trauma Management (EVTM) that takes into considerations early vascular arterial access, REBOA, embolization and stent-grafts for bleeding control with hybrid (Open and endovascular) procedures. This concept takes into consideration all the above in the initial treatment of trauma patients and can finally suggest to take into account the presence of a vascular surgeon in the team managing selected politraumatized patients [52, 69, 70].

Role of Pre-peritoneal Pelvic Packing in hemodynamically unstable pelvic fractures

- - *Patients with pelvic fracture-related hemodynamic instability should always be considered for pre-peritoneal pelvic packing, especially in hospitals with no angiography service [Grade 1C].*
- - *Direct preperitoneal pelvic packing represents an effective surgical measure of early haemorrhage control in hypotensive patients with bleeding pelvic ring disruptions [Grade 1B].*
- - *Pelvic packing should be performed in conjunction with pelvic stabilization to maximize the effectiveness of bleeding control [Grade 2A].*
- - *Patients with pelvic fracture-related hemodynamic instability with persistent bleeding after angiography should always be considered for pre-peritoneal pelvic packing [Grade 2A].*
- - *Pre-peritoneal pelvic packing is an effective technique in controlling hemorrhage in patients with pelvic fracture-related hemodynamic instability undergone prior anterior/C-clamp fixation [Grade 2A].*

The main source of acute retroperitoneal hemorrhage in patients with hemodynamically unstable pelvic ring disruptions is attributed to venous bleeding in 80%–90% of all cases, originating from presacral and paravesical venous plexus and from bleeding cancellous bone surfaces from sacral and iliac fractures and sacro-iliac joint disruptions [77]. Only 10%–20% of all pelvic bleeding sources are arterial [77]. Arterial bleeding may be predominant in patients with persistent hemodynamic instability after mechanical stabilization [78]. Moreover, when arterial bleeding is present, the likelihood of concomitant venous bleeding is close to 100% [46, 79]. Since venous bleeding sources are inadequately managed by angio-embolization, studies have shown that the traditional ATLS-guided management of hemodynamically unstable pelvic ring injuries with angio-embolization results in poor patient outcomes with high post-injury mortality rates greater than 40% [80, 81]. The notion of a mainly venous retroperitoneal bleeding source in pelvic fractures provides the main rationale for pelvic packing for acute surgical hemorrhage control [4, 82].

Pre-peritoneal pelvic packing (PPP) has become a commonly used technique to control bleeding in hemodinamically unstable pelvic fractures in recent years. PPP has been reported to be a quick and easy-to-perform technique [4, 79] and it could be accomplished both in the emergency department (ED) and the operating room [4]. In experienced hands it can be completed with a minimal operative blood loss in less than 20 min [79, 83]. Since its first description by Hannover and Zurich groups in patients with pelvic ring injuries, outcomes have been improved by early surgical "damage control" intervention, including temporary external stabilization of unstable pelvic fractures, transabdominal pelvic packing, and surgical bleeding control [84–86].

More recently, the concept of "direct" preperitoneal pelvic packing (PPP) was described in Denver using a distinct surgical technique by a separate suprapubic midline incision that allows a direct retroperitoneal approach to the space of Retzius [83]. The modified PPP technique allows for more effective packing within the concealed preperitoneal space with three laparotomy pads for each side of the bladder in the retroperitoneal space packed below the pelvic brim towards the iliac vessels [79, 83, 87], without the necessity of opening the retroperitoneal space [82, 83]. With this technique, a midline laparotomy can be performed through a separate incision proximal to the suprapubic approach, if indicated for associated intra-abdominal injuries [88]. The separate incision technique has been shown to be safe with regard to preventing cross-contamination from intra-abdominal injuries to the retroperitoneal space and thereby decreasing the risk of postoperative infections after pelvic packing and subsequent pelvic fracture fixation [88]. PPP revision should be done within 48–72 h.

Retrospective observational studies revealed that the implementation of standardized multidisciplinary clinical guidelines that include early surgical management with pelvic external fixation and direct PPP for hypotensive patients with hemodynamical and mechanical unstable

pelvic ring injuries led to a significant decrease of transfused blood products and to a significantly decreased post-injury mortality [5, 6, 87]. More recent observational studies confirmed the notion that extraperitoneal pelvic packing is a safe and fast procedure associated with a significantly reduced mortality in hemodynamically unstable patients with pelvic fractures, compared to patients managed by conventional measures without pelvic packing [89–91].

In hemodynamically and mechanically unstable pelvic fractures, PPP should be performed along with external fixation [46, 56, 79]. Cothren et al. showed that external fixation and PPP could be sufficient to control bleeding in severely injured patients with pelvic fractures, reporting that only 13% of patients required a subsequent angioembolization for an arterial blush [82]. In very sick patients, pelvic ring stabilization can be rapidly obtained by pelvic binder, with posterior compression using rolled surgical towels under the binder in sacro-iliac disruption [92].

Subsequent (secondary) angioembolization is recommended in the selected cohort of patients with ongoing hemorrhage and/or transfusion requirements after the pelvic packing procedure [4, 29, 56, 79, 87, 93]. The need for angioembolization following PPP has been reported to be between 13 and 20% [56, 87, 91]. However, Totterman et al. reported that 80% of patients who underwent PPP had positive findings for arterial injury at angiography [94].

PPP has been proposed as an alternative to angiography [79, 87, 91, 93]. Some papers [87, 91, 93] compared the use of PPP vs. Angioembolization. In a recent a prospective quasi-randomized trial Li et al. [91] showed that time-to-procedure and procedure time were significantly shorter in the PACK group than in the ANGIO one. The need for packed red cells in the first 24 h after procedure, the need for complementary procedures (angiography or PPP), mortality rates did not differ between the two groups [91]. Present guidelines recommend considering angiography and PPP as complementary procedures.

Role of external pelvic fixation in hemodynamic unstable pelvic ring injuries

- - *External pelvic fixation provides rigid temporary pelvic ring stability and serves as an adjunct to early haemorrhage control in hemodynamically unstable pelvic ring disruptions [Grade 1A].*
- - *External pelvic fixation is a required adjunct to preperitoneal pelvic packing to provide a stable counterpressure for effective packing [Grade 2A].*
- - *Anterior "resuscitation frames" through iliac crest or supra-acetabular route provide adequate temporary*

pelvic stability in APC-II/-III and LC-II/-III injury patterns. A posterior pelvic C-clamp can be indicated for hemorrhage control in "vertical shear" injuries with sacroiliac joint disruptions [Grade 2A].
- *- Pelvic C-clamp application is contraindicated in comminuted and transforaminal sacral fractures, iliac wing fractures, and LC-type pelvic ring disruptions [Grade 2B].*

The biomechanics of pelvic ring injuries and the underlying trauma mechanism dictate the need for external fixation [58, 95]. Pelvic ring disruptions in hemodynamically unstable patients should be temporarily stabilized to prevent further hemorrhage and to support measures of hemorrhage control, including angiography and pelvic packing [28, 46, 58, 96, 97]. The rationale for acute external pelvic fixation consists of (1) reducing the intrapelvic volume in "open book" equivalent injuries to decrease the retroperitoneal bleeding space, and (2) to provide a stable counter-pressure to the "packed" lap sponges for effective pelvic packing. For example, pelvic packing is not effective in absence of adequate counterpressure by posterior pelvic elements, which requires external fixation for unstable pelvic ring disruptions [56, 87, 98]. The technical aspects of decision-making for the modality of "damage control" external fixation for unstable pelvic ring injuries have been described elsewhere [58]. In essence, the indication and technique of pelvic external fixation can be guided by the Young & Burgess fracture classification [58, 99]. Unstable antero-posterior compression (APC-II/APC-III) and lateral compression injuries (LC-II/LC-III) injuries are ideally managed by anterior resuscitation frames, using iliac crest or supra-acetabular Schanz pin application. While the iliac crest route is technically less demanding and allows a faster "damage control" application, the pull-out resistance of Schanz pins in the iliac crest is very low and therefore associated with a higher risk of failure of reduction and fixation. In contrast, supra-acetabular frames require diligent pin placement under radiographic control using a C-arm, however, these frames have a very high pull-out resistance due to the solid supra-acetabular surgical corridor [58]. In contrast to rotationally unstable APC and LC-type injuries, vertically unstable pelvic ring disruptions, such as "vertical shear" (VS) injuries, are best stabilized by a posterior C-clamp [84, 86, 100–103]. Of note, the trauma surgeon must be aware of inherent risks and potential technical complications using the C-clamp due to the learning curve and required experience for safe application [104, 105]. Contraindications for the application of a pelvic C-clamp include comminuted and transforaminal sacral fractures, fractures of the iliac wing, and lateral compression-type injuries [58]. For

these reasons, C-clamp is not used in many trauma centers.

Role of Angioembolization in hemodynamic unstable pelvic fractures

- *- Angioembolization is an effective measure of haemorrhage control in patients with arterial sources of retroperitoneal pelvic bleeding [Grade 1A].*
- *- CT-scan demonstrating arterial contrast extravasation in the pelvis and the presence of pelvic hematoma are the most important signs predictive of the need for angioembolization [Grade 1C].*
- *- After pelvic stabilization, initiation of aggressive hemostatic resuscitation and exclusion of extra-pelvic sources of blood loss, patients with pelvic fractures and hemodynamic instability or evidence of ongoing bleeding should be considered for pelvic angiography/angioembolization [Grade 2A].*
- *- Patients with CT-scan demonstrating arterial contrast extravasation in the pelvis may benefit from pelvic angiography/angioembolization regardless of hemodynamic status [Grade 2A].*
- *- After extra-pelvic sources of blood loss have been ruled out, patients with pelvic fractures who have undergone pelvic angiography with or without angioembolization, with persisting signs of ongoing bleeding, should be considered for repeat pelvic angiography/angioembolization [Grade 2B].*
- *- Elderly patients with pelvic fractures should be considered for pelvic angiography/angioembolization regardless of hemodynamic status [Grade 2C].*

Since the 1980s, percutaneous trans-catheter angioembolization has been shown to represent an effective non-surgical measure of acute bleeding control in hemodynamically unstable pelvic fractures [106–109]. Most published clinical guidelines recommend the use of early angioembolization, in conjunction with external pelvic fixation if indicated, as the main measure of acute bleeding control [10, 46, 93, 110–117]. As a counterpart it is important to consider a number of factors that are critical to decision-making. The exclusive use of angioembolization has been associated with a high mortality in patients with bleeding pelvic fractures [118], which was significantly reduced by application of a combined protocol with initial preperitoneal pelvic packing and subsequent (secondary) angioembolization, if indicated [28, 56, 79, 86, 89]. It has been estimated that 85% of pelvic bleeding originates from bone, soft tissues, or major venous structures [2]. In addition, as many as 90% of patients with unstable pelvic fractures will have significant associated injuries. Bleeding in the abdomen, chest, or extremities will contribute to shock and may require more urgent control than the pelvic bleeding. Thus, the fundamental management principles include aggressive hemostatic resuscitation, bony stabilization of the pelvis, and identification and management of extrapelvic bleeding. Management guidelines that emphasize these principles demonstrate improved outcomes [6, 16, 46, 116]. Pelvic Angiography/Angioembolization (AG/AE) is expected to benefit only a small minority of patients, and therefore should be employed once extrapelvic and non-arterial sources of bleeding are controlled [2]. Arterial contrast extravasation seen on CT scan is a good indicator of the need for pelvic AG/AE [114]. In contrast, fracture pattern alone has not been predictive of who will require angiography [119]. Pelvic AG/AE is very effective in controlling hemorrhage. However, some patients will continue to bleed and repeat AG/AE has been found to be an effective strategy [115]. Elderly patients have been found to require AG/AE more frequently than younger adults, regardless of apparently normal hemodynamics at presentation, even in mechanical stable-low risk fractures. Therefore, AG/AE should be considered in these patients even when there is low suspicion of pelvic bleeding [120].

Indications for definitive surgical fixation of pelvic ring injuries

- - *Posterior pelvic ring instability represents a surgical indication for anatomic fracture reduction and stable internal fixation. Typical injury patterns requiring surgical fixation include rotationally unstable (APC-II, LC-II) and/or vertically unstable pelvic ring disruptions (APC-III, LC-III, VS, CM) [Grade 2A].*
- - *Selected lateral compression patterns with rotational instability (LC-II, L-III) benefit from adjunctive, temporary external fixation, in conjunction to posterior pelvic ring fixation [Grade 2A].*
- - *Pubic symphysis plating represents the modality of choice for anterior fixation of "open book" injuries with a pubic symphysis diastasis > 2.5 cm (APC-II, APC-III) [Grade 1A].*
- - *The technical modality of posterior pelvic ring fixation remains a topic of debate, and individual decision-making is largely guided by surgeons' preference. Spinopelvic fixation has the benefit of immediate weight bearing in patients with vertically unstable sacral fractures [Grade 2C].*
- - *Patients hemodynamically stable and mechanically unstable with no other lesions requiring treatment and with a negative CT-scan can proceed directly to definitive mechanical stabilization [Grade 2B].*

Pelvic ring injuries with rotational or vertical instability require surgical fixation with the goal of achieving anatomic reduction and stable fixation as a prerequisite for early functional rehabilitation. There is general consensus that pelvic ring disruptions with instability of posterior elements require internal fixation [95, 121]. Trauma mechanism-guided fracture classifications, including the widely used Young & Burgess system, provide guidance for surgical indications for pelvic fracture fixation [58, 122]. For example, stable fracture patterns, such as antero-posterior compression type 1 (APC-I) and lateral compression type 1 (LC-I) injuries are managed non-operatively, allowing functional rehabilitation and early weight bearing [123, 124]. In contrast, rotationally unstable APC-II/APC-III ("open book") injuries and LC-II fracture patterns ("crescent fracture"), as well as rotationally and vertically unstable LC-III ("windswept pelvis"), "vertical shear" (VS), and "combined mechanism" (CM) fracture patterns require definitive internal fixation [123, 124]. Multiple technical modalities of surgical fixation have been described, including open reduction and anterior plating of pubic symphysis disruptions, minimal-invasive percutaneous iliosacral screw fixation for unstable sacral fractures and iliosacral joint disruptions, plating of iliac wing fractures, and spino-pelvic fixation (named "triangular osteosynthesis" in conjunction with iliosacral screw fixation) or tension band plating for posterior pelvic ring injuries, including vertically unstable sacral fractures [125–133]. In addition, selected lateral compression (LC) type injuries are occasionally managed with temporary adjunctive external fixators for 6 weeks post injury, to protect from rotational instability of the anterior pelvic ring [58, 134]. Minimal invasive anterior "internal fixators" have been recently described as an alternative technical option [135]. The ultimate goal of internal fixation of unstable pelvic ring injuries is to allow early functional rehabilitation and to decrease long-term morbidity, chronic pain and complications that have been historically associated with prolonged immobilization [136, 137].

Ideal time-window to proceed with definitive pelvic fixation

- - *Hemodynamically unstable patients and coagulopathic patients "in extremis" should be successfully resuscitated prior to proceeding with definitive pelvic fracture fixation [Grade 1B].*
- - *Hemodynamically stable patients and "borderline" patients can be safely managed by early definitive pelvic fracture fixation within 24 h post injury [Grade 2A].*
- - *Definitive pelvic fracture fixation should be postponed until after day 4 post injury in physiologically deranged politrauma patients [Grade 2A].*

The timing of definitive internal fixation of unstable pelvic ring injuries remains a topic of debate [138–145]. Most authors agree that patients in severe traumatic-hemorrhagic shock from bleeding pelvic ring disruptions are unlikely candidates for early definitive pelvic fracture fixation, due to the inherent risk of increased mortality from exsanguinating hemorrhage and the "lethal triad" of coagulopathy, acidosis and hypothermia [22, 146]. A prospective multicenter cohort study revealed a significantly increased extent of blood loss and increased interleukin (IL-6 and IL-8) serum levels, reflective of an exacerbated systemic inflammatory response, in politrauma patients who underwent early pelvic fracture fixation on the first or second day post injury [147]. The early timing and short duration of initial pelvic stabilization revealed to have a positive impact on decreasing the incidence of multiple organ failure (MOF) and mortality [148]. Furthermore, post-injury complication rates were shown to be significantly increased when definitive pelvic ring fixation was performed between days 2 and 4, and decreased when surgery was delayed to days 6 to 8 post injury [149]. Many authors concur with the traditional concept of initial "damage control" external fixation of hemodynamically unstable pelvic ring injuries, and delayed definitive internal fixation after day 4, subsequent to successful resuscitative measures [28, 41, 58, 95, 118, 150–152]. The use of such definitions and classification systems can provide guidance for future stratification of unstable politrauma patients with pelvic ring injuries requiring "damage control" resuscitative measures compared to stable or "borderline" patients who may be safely amenable to early total care by definitive pelvic fracture fixation [141, 146]. In this regard, multiple observational cohort studies from the orthopedic trauma group at MetroHealth in Cleveland have shown that early pelvic fracture fixation in stable or borderline resuscitated patients within 24 h of admission reduces the risk of complications and improves outcomes [139, 141, 144, 145]. Recently, a new definition of politrauma has been proposed by an international consensus group, which is based on injury severity and derangement of physiological parameters [153]. This new politrauma definition in conjunction with recently established grading systems [141] may provide further guidance towards the "ideal" timing of definitive pelvic fracture fixation, pending future validation studies.

Damage Control Orthopedics in Severe Head Injuries

Severe head injuries are common in politrauma patients with concomitant pelvic injuries. No definitive guidelines exist regarding severe head injuries and pelvic fixation. One of the main issues is that pelvic fracture associated bleeding and consequent coagulopathy leads to a deterioration of the head injury through secondary bleeding and subsequent progression of hemorrhagic contusions in a risky vicious circle. For these reasons the acute definitive hemorrhage control and prevention and prompt reversal of coagulopathy is essential. Careful monitoring of brain injuries, potential early re-scanning with perfusion CT-scan is helpful. In the major part of the trauma centers patients are treated according to the indications of the neurosurgery team [150]. On one hand several articles suggested that early fracture fixation might be deleterious in patients with brain injury especially if old-aged, on the other hand however some trials didn't confirm these concerns suggesting that outcomes are worse in patients who do not have early skeletal stabilization [44, 154–156]. Usually neurosurgeons are very concerned for the possible additional brain injury deriving from blood pressure fluctuations during orthopedic fixative surgery [150]. This in general leads to several doubts and additional delay to let the patients being considered suitable for operating room [150]. The potential benefit of damage control orthopedics interventions and the minimal physiologic insult of placing an external fixator allows for almost all patients with closed head injuries to be appropriate for at least external fixation [150]. However no definitive indications can be obtained from the literature.

Morbidity, mortality and outcomes

Complications with important functional limitations are present especially in patients with open PT who may have chronic sequelae as fecal and urinary incontinence, impotence, dyspareunia, residual disability in physical functions, perineal and pelvic abscess, chronic pain and vascular complications as embolism or thrombosis [1, 3].

The majority of deaths (44.7%) occurred on the day of trauma and the main factors that correlate with mortality are increasing age, ISS, pelvic ring instability, size and contamination of the open wound, rectal injury, fecal diversion, numbers of blood units transfused, head Abbreviated Injury Scale (AIS), admission base deficit [3, 5].

Lastly, a recent study reported the impact given by the multidisciplinary approach resulting in an improvement in performance and in patient outcomes [5]. At first a defined decision making algorithm reduce significantly ($p = 0.005$) the time from hospital arrival and bleeding control in the theatre with PPP [5]. Furthermore the definition of a massive hemorrhage protocol reduced significantly the use of liquids administered prior blood transfusions and rationalized the use of packed red cells and fresh frozen plasma (ratio 2:1) starting within the first hours following injury [5]. Moreover a dedicated pelvic orthopedic surgeons can improve ($p = 0.004$) the number of patients that undergoing definitive unstable pelvic fractures repair with a consequently improvement in outcome [5]. Similar data about the importance of the adherence to defined guidelines have been reported by Balogh et al. [16] and recently confirmed by the multi-institutional trial by Costantini et al. [10].

Conclusions

the management of pelvic trauma must keep into consideration the physiological and mechanical derangement. Critical and operative decisions can be taken more effectively if both anatomy of injury and its physiological and mechanical effects are considered.

Abbreviations

ABO: Aortic Balloon Occlusion; AE: Angioembolization; AG: Angiography; AIS: Abbreviated Injury Score; APC: Antero Posterior Compression; ATLS: Advanced Trauma Life Support; BD: Base Deficit; BPM: Beat Per Minute; CM: Combined Mechanism; CT: Computed Tomography; DSA: Digital Subtraction Angiography; ED: Emergency Department; E-FAST: Extended-Focused Assessment with Sonography for Trauma; EVTM: Endovascular Trauma Management; ICU: Intensive Care Unit; IREBOA: Intermittent Resuscitative Endo Vascular Balloon Occlusion; ISS: Injury Severity Score; LC: Lateral Compression; LE: Level of Evidence; MOF: Multi-Organ Failure; NOM: Non-Operative Management; OM: Operative Management; PB: Pelvic Binder; PPP: Pre-peritoneal Pelvic Packing; PREBOA: Partial Resuscitative Endo Vascular Balloon Occlusion; PT: Pelvic Trauma; PXR: Pelvic X-ray; RCT: Randomized Controlled Tria; REBOA: Resuscitative Endo Vascular Balloon Occlusion; ROTEM: Rotational Thromboelastometry; RUG: Retrograde Urethrogram; TEG: Thromboelastography; VS: Vertical Shear; WSES: World Society of Emergency Surgery

Acknowledgements
Special thanks to Ms. Franca Boschini (Bibliographer, Medical Library, Papa Giovanni XXIII Hospital, Bergamo, Italy) for the precious bibliographical work.

Authors' contribution
FC, PS, GM, WB, TH, FaCa, YK, EM, AP, RI, RC, GPF, BP, SR, AK, AL, RM, SM, OC, CA, GV, ZB, NN, DW, FAZ, LS, MC, NA, MS, LA, manuscript conception and draft critically revised the manuscript and contribute with important scientific knowledge giving the final approval.

Competing interest
All authors declare to have no competing interests.

Author details
[1]General, Emergency and Trauma Surgery, Papa Giovanni XXIII Hospital, P.zza OMS 1, 24128 Bergamo, Italy. [2]Department of Orthopedic Surgery and Department of Neurosurgery, Denver Health Medical Center and University of Colorado School of Medicine, Denver, CO, USA. [3]Acute Care Surgery, The Queen's Medical Center, Honolulu, HI, USA. [4]Dept. of Cardiothoracic and Vascular Surgery & Dept. Of Surgery Örebro University Hospital and Örebro University, Örebro, Sweden. [5]Emergency and Trauma Surgery, Maggiore Hospital, Parma, Italy. [6]Division of General Surgery Rambam Health Care Campus Haifa, Haifa, Israel. [7]Trauma Surgery, Denver Health, Denver, CO, USA. [8]Surgery Department, University of Pittsburgh, Pittsburgh, Pensylvania, USA. [9]Virginia Commonwealth University, Richmond, VA, USA. [10]Department of Surgery, UC San Diego Health System, San Diego, USA. [11]Faculdade de Ciências Médicas (FCM) – Unicamp, Campinas, SP, Brazil. [12]Trauma & Acute Care Service, St Michael's Hospital, Toronto, ON, Canada. [13]General, Acute Care, Abdominal Wall Reconstruction, and Trauma Surgery Foothills Medical Centre, Calgary, AB, Canada. [14]Abdominal Center, University Hospital Meilahti, Helsinki, Finland. [15]Emergency and Trauma Surgery, Niguarda Hospital, Milan, Italy. [16]Digestive and Emergency Surgery, UGA-Université Grenoble Alpes, Grenoble, France. [17]Harvard Medical School, Division of Trauma, Emergency Surgery and Surgical Critical Care Massachusetts General Hospital, Boston, MA, USA. [18]Department of Traumatology, John Hunter Hospital and University of Newcastle, Newcastle, NSW, Australia. [19]Department of Surgery, University of KwaZulu-Natal, Durban, South Africa. [20]Department of General Surgery, Royal Perth Hospital, Perth, Australia. [21]Department of Surgery, College of Medicine and Health Sciences, UAE University, Al-Ain, United Arab Emirates. [22]General and Emergency Surgery, Macerata Hospital, Macerata, Italy.

References
1. Arvieux C, Thony F, Broux C, et al. Current management of severe pelvic and perineal trauma. J Visc Surg. 2012;149:e227–38.
2. Cullinane DC, Schiller HJ, Zielinski MD, et al. Eastern Association for the Surgery of Trauma practice management guidelines for hemorrhage in pelvic fracture–update and systematic review. J Trauma. 2011;71:1850–68.
3. Grotz MR, Allami MK, Harwood P, Pape HC, Krettek C, Giannoudis PV. Open pelvic fractures: epidemiology, current concepts of management and outcome. Injury. 2005;36:1–13.
4. Magnone S, Coccolini F, Manfredi R, et al. Management of hemodynamically unstable pelvic trauma: results of the first Italian consensus conference (cooperative guidelines of the Italian Society of Surgery, the Italian Association of Hospital Surgeons, the Multi-specialist Italian Society of Young Surgeons, the Italian Society of Emergency Surgery and Trauma, the Italian Society of Anesthesia, Analgesia, Resuscitation and Intensive Care, the Italian Society of Orthopaedics and Traumatology, the Italian Society of Emergency Medicine, the Italian Society of Medical Radiology -Section of Vascular and Interventional Radiology- and the World Society of Emergency Surgery). World J Emerg Surg. 2014;9:18.
5. Perkins ZB, Maytham GD, Koers L, Bates P, Brohi K, Tai NR. Impact on outcome of a targeted performance improvement programme in haemodynamically unstable patients with a pelvic fracture. Bone Joint J. 2014;96-B:1090–7.
6. Biffl WL, Smith WR, Moore EE, et al. Evolution of a multidisciplinary clinical pathway for the management of unstable patients with pelvic fractures. Ann Surg. 2001;233:843–50.
7. Goslings JC, Ponsen KJ, van Delden OM. Injuries to the pelvis and extremities. In: ACS Surgery: Principles and Practice: Decker Intellectual Properties. 2013.
8. Coccolini F, Montori G, Catena F, et al. Liver trauma: WSES position paper. World J Emerg Surg. 2015;10:39.
9. Oxford Centre for Evidence-based Medicine – Levels of Evidence (March 2009). 2009. (Accessed at http://www.cebm.net/ocebm-levels-of-evidence/).
10. Costantini TW, Coimbra R, Holcomb JB, et al. Current management of hemorrhage from severe pelvic fractures: Results of an American Association for the Surgery of Trauma multi-institutional trial. J Trauma Acute Care Surg. 2016;80:717–23. discussion 23–5.
11. Pereira SJ, O'Brien DP, Luchette FA, et al. Dynamic helical computed tomography scan accurately detects hemorrhage in patients with pelvic fracture. Surgery. 2000;128:678–85.
12. Burgess AR, Eastridge BJ, Young JW, et al. Pelvic ring disruptions: effective classification system and treatment protocols. J Trauma. 1990;30:848–56.
13. Huittinen VM, Slatis P. Postmortem angiography and dissection of the hypogastric artery in pelvic fractures. Surgery. 1973;73:454–62.
14. Luckhoff C, Mitra B, Cameron PA, Fitzgerald M, Royce P. The diagnosis of acute urethral trauma. Injury. 2011;42:913–6.
15. Blackmore CC, Cummings P, Jurkovich GJ, Linnau KF, Hoffer EK, Rivara FP. Predicting major hemorrhage in patients with pelvic fracture. J Trauma. 2006;61:346–52.
16. Balogh Z, Caldwell E, Heetveld M, et al. Institutional practice guidelines on management of pelvic fracture-related hemodynamic instability: do they make a difference? J Trauma. 2005;58:778–82.

17. Da Luz LT, Nascimento B, Shankarakutty AK, Rizoli S, Adhikari NK. Effect of thromboelastography (TEG(R)) and rotational thromboelastometry (ROTEM(R)) on diagnosis of coagulopathy, transfusion guidance and mortality in trauma: descriptive systematic review. Crit Care. 2014;18:518.

18. Duane TM, Tan BB, Golay D, Cole Jr FJ, Weireter Jr LJ, Britt LD. Blunt trauma and the role of routine pelvic radiographs: a prospective analysis. J Trauma. 2002;53:463–8.

19. Gonzalez E, Moore EE, Moore HB, et al. Goal-directed Hemostatic Resuscitation of Trauma-induced Coagulopathy: A Pragmatic Randomized Clinical Trial Comparing a Viscoelastic Assay to Conventional Coagulation Assays. Ann Surg. 2016;263:1051–9.

20. Kashuk JL, Moore EE, Sawyer M, et al. Postinjury coagulopathy management: goal directed resuscitation via POC thrombelastography. Ann Surg. 2010; 251:604–14.

21. Rossaint R, Cerny V, Coats TJ, et al. Key issues in advanced bleeding care in trauma. Shock. 2006;26:322–31.

22. Stahel PF, Moore EE, Schreier SL, Flierl MA, Kashuk JL. Transfusion strategies in postinjury coagulopathy. Curr Opin Anaesthesiol. 2009;22:289–98.

23. Paydar S, Ghaffarpasand F, Foroughi M, et al. Role of routine pelvic radiography in initial evaluation of stable, high-energy, blunt trauma patients. Emerg Med J. 2013;30:724–7.

24. Mutschler M, Nienaber U, Brockamp T, et al. Renaissance of base deficit for the initial assessment of trauma patients: a base deficit-based classification for hypovolemic shock developed on data from 16,305 patients derived from the TraumaRegister DGU(R). Crit Care. 2013;17:R42.

25. Mutschler M, Nienaber U, Munzberg M, et al. The Shock Index revisited - a fast guide to transfusion requirement? A retrospective analysis on 21,853 patients derived from the TraumaRegister DGU. Crit Care. 2013;17:R172.

26. Committee of trauma of ACS. Advanced Trauma Life Support (ATLS) Student manual 9th ed. ACS. Chicago. 2012.

27. Salim A, Teixeira PG, DuBose J, et al. Predictors of positive angiography in pelvic fractures: a prospective study. J Am Coll Surg. 2008;207:656–62.

28. Marzi I, Lustenberger T. Management of Bleeding Pelvic Fractures. Scand J Surg. 2014;103:104–11.

29. Rossaint R, Bouillon B, Cerny V, et al. Management of bleeding following major trauma: an updated European guideline. Crit Care. 2010;14:R52.

30. Kirkpatrick AW, Sirois M, Laupland KB, et al. Hand-held thoracic sonography for detecting post-traumatic pneumothoraces: the Extended Focused Assessment with Sonography for Trauma (EFAST). J Trauma. 2004;57:288–95.

31. Volpicelli G, Elbarbary M, Blaivas M, et al. International evidence-based recommendations for point-of-care lung ultrasound. Intensive Care Med. 2012;38:577–91.

32. Gonzalez RP, Fried PQ, Bukhalo M. The utility of clinical examination in screening for pelvic fractures in blunt trauma. J Am Coll Surg. 2002;194:121–5.

33. Yugueros P, Sarmiento JM, Garcia AF, Ferrada R. Unnecessary use of pelvic x-ray in blunt trauma. J Trauma. 1995;39:722–5.

34. Guillamondegui OD, Pryor JP, Gracias VH, Gupta R, Reilly PM, Schwab CW. Pelvic radiography in blunt trauma resuscitation: a diminishing role. J Trauma. 2002;53:1043–7.

35. Hallinan JT, Tan CH, Pua U. Emergency computed tomography for acute pelvic trauma: where is the bleeder? Clin Radiol. 2014;69:529–37.

36. Chen B, Zhang Y, Xiao S, Gu P, Lin X. Personalized image-based templates for iliosacral screw insertions: a pilot study. Int J Med Robot. 2012;8:476–82.

37. Fleiter N, Reimertz C, Lustenberger T, et al. Importance of the correct placement of the pelvic binder for stabilisation of haemodynamically compromised patients. Z Orthop Unfall. 2012;150:627–9.

38. Bottlang M, Krieg JC, Mohr M, Simpson TS, Madey SM. Emergent management of pelvic ring fractures with use of circumferential compression. J Bone Joint Surg Am. 2002;84-A Suppl 2:43–7.

39. DeAngelis NA, Wixted JJ, Drew J, Eskander MS, Eskander JP, French BG. Use of the trauma pelvic orthotic device (T-POD) for provisional stabilisation of anterior-posterior compression type pelvic fractures: a cadaveric study. Injury. 2008;39:903–6.

40. Hedrick-Thompson JK. A review of pressure reduction device studies. J Vasc Nurs. 1992;10:3–5.

41. Spanjersberg WR, Knops SP, Schep NW, van Lieshout EM, Patka P, Schipper IB. Effectiveness and complications of pelvic circumferential compression devices in patients with unstable pelvic fractures: a systematic review of literature. Injury. 2009;40:1031–5.

42. Croce MA, Magnotti LJ, Savage SA, Wood 2nd GW, Fabian TC. Emergent pelvic fixation in patients with exsanguinating pelvic fractures. J Am Coll Surg. 2007;204:935–9. discussion 40–2.

43. Krieg JC, Mohr M, Ellis TJ, Simpson TS, Madey SM, Bottlang M. Emergent stabilization of pelvic ring injuries by controlled circumferential compression: a clinical trial. J Trauma. 2005;59:659–64.

44. Tinubu J, Scalea TM. Management of fractures in a geriatric surgical patient. Surg Clin North Am. 2015;95:115–28.

45. Bakhshayesh P, Boutefnouchet T, Totterman A. Effectiveness of non invasive external pelvic compression: a systematic review of the literature. Scand J Trauma Resusc Emerg Med. 2016;24:73.

46. Abrassart S, Stern R, Peter R. Unstable pelvic ring injury with hemodynamic instability: what seems the best procedure choice and sequence in the initial management? Orthop Traumatol Surg Res. 2013;99:175–82.

47. Amorosa LF, Amorosa JH, Wellman DS, Lorich DG, Helfet DL. Management of pelvic injuries in pregnancy. Orthop Clin North Am. 2013;44:301–15. viii.

48. Stannard A, Eliason JL, Rasmussen TE. Resuscitative Endovascular Balloon Occlusion of the Aorta (REBOA) as an Adjunct for Hemorrhagic Shock. J Trauma. 2011;71:1869–72.

49. Morrison JJ, Galgon RE, Jansen JO, Cannon JW, Rasmussen TE, Eliason JL. A systematic review of the use of resuscitative endovascular balloon occlusion of the aorta in the management of hemorrhagic shock. The journal of trauma and acute care surgery. 2016;80:324–34.

50. Biffl WL, Fox CJ, Moore EE. The role of REBOA in the control of exsanguinating torso hemorrhage. J Trauma Acute Care. 2015;78:1054–8.

51. Delamare L, Crognier L, Conil JM, Rousseau H, Georges B, Ruiz S. Treatment of intra-abdominal haemorrhagic shock by Resuscitative Endovascular Balloon Occlusion of the Aorta (REBOA). Anaesthesia, critical care & pain medicine. 2015;34:53–5.

52. Hörer TM, Skoog P, Pirouzram A, Nilsson KF, Larzon T. A small case series of aortic balloon occlusion in trauma: lessons learned from its use in ruptured abdominal aortic aneurysms and a brief review. Eur J Trauma Emerg Surg. 2016;42(5):585–92.

53. Ogura T, Lefor AT, Nakano M, Izawa Y, Morita H. Nonoperative management of hemodynamically unstable abdominal trauma patients with angioembolization and resuscitative endovascular balloon occlusion of the aorta. J Trauma Acute Care. 2015;78:132–5.

54. DuBose JJ, Scalea TM, Brenner M, Skiada D, Inaba K, Cannon J, et al; AAST AORTA Study Group. The AAST prospective Aortic Occlusion for Resuscitation in Trauma and Acute Care Surgery (AORTA) registry: data on contemporary utilization and outcomes of aortic occlusion and resuscitative balloon occlusion of the aorta (REBOA). J Trauma Acute Care Surg. 2016;81(3):409-19.

55. Burlew CC, Moore EE, Moore FA, et al. Western Trauma Association Critical Decisions in Trauma: Resuscitative thoracotomy. J Trauma Acute Care. 2012; 73:1359–64.

56. Burlew CC, Moore EE, Smith WR, et al. Preperitoneal pelvic packing/external fixation with secondary angioembolization: optimal care for life-threatening hemorrhage from unstable pelvic fractures. J Am Coll Surg. 2011;212:628–35. discussion 35–7.

57. Martinelli T, Thony F, Declety P, et al. Intra-Aortic Balloon Occlusion to Salvage Patients With Life-Threatening Hemorrhagic Shocks From Pelvic Fractures. J Trauma. 2010;68:942–8.

58. Stahel PF, Mauffrey C, Smith WR, et al. External fixation for acute pelvic ring injuries: decision making and technical options. J Trauma Acute Care Surg. 2013; 75:882–7.

59. Brenner ML, Moore LJ, DuBose JJ, et al. A clinical series of resuscitative endovascular balloon occlusion of the aorta for hemorrhage control and resuscitation. J Trauma Acute Care. 2013;75:506–11.

60. Norii T, Crandall C, Terasaka Y. Survival of severe blunt trauma patients treated with resuscitative endovascular balloon occlusion of the aorta compared with propensity score-adjusted untreated patients. J Trauma Acute Care. 2015;78:721–8.

61. Mayer D, Aeschbacher S, Pfammatter T, et al. Complete Replacement of Open Repair for Ruptured Abdominal Aortic Aneurysms by Endovascular Aneurysm Repair A Two-Center 14-Year Experience. Ann Surg. 2012;256:688–96.

62. Malina M, Holst J. Balloon control for ruptured AAAs: when and when not to use? J Cardiovasc Surg. 2014;55:161–7.

63. Malina M, Veith F, Ivancev K, Sonesson B. Balloon occlusion of the aorta during endovascular repair of ruptured abdominal aortic aneurysm. Journal of endovascular therapy : an official journal of the International Society of Endovascular Specialists. 2005;12:556–9.

64. Larzon T, Skoog P. One hundred percent of ruptured aortic abdominal aneurysms can be treated endovascularly if adjunct techniques are used such as chimneys, periscopes and embolization. J Cardiovasc Surg. 2014;55:169–78.

65. Morrison J, Ross J, Houston R, Watson D, Rasmussen T. Resuscitative endovascular balloon occlusion of the aorta reduces mortality in a lethal model of non-compressible torso hemorrhage. Brit J Surg. 2013;100:8.

66. Morrison JJ, Ross JD, Houston R, Watson DB, Sokol KK, Rasmussen TE. Use of Resuscitative Endovascular Balloon Occlusion of the Aorta in a Highly Lethal Model of Noncompressible Torso Hemorrhage. Shock. 2014;41:130–7.

67. Russo RM, Neff LP, Lamb CM, Cannon JW, Galante JM, Clement NF, Grayson JK, Williams TK. Partial resuscitative endovascular balloon occlusion of the aorta in swine model of hemorrhagic shock. J Am Coll Surg. 2016;223(2): 359–68.

68. White JM, Cannon JW, Stannard A, Markov NP, Spencer JR, Rasmussen TE. Endovascular balloon occlusion of the aorta is superior to resuscitative thoracotomy with aortic clamping in a porcine model of hemorrhagic shock. Surgery. 2011;150:400–9.

69. Horer TM, Hebron D, Swaid F, et al. Aorta Balloon Occlusion in Trauma: Three Cases Demonstrating Multidisciplinary Approach Already on Patient's Arrival to the Emergency Room. Cardiovascular and interventional radiology 2015.BRS

70. EndoVascular hybrid Trauma and bleeding Management (EVTM) declaration. (Accessed at www.jevtm.com).

71. Morrison JJ, Ross JD, Markov NP, Scott DJ, Spencer JR, Rasmussen TE. The inflammatory sequelae of aortic balloon occlusion in hemorrhagic shock. J Surg Res. 2014;191:423–31.

72. Horer TM, Skoog P, Nilsson KF, et al. Intraperitoneal metabolic consequences of supraceliac aortic balloon occlusion in an experimental animal study using microdialysis. Ann Vasc Surg. 2014;28:1286–95.

73. Markov NP, Percival TJ, Morrison JJ, et al. Physiologic tolerance of descending thoracic aortic balloon occlusion in a swine model of hemorrhagic shock. Surgery. 2013;153:848–56.

74. Park TS, Batchinsky AI, Belenkiy SM, Jordan BS, Baker WL, Necsoiu CN, et al. Resuscitative endovascular balloon occlusion of the aorta (REBOA): comparison with immediate transfusion following massive hemorrhage in swine. J Trauma Acute Care Surg. 2015;79(6):930–6.

75. Hörer TMCP, Jans A, Nilsson K. A case of partial aortic ballon occlusion in an unstable multi-trauma patient. Trauma. 2016;18:150–4.

76. Johnson MA, Neff LP, Williams TK, DuBose JJ; EVAC Study Group. Partial resuscitative balloon occlusion of the aorta (P-REBOA): clinical technique and rationale. J Trauma Acute Care Surg. 2016;81(5 Suppl 2 Proceedings of the 2015 Military Health System Research Symposium):S133–7.

77. Gansslen A, Hildebrand F, Pohlemann T. Management of hemodynamic unstable patients "in extremis" with pelvic ring fractures. Acta Chir Orthop Traumatol Cech. 2012;79:193–202.

78. Lustenberger T, Wutzler S, Stormann P, Laurer H, Marzi I. The role of angio-embolization in the acute treatment concept of severe pelvic ring injuries. Injury. 2015;46 Suppl 4:S33–8.

79. Suzuki T, Smith WR, Moore EE. Pelvic packing or angiography: competitive or complementary? Injury. 2009;40:343–53.

80. Agnew SG. Hemodynamically unstable pelvic fractures. Orthop Clin North Am. 1994;25:715–21.

81. Hou Z, Smith WR, Strohecker KA, et al. Hemodynamically unstable pelvic fracture management by advanced trauma life support guidelines results in high mortality. Orthopedics. 2012;35:e319–24.

82. Cothren CC, Osborn PM, Moore EE, Morgan SJ, Johnson JL, Smith WR. Preperitonal pelvic packing for hemodynamically unstable pelvic fractures: a paradigm shift. J Trauma. 2007;62:834–9. discussion 9–42.

83. Smith WR, Moore EE, Osborn P, et al. Retroperitoneal packing as a resuscitation technique for hemodynamically unstable patients with pelvic fractures: report of two representative cases and a description of technique. J Trauma. 2005;59:1510–4.

84. Ertel W, Eid K, Keel M, Trentz O. Therapeutic Strategies and Outcome of Polytraumatized Patients with Pelvic InjuriesA Six-Year Experience. European Journal of Trauma. 2000;26:278–86.

85. Giannoudis PV, Pape HC. Damage control orthopaedics in unstable pelvic ring injuries. Injury. 2004;35:671–7.

86. Lustenberger T, Fau MC, Benninger E, Fau BE, Lenzlinger PM, Lenzlinger Pm F, Keel MJB, Keel MJ. C-clamp and pelvic packing for control of hemorrhage in patients with pelvic ring disruption. J Emerg Trauma Shock. 2011;4:477–82.

87. Osborn PM, Smith WR, Moore EE, et al. Direct retroperitoneal pelvic packing versus pelvic angiography: A comparison of two management protocols for haemodynamically unstable pelvic fractures. Injury. 2009;40:54–60.

88. Burlew CC, Moore EE, Smith WR, Johnson JL, Biffl WL, Barnett CC, Stahel PF. Preperitoneal pelvic packing/external fixation with secondary angioembolization: optimal care for life-threatening haemorrhage from unstable pelvic fractures. J Am Coll Surg. 2011;212(4):628–35.

89. Chiara O, di Fratta E, Mariani A, et al. Efficacy of extra-peritoneal pelvic packing in hemodynamically unstable pelvic fractures, a Propensity Score Analysis. World J Emerg Surg. 2016;11:22.

90. Jang JY, Shim H, Jung PY, Kim S, Bae KS. Preperitoneal pelvic packing in patients with hemodynamic instability due to severe pelvic fracture: early experience in a Korean trauma center. Scand J Trauma Resusc Emerg Med. 2016;24:3.

91. Li Q, Dong J, Yang Y, Wang G, Wang Y, Liu P, Robinson Y, Zhou D. Retroperitoneal packing or angioembolization for haemorrhage control of pelvic fractures–Quasi-randomized clinical trial of 56 haemodynamically unstable patients with Injury Severity Score ≥33. Injury. 2016;47(2):395–401.

92. Brenner ML, Moore LJ, DuBose JJ, et al. A clinical series of resuscitative endovascular balloon occlusion of the aorta for hemorrhage control and resuscitation. J Trauma Acute Care Surg. 2013;75:506–11.

93. Tai DK, Li WH, Lee KY, et al. Retroperitoneal pelvic packing in the management of hemodynamically unstable pelvic fractures: a level I trauma center experience. J Trauma. 2011;71:E79–86.

94. Totterman A, Madsen JE, Skaga NO, Roise O. Extraperitoneal pelvic packing: a salvage procedure to control massive traumatic pelvic hemorrhage. J Trauma. 2007;62:843–52.

95. Halawi MJ. Pelvic ring injuries: Emergency assessment and management. J Clin Orthop Trauma. 2015;6:252–8.

96. Esmer E, Esmer E, Derst P, Schulz M, Siekmann H, Delank KS; das TraumaRegister DGU®. Influence of external pelvic stabilization on hemodynamically unstable pelvic fractures. Unfallchirurg. 2015. [Epub ahead of print].

97. Poenaru DV, Popescu M, Anglitoiu B, Popa I, Andrei D, Birsasteanu F. Emergency pelvic stabilization in patients with pelvic posttraumatic instability. Int Orthop. 2015;39:961–5.

98. Rommens PM, Hofmann A, Hessmann MH. Management of Acute Hemorrhage in Pelvic Trauma: An Overview. Eur J Trauma Emerg Surg. 2010;36:91–9.

99. Burgess A. Invited commentary: Young-Burgess classification of pelvic ring fractures: does it predict mortality, transfusion requirements, and non-orthopaedic injuries? J Orthop Trauma. 2010;24:609.

100. Heini PF, Witt J, Ganz R. The pelvic C-clamp for the emergency treatment of unstable pelvic ring injuries. A report on clinical experience of 30 cases. Injury. 1996;27 Suppl 1:S-A38–45.

101. Pohlemann T, Culemann U, Tosounidis G, Kristen A. Application of the pelvic C-clamp. Unfallchirurg. 2004;107:1185–91.

102. Tiemann AH, Schmidt C, Gonschorek O, Josten C. Use of the "c-clamp" in the emergency treatment of unstable pelvic fractures. Zentralbl Chir. 2004; 129:245–51.

103. Witschger P, Heini P, Ganz R. Pelvic clamps for controlling shock in posterior pelvic ring injuries. Application, biomechanical aspects and initial clinical results. Orthopade. 1992;21:393–9.

104. Koller H, Balogh ZJ. Single training session for first time pelvic C-clamp users: correct pin placement and frame assembly. Injury. 2012;43:436–9.

105. Koller H, Keil P, Seibert F. Individual and team training with first time users of the Pelvic C-Clamp: do they remember or will we need refresher trainings? Arch Orthop Trauma Surg. 2013;133:343–9.

106. Metsemakers WJ, Vanderschot P, Jennes E, Nijs S, Heye S, Maleux G. Transcatheter embolotherapy after external surgical stabilization is a valuable treatment algorithm for patients with persistent haemorrhage from unstable pelvic fractures: outcomes of a single centre experience. Injury. 2013;44:964–8.

107. Panetta T, Sclafani SJ, Goldstein AS, Phillips TF, Shaftan GW. Percutaneous transcatheter embolization for massive bleeding from pelvic fractures. J Trauma. 1985;25:1021–9.

108. Rossaint R, Duranteau J, Stahel PF, Spahn DR. Nonsurgical treatment of major bleeding. Anesthesiol Clin. 2007;25:35–48. viii.

109. Velmahos GC, Toutouzas KG, Vassiliu P, et al. A prospective study on the safety and efficacy of angiographic embolization for pelvic and visceral injuries. J Trauma. 2002;53:303–8. discussion 8.

110. Agolini SF, Shah K, Jaffe J, Newcomb J, Rhodes M, Reed 3rd JF. Arterial embolization is a rapid and effective technique for controlling pelvic fracture hemorrhage. J Trauma. 1997;43:395–9.

111. Eastridge BJ, Starr A, Minei JP, O'Keefe GE, Scalea TM. The importance of fracture pattern in guiding therapeutic decision-making in patients with

hemorrhagic shock and pelvic ring disruptions. J Trauma. 2002;53:446–50. discussion 50–1.

112. Hagiwara A, Minakawa K, Fukushima H, Murata A, Masuda H, Shimazaki S. Predictors of death in patients with life-threatening pelvic hemorrhage after successful transcatheter arterial embolization. J Trauma. 2003;55:696–703.

113. Heetveld MJ, Harris I, Schlaphoff G, Sugrue M. Guidelines for the management of haemodynamically unstable pelvic fracture patients. ANZ J Surg. 2004;74:520–9.

114. Miller PR, Moore PS, Mansell E, Meredith JW, Chang MC. External fixation or arteriogram in bleeding pelvic fracture: initial therapy guided by markers of arterial hemorrhage. J Trauma. 2003;54:437–43.

115. Shapiro M, McDonald AA, Knight D, Johannigman JA, Cuschieri J. The role of repeat angiography in the management of pelvic fractures. J Trauma. 2005;58:227–31.

116. Thorson CM, Ryan ML, Otero CA, et al. Operating room or angiography suite for hemodynamically unstable pelvic fractures? J Trauma Acute Care Surg. 2012;72:364–70. discussion 71–2.

117. Verbeek DO, Sugrue M, Balogh Z, et al. Acute management of hemodynamically unstable pelvic trauma patients: time for a change? Multicenter review of recent practice. World J Surg. 2008;32:1874–82.

118. Chu CH, Tennakoon L, Maggio PM, Weiser TG, Spain DA, Staudenmayer KL. Trends in the management of pelvic fractures, 2008–2010. J Surg Res. 2016; 202:335–40.

119. Sarin EL, Moore JB, Moore EE, et al. Pelvic fracture pattern does not always predict the need for urgent embolization. J Trauma. 2005;58:973–7.

120. Kimbrell BJ, Velmahos GC, Chan LS, Demetriades D. Angiographic embolization for pelvic fractures in older patients. Arch Surg. 2004;139:728–32. discussion 32–3.

121. Jones CB. Posterior pelvic ring injuries: when to perform open reduction and internal fixation. Instr Course Lect. 2012;61:27–38.

122. Bazylewicz D, Konda S. A Review of the Definitive Treatment of Pelvic Fractures. Bull Hosp Jt Dis (2013). 2016;74:6–11.

123. Sembler Soles GL, Lien J, Tornetta 3rd P. Nonoperative immediate weightbearing of minimally displaced lateral compression sacral fractures does not result in displacement. J Orthop Trauma. 2012;26:563–7.

124. Suzuki T, Morgan SJ, Smith WR, Stahel PF, Flierl MA, Hak DJ. Stress radiograph to detect true extent of symphyseal disruption in presumed anteroposterior compression type I pelvic injuries. J Trauma. 2010;69:880–5.

125. Hak DJ, Baran S, Stahel P. Sacral fractures: current strategies in diagnosis and management. Orthopedics. 2009;32(10).

126. Kach K, Trentz O. Distraction spondylodesis of the sacrum in "vertical shear lesions" of the pelvis. Unfallchirurg. 1994;97:28–38.

127. Lindahl J, Makinen TJ, Koskinen SK, Soderlund T. Factors associated with outcome of spinopelvic dissociation treated with lumbopelvic fixation. Injury. 2014;45:1914–20.

128. Min KS, Zamorano DP, Wahba GM, Garcia I, Bhatia N, Lee TQ. Comparison of two-transsacral-screw fixation versus triangular osteosynthesis for transforaminal sacral fractures. Orthopedics. 2014;37:e754–60.

129. Putnis SE, Pearce R, Wali UJJ, Bircher MD, Rickman MS. Open reduction and internal fixation of a traumatic diastasis of the pubic symphysis: one-year radiological and functional outcomes. J Bone Joint Surg (Br). 2011;93:78–84.

130. Sagi HC. Technical aspects and recommended treatment algorithms in triangular osteosynthesis and spinopelvic fixation for vertical shear transforaminal sacral fractures. J Orthop Trauma. 2009;23:354–60.

131. Sagi HC, Militano U, Caron T, Lindvall E. A comprehensive analysis with minimum 1-year follow-up of vertically unstable transforaminal sacral fractures treated with triangular osteosynthesis. J Orthop Trauma. 2009;23: 313–9. discussion 9–21.

132. Schildhauer TA, Josten C, Muhr G. Triangular osteosynthesis of vertically unstable sacrum fractures: a new concept allowing early weight-bearing. J Orthop Trauma. 2006;20:S44–51.

133. Suzuki T, Hak DJ, Ziran BH, et al. Outcome and complications of posterior transiliac plating for vertically unstable sacral fractures. Injury. 2009;40:405–9.

134. Scaglione M, Parchi P, Digrandi G, Latessa M, Guido G. External fixation in pelvic fractures. Musculoskelet Surg. 2010;94:63–70.

135. Vaidya R, Colen R, Vigdorchik J, Tonnos F, Sethi A. Treatment of unstable pelvic ring injuries with an internal anterior fixator and posterior fixation: initial clinical series. J Orthop Trauma. 2012;26:1–8.

136. Barei DP, Shafer BL, Beingessner DM, Gardner MJ, Nork SE, Routt ML. The impact of open reduction internal fixation on acute pain management in unstable pelvic ring injuries. J Trauma. 2010;68:949–53.

137. Stahel PF, Hammerberg EM. History of pelvic fracture management: a review. World J Emerg Surg. 2016;11:18.

138. Balbachevsky D, Belloti JC, Doca DG, et al. Treatment of pelvic fractures - a national survey. Injury. 2014;45 Suppl 5:S46–51.

139. Childs BR, Nahm NJ, Moore TA, Vallier HA. Multiple Procedures in the Initial Surgical Setting: When Do the Benefits Outweigh the Risks in Patients With Multiple System Trauma? J Orthop Trauma. 2016;30:420–5.

140. Enninghorst N, Toth L, King KL, McDougall D, Mackenzie S, Balogh ZJ. Acute definitive internal fixation of pelvic ring fractures in polytrauma patients: a feasible option. J Trauma. 2010;68:935–41.

141. Nahm NJ, Moore TA, Vallier HA. Use of two grading systems in determining risks associated with timing of fracture fixation. J Trauma Acute Care Surg. 2014;77:268–79.

142. Pape HC, Tornetta 3rd P, Tarkin I, Tzioupis C, Sabeson V, Olson SA. Timing of fracture fixation in multitrauma patients: the role of early total care and damage control surgery. J Am Acad Orthop Surg. 2009;17:541–9.

143. Schreiber VM, Tarkin IS, Hildebrand F, et al. The timing of definitive fixation for major fractures in polytrauma–a matched-pair comparison between a US and European level I centres: analysis of current fracture management practice in polytrauma. Injury. 2011;42:650–4.

144. Vallier HA, Cureton BA, Ekstein C, Oldenburg FP, Wilber JH. Early definitive stabilization of unstable pelvis and acetabulum fractures reduces morbidity. J Trauma. 2010;69:677–84.

145. Vallier HA, Moore TA, Como JJ, et al. Complications are reduced with a protocol to standardize timing of fixation based on response to resuscitation. J Orthop Surg Res. 2015;10:155.

146. Pape HC, Giannoudis PV, Krettek C, Trentz O. Timing of fixation of major fractures in blunt polytrauma: role of conventional indicators in clinical decision making. J Orthop Trauma. 2005;19:551–62.

147. Pape HC, Griensven MV, Hildebrand FF, et al. Systemic inflammatory response after extremity or truncal fracture operations. J Trauma. 2008;65: 1379–84.

148. Probst C, Probst T, Gaensslen A, Krettek C, Pape HC. Timing and duration of the initial pelvic stabilization after multiple trauma in patients from the German trauma registry: is there an influence on outcome? J Trauma. 2007; 62:370–7. discussion 6–7.

149. Pape H, Stalp M, v Griensven M, Weinberg A, Dahlweit M, Tscherne H. [Optimal timing for secondary surgery in polytrauma patients: an evaluation of 4,314 serious-injury cases]. Chirurg. 1999;70:1287–92.

150. D'Alleyrand JC, O'Toole RV. The evolution of damage control orthopedics: current evidence and practical applications of early appropriate care. Orthop Clin North Am. 2013;44:499–507.

151. Katsoulis E, Giannoudis PV. Impact of timing of pelvic fixation on functional outcome. Injury. 2006;37:1133–42.

152. Pape HC, Giannoudis P, Krettek C. The timing of fracture treatment in polytrauma patients: relevance of damage control orthopedic surgery. Am J Surg. 2002;183:622–9.

153. Pape HC, Lefering R, Butcher N, et al. The definition of polytrauma revisited: An international consensus process and proposal of the new 'Berlin definition'. J Trauma Acute Care Surg. 2014;77:780–6.

154. Scalea TM. Optimal timing of fracture fixation: have we learned anything in the past 20 years? J Trauma. 2008;65:253–60.

155. Scalea TM, Boswell SA, Scott JD, Mitchell KA, Kramer ME, Pollak AN. External fixation as a bridge to intramedullary nailing for patients with multiple injuries and with femur fractures: damage control orthopedics. J Trauma. 2000;48:613–21. discussion 21–3.

156. Scalea TM, Scott JD, Brumback RJ, et al. Early fracture fixation may be "just fine" after head injury: no difference in central nervous system outcomes. J Trauma. 1999;46:839–46.

26

Non operative management of traumatic esophageal perforation leading to esophagocutaneous fistula in pediatric age group

Biplab Mishra[1], Saurabh Singhal[2*], Divya Aggarwal[3], Nitesh Kumar[2] and Subodh Kumar[1]

Abstract

Management of delayed presenting esophageal perforations has long been a topic of debate. Most authors consider definitive surgery being the management of choice. Management, however, differs in pediatric patients in consideration with better healing of younger tissues. We extensively review the role of aggressive non-operative management in pediatric esophageal perforations, especially with delayed presentation and exemplify with case of a young boy with esophageal perforation and esophago-cutaneous fistula. We also lay down the protocol to manage such patients based on our institutional recommendations.

Keywords: Esophageal perforation, Perforation, Pediatric, Traumatic, Non-operative, Conservative, Protocol, Thoracic, Iatrogenic

Background

Management of esophageal perforations (EPs) has long been a topic of debate. The management protocols are chiefly governed by symptom severity, perforation site, time elapsed since perforation and cause of perforation. Esophageal perforations can be iatrogenic, traumatic, spontaneous or following forceful vomiting. Penetrating non-iatrogenic EP is a rare, life-threatening condition [1-4]. Surgical interventions including primary repair with tissue reinforcement or resection-reconstruction have long been the preferred approach [4]. Non operative management is generally advocated in contained leaks, iatrogenic injuries and hemodynamically stable patients. It is not recommended in delayed EPs (presenting after 24 hours) [5]. We review the literature on the role of non-operative management in EPs and describe management of a pediatric case with delayed traumatic thoracic EP with esophago-cutaneous fistula.

Case presentation

An 11 year old male with alleged history of penetrating trauma to lower chest presented to a local community

* Correspondence: drsaurabhsinghal@gmail.com
[2]All India Institute of Medical Sciences, New Delhi, India
Full list of author information is available at the end of the article

hospital. While playing at a construction site, the child fell on a sharp iron rod which inflicted the injury. He was managed with fluid resuscitation followed by removal of the rod through the entry wound. The wound was thoroughly irrigated and dressed. No other surgical intervention was done. On day 1, the child developed lower chest pain, dyspnea and low grade fever. Chest x-ray revealed right sided moderate hydropneumothorax for which intercostal drain (ICD) was placed. No further imaging studies were done. Child was kept nil per oral (NPO) with intravenous (IV) fluids and nutritional supplements for first two days; analgesics and IV amoxicillin-clavulanate were given for five days. No naso-gastric (NG) tube insertion was done during the hospital stay. There were no further fever episodes. Local wound care and regular dressings were done.

Child was allowed oral liquids on day 4. Ingested liquids were found to be coming out of the entry wound. There was no associated chest pain or dysphagia. Patient was again kept NPO for another ten days with repeat trials of oral feeds thrice in this duration. On similar observation, possibility of esophageal perforation with esophago-cutaneous fistula was made and feeding gastrostomy (FG) was done for enteral nutrition. Patient was then referred to our tertiary care level-I trauma centre.

Child presented to our emergency department on day 13 following injury. He was lethargic and malnourished with a GCS of 15/15, though did not appear to be in any acute distress. Airway was patent, with reduced air entry and crepitation in right lower zone and saturation >97% on room air. Chest compression test was negative. He was afebrile with a pulse rate of 104 per minute and blood pressure of 102/60 mmHg. Capillary filling time was normal. Child weighed 10 kg with height of 98 cm. He was afebrile to touch.

On examination, a 3×3 cm entry wound was noted 2 cm lateral to the right border of sternum, in 6th intercostal space, about 3.5 cm below right nipple. Wound was healthy with granulation tissue and sero-mucoid discharge. There was 24 Fr ICD in situ in right 4th intercostal space and a feeding gastrostomy in place. Total ISS score and Braden score at presentation were 18 and 19 respectively.

Chest roentgenogram revealed right lower lobe consolidation and right sided pleural effusion with ICD in situ. A contrast enhanced CT scan (CECT) of chest and abdomen was done with additional non-ionic contrast given orally (Figure 1). It revealed right sided hydropneumothorax with contrast leak from thoracic esophagus, pooling of contrast in right pleural cavity, draining through entry wound and ICD, and right sided mid and lower lobe lung contusions with consolidation of right lower lobe. Left lung was healthy with no significant radiologic abnormalities detected. There was visible contrast leak from the skin wound as well.

Patient was admitted and managed conservatively with IV fluids, IV antibiotics (cefoperazone-sulbactam for 10 days and metronidazole for 6 days), adequate wound care and nutritional care. He was kept NPO on parenteral nutrition with vitamin K supplements. No NG tube insertion was done. FG feeding, alongwith electrolyte and vitamin C supplements, was initiated on day 2 of admission at 30 mL/hour and gradually increased to 50 ml/hour as it was well tolerated. ICD was kept on under water seal drainage. Patient's progress records have been charted in Table 1.

On day 20 of admission, ICD removal was done as drain output was minimal (serous) and ICD fluid cultures were consistently negative. Repeat CECT chest with oral contrast revealed no leak (Figure 2). Full oral diet was initiated.

Child was discharged on day 22 of admission after removing FG. On discharge, child was in good health, accepting orally with stable vitals, bilaterally clear chest and soft, non-tender abdomen. He gained 3.2 kg during hospital stay and total leucocyte count fell from 15,500/cumm to 9,800/cumm. Braden risk score remained above 19 throughout hospital stay. Wound healed with secondary intention.

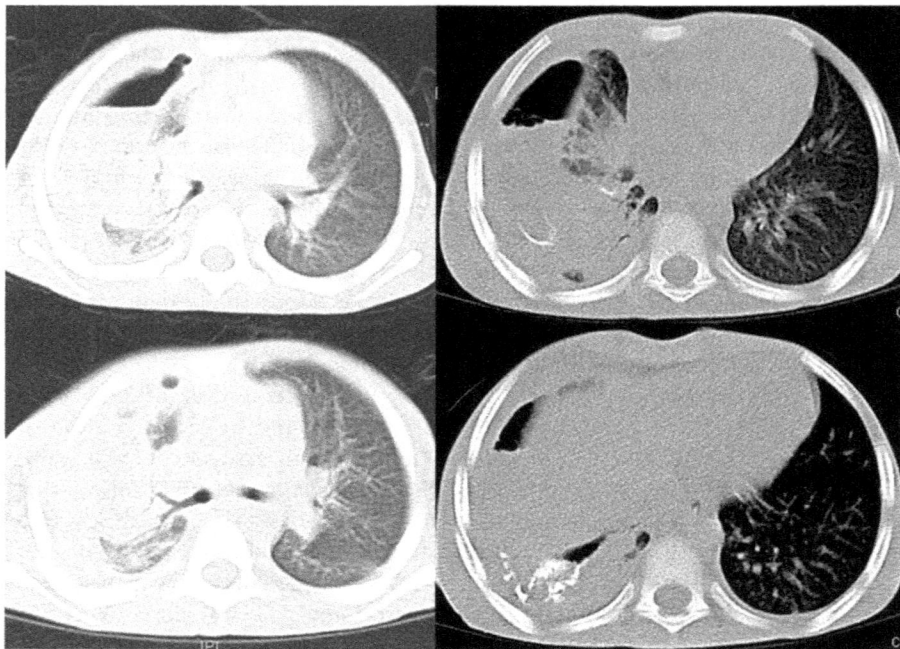

Figure 1 CECT chest showing contrast leak from thoracic esophagus with pooling of contrast in right pleural cavity. Lung consolidation may be appreciated.

Table 1 Progress chart of patient during in-hospital stay

	Presentation	Day 2 of admission	Day 10 of admission	Discharge
Weight (kg)	10	10.3	12.8	13.2
Pulse rate (per minute)	104	92	94	91
Temperature (°F)	99.1	97.4	98.1	98.6
Braden risk	19	20	20	21
Hemogram				
Hb (gm%)	9.5	10.1	11.5	10.9
Hct (%)	27.3	32.7	37	36.8
Plt (per cumm)	567,000	805,000	796,000	512,000
TLC (per cumm)	15,500	14,100	11,800	9,800
Blood biochemistry				
U/Cr/Na/K	15/0.3/137/4.1	15/0.3/135/4.8	26/0.2/137/5.5	24/0.4/133/4.2
Serum Protein	4.2	4.3	6.6	6.8
Serum Albumin	2.3	2.6	3.3	3.5

Hb- Haemoglobin; Hct- Haematocrit; Plt- Platelet count; TLC- Total leucocyte count; U- Urea; Cr- Creatinine; Na- Sodium; K- Potassium.

Repeat barium swallow on two month follow-up revealed no leak (Figure 3). Chest x-ray revealed clear lung fields bilaterally. Patient is doing fine on 18 month follow-up, with weight and height appropriate for age, and is accepting oral feeds. There are no respiratory symptoms, dysphagia or chest pain. Scar at wound site is healthy.

Review and discussion

Esophageal perforation (EP); traumatic, iatrogenic or due to any other cause; has long been a dreaded condition with high morbidity and mortality rates. The first account of EP comes from late 18th Century as described by Boerhaave [6]. First pediatric perforation was described by Fryfogle in 1952 [7].

EP is a life threatening condition associated with mortality rates reaching upto 20-50% [7-10]. Contamination with oral and gastro-intestinal contents can cause mediastinitis and generalized sepsis leading to multi-organ dysfunction and death [11]. Delay in diagnosis is not uncommon owing to the more common differentials with similar presentation and is dreadful, unless there is a

temporal relationship present with esophageal instrumentation or trauma to have high suspicion of EP [12]. With advent of esophago-gastric instrumentation, iatrogenic causes have replaced the other causes as the most common etiology. Traumatic perforations are very rare but demand a high index of suspicion owing to their high morbidity and mortality [4] (Table 2).

Historically, early surgical intervention (within 24 hours of presentation), with intent of definitive repair, used to be the mainstay of treatment owing to the reported mortality rates as high as 69% in patients managed non-operatively or in whom surgeries were delayed. Early surgical interventions were considered to bring down mortality rates to less than half [13]. Primary surgery had since been considered the management of choice for EP in adults and most children except for few early presenting cases [13-18]. Okanta et al [5] reviewed seven major studies describing management of delayed benign esophageal perforations and concluded esophagectomy as better management approach compared with primary repair and conservative management. Their review, however, mostly included retrospective studies, lacked randomized controlled trials

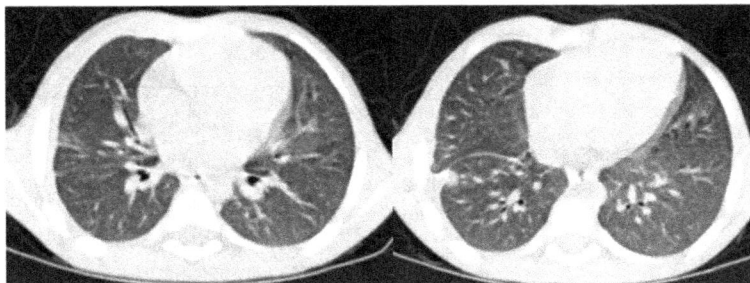

Figure 2 Repeat CECT chest on day 20 of admission revealed no contrast leak.

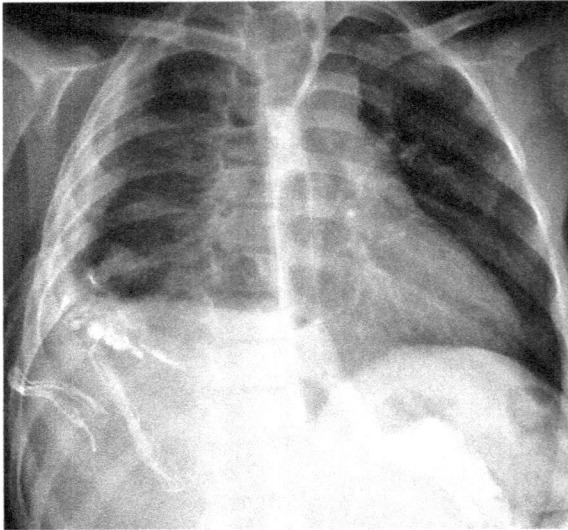

Figure 3 Barium swallow at 2 months follow-up revealed no contrast leak.

and adequate follow-up and did not differentiate between mortalities for early and delayed EPs in many of the studies.

First published account of successful non operative management for EPs came from work of Mengoli and Klassen in 1965. They achieved mortality rates of about 6% in 18 cases of iatrogenic esophageal perforations (following diagnostic or therapeutic esophagoscopy) managed conservatively. Two-third of their patients had perforation in distal third of the esophagus. They relied on massive use of antibiotics, nasoesophageal suction and intercostal drainage [19-21]. Brinster et al [4] reviewed various series published between 1990 and 2003 for management options for EPs and concluded a total mortality of 18% with any kind of treatment. Mortality with non-operative management (17%) was slightly higher than the primary repair (12%) whereas it was much higher with drainage (36%) and exclusion (24%).

Table 2 Aetiology of esophageal perforation (in descending order of incidence) [4,14-16]

Children	Adults
1) Iatrogenic (diagnostic or therapeutic instrumentation)	1) Iatrogenic (diagnostic or therapeutic instrumentation)
2) Lye burns	2) Spontaneous (Boerhaave's syndrome)
3) Direct/Indirect trauma	3) Foreign bodies
4) Foreign bodies	4) Penetrating trauma (m.c.- gunshot)
5) Operative procedures in the area	5) Malignant perforations
6) Idiopathic	6) Operative injury
	7) Idiopathic

m.c. – most common.

Increasing incidence of iatrogenic injuries, which are earlier diagnosed and are associated with less mediastinal contamination, are ideal for non-operative management. Less contamination is due to nil per oral status of patient prior to endoscopic procedures and injuries mostly being limited. Traumatic injuries have lesser evidence but yet have been proven to show successful healing with the latter, as was in our patient. Not to forget the younger age, which has a positive impact in healing of tissues.

Thoracic EPs are more amenable to successful non-operative management owing to ease of pleural drainage for esophageal leaks [14]. With adequate pleural toilet, proper antibiotic coverage and nutritional support, the thoracic esophageal perforations as well as esophagocutaneous fistulas heal spontaneously, just like any other gastrointestinal fistulas [15].

EP in children have special relevance in view of inability of very young children to present with early signs and symptoms. Most perforations in pediatric age group are iatrogenic following upper airway or esophageal corrosive esophageal injuries [7] (Table 2). Children developing chest or abdominal pain, nausea, dyspnea, fever, leucocytosis, subcutaneous emphysema and other signs and symptoms following esophageal instrumentation or trauma to lower neck, chest or upper abdomen should be dealt with high index of suspicion [4,12,22]. Early diagnosis is vital. Prognosis is better with diagnosis within 24 hours of perforation. Chest X-rays, water soluble or non-ionic contrast studies of esophagus and contrast enhanced CT scan with oral contrast should be utilised for early and accurate diagnosis [4]. Endoscopy may be combined with contrast studies for accurate diagnosis and can play a therapeutic role in the same sitting. Raised drain amylase is another sensitive but non-specific indicator of esophageal injury [22]. Favourable prognostic factors are listed in Table 3.

Table 3 Favourable prognostic predictors after EP* [17,39]

1.	Early diagnosis and treatment
2.	Iatrogenic origin
3.	Young age
4.	Absence of concomitant esophageal disease
5.	Benign perforations
6.	Absence of co-morbidities
7.	Good nutritional and hemodynamic status
8.	Site- Cervical > Thoracic (Abdominal EP generally has poor outcome)
9.	Sharp penetrating injuries better than blunt and thermal puncture (gunshot) injuries

*Apply to both operative and non-operative management.

Non-operative approach to pediatric EPs stem from the unparalleled healing capacity of tissues at younger age [23]. Martinez et al [13] published an elaborate case series of non-operative management of EPs in children. They successfully managed 17 of 18 pediatric cases of thoracic esophageal perforations. They had 100% survival rate with only one patient developing long term esophageal stricture requiring dilatation. Their results emphasize the importance of non-operative management in pediatric age-group. Children with caustic injury are prone to iatrogenic esophageal injuries during endoscopic balloon dilatation

for strictures. A conservative approach with or without cervical esophagostomy and gastrostomy has been found to be adequate in such patients. Resection anastomosis and colonic interpositions may be considered in patients with long segment strictures following perforation [24]. Delayed EPs, extensive involvements and esophago-cutaneous fistulas, which are relatively contraindicate conservative management, can still be managed successfully by active and aggressive non-operative approach in children.

A recently published position paper on esophageal injuries recommends non-operative management to be

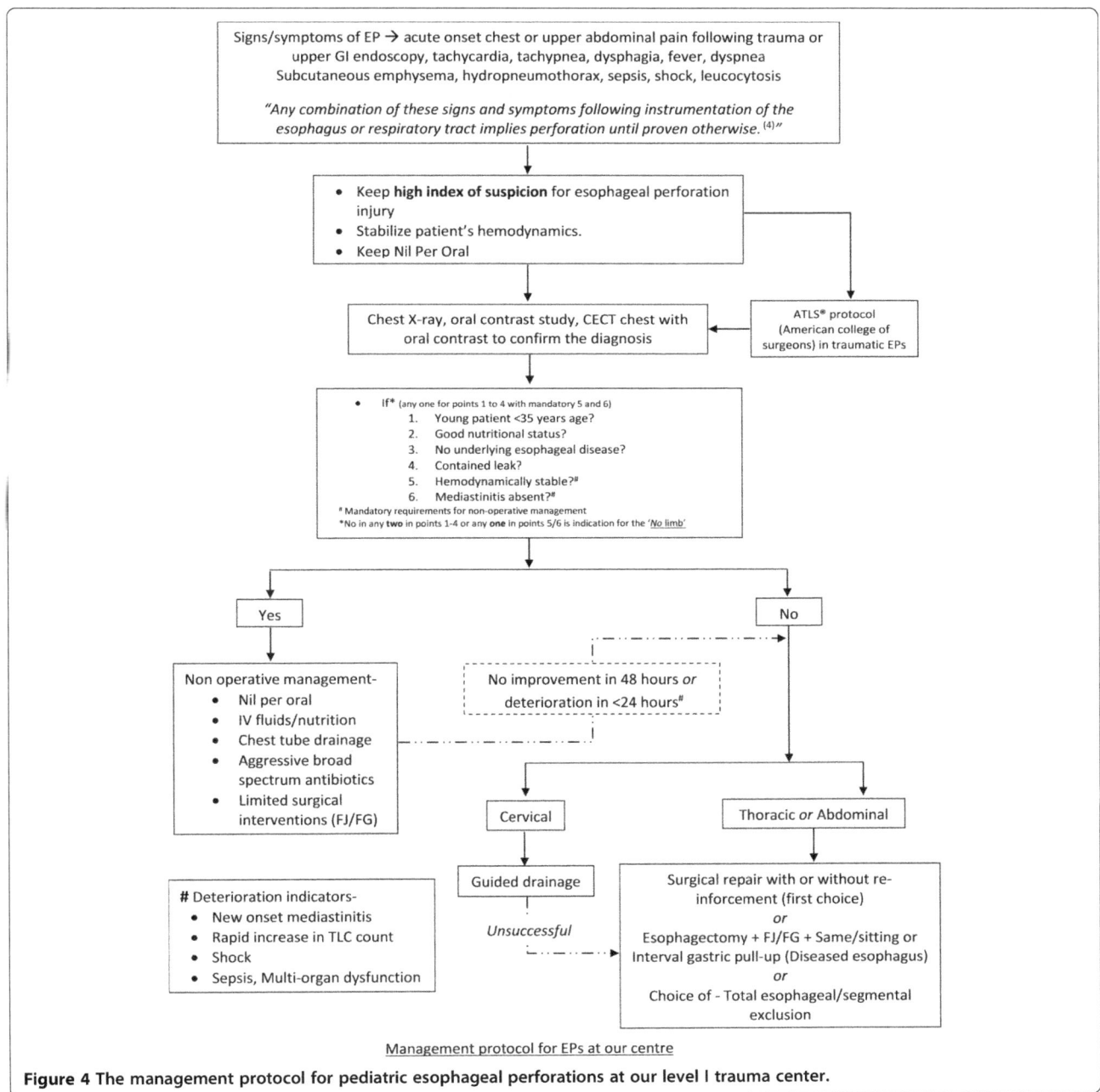

Figure 4 The management protocol for pediatric esophageal perforations at our level I trauma center.

done in hemodynamically stable patients with small perforations presenting within 48 hours of injury [22]. We agree with the recommendations and emphasize the importance of aggressive conservative management in pediatric population (as per our protocol flowchart).

Neonatal esophageal perforation is mostly seen in premature new-borns with history of multiple attempts at intubation or forceful oropharyngeal suctioning. Various authors have shown the successful non-operative approach with minimal surgical interventions for such patients [25,26].

Adequate nutritional support is of prime concern in children. Enteral feeding is always considered superior to prolonged parenteral support, which has its own drawbacks. Feeding gastrostomy and jejunostomy are considered limited surgical interventions and should be included in non-operative approach to pediatric EPs. Apart from providing nutritional support, they help in preventing retrograde contamination of mediastinum with gastric secretions [20].

To prevent mediastinal contamination, nasogastric drainage is suggested and practised by some physicians, though its role has long been debated. While many authors include it in the non-operative regime [27], Cameron et al. achieved uncomplicated spontaneous closure of esophageal leaks in all eight patients without even pleural drainage, seven of whom did not undergo nasogastric drainage as well. They claim that latter only increases gastro-esophageal reflux which will further aggravate mediastinal contamination [28,29]. We do not recommend nasogastric drainage in our protocol, especially in pediatric age group. Our patient, without nasogastric drainage, achieved successful outcome which further affirms our recommendations.

There are some recent studies addressing uses of endoscopically placed self-expandable metallic stents with or without chest drainage in patients with esophageal perforations and post-operative esophageal anastomotic leaks [8,30-34]. However, none of the studies have sufficiently large sample size and long term follow-ups to look at possibility of esophageal strictures associated with metallic stents in situ [8,24,35-37]. Also, there are very few cases among pediatric age group. While stent placement can act as a bridging option to definitive surgeries like esophagectomy and colonic interposition, however, there are reports of esophageal stents themselves causing esophageal injury [8,22,24]. Displaced stents may also be of concern in younger children. We recommend more studies on their usage. We, currently, do not include esophageal stent placement in the management protocol of pediatric or adult esophageal perforations at our institution.

Use of endoscopically placed clips and endoscopic vacuum sponge are the other newer modalities being

Table 4 Non-operative management protocol for pediatric esophageal perforations (at our centre)

Intervention	Significance
1) Nil per oral (minimum of 7–10 days)	+++
2) Adequate enteral/parenteral hyperalimentation	+++
3) Aggressive broad spectrum antibiotic therapy (minimum 7 days)	+++
4) Early limited surgical interventions (gastrostomy/jejunostomy)	+
5) Chest drainage with wide bore intercostal drain	++
6) Nasogastric suction/drainage	+/−
7) Intravenous proton pump inhibitors (minimum 7 days)	+/−

introduced with promising results. The adequately powered randomised and blinded trials are required to prove their efficacy in children [38].

Overall, non-operative management protocols, with advent of early diagnostic modalities and close monitoring in delayed presentations, are useful and should be implemented in carefully chosen patients. Our protocol for management of esophageal perforations is shown in the form of a flowchart in Figure 4. Non-operative management protocol has been described in Table 4.

Conclusion

EPs are rare in children and traumatic EPs are even rarer. We conclude that they can successfully be managed by an active and aggressive non-operative approach. A good antibiotic coverage, nutritional support, downstream drainage of leaks via intercostal drains and occasional need for limited surgical interventions as gastrostomy and jejunostomy are vital and may even be employed in extensive and delayed EPs. Authors still recommend attending physician's discretion in planning the management and deciding for early definite surgical interventions depending on individual presentations.

Consent

Informed and written consent was taken from the patient's parents to publish this case report, investigation reports and images.

Abbreviations
EP: Esophageal Perforation; CECT: Contrast enhanced computed tomography; ICD: Intercostal drain; IV: Intravenous; FG: Feeding gastrostomy; FJ: Feeding jejunostomy.

Competing interests
The authors declare that they have no competing interests.

Authors' contributions
BM and SK headed the team managing this patient. SS was the primary physician in-charge for the patient. All authors were involved in management and follow-up of the patient. SS wrote the manuscript. SS, BM and NK reviewed the literature. SS and DA proof-read the manuscript, reviewed the corrections and revised the manuscript. All authors read and approved the manuscript prior to submission. SS is the corresponding author.

Authors' information
All authors except DA are affiliated to All India Institute of Medical Sciences (AIIMS), New Delhi and Jai Prakash Narayan Apex Trauma Centre, AIIMS, New Delhi. DA is affiliated to University College of Medical Sciences, New Delhi.

Author details
[1]Jai Prakash Narayan Apex Trauma Center, All India Institute of Medical Sciences, New Delhi, India. [2]All India Institute of Medical Sciences, New Delhi, India. [3]University College of Medical Sciences, New Delhi, India.

References
1. Weiman DS, Walker WA, Brosnan KM, Pate JW, Fabian TC. Noniatrogenic esophageal trauma. Ann Thorac Surg. 1995;59(4):845–50.
2. Asensio JA, Chahwan S, Forno W, MacKersie R, Wall M, Lake J, et al. Penetrating esophageal injuries. multicenter study of the American Association for the Surgery of Trauma. J Trauma. 2001;50(2):289–96.
3. Plott E, Jones D, McDermott D, Levoyer T. A state-of-the-art review of esophageal trauma: where do we stand? Dis Esophagus. 2007;20(4):279–89.
4. Brinster CJ, Singhal S, Lee L, Marshall MB, Kaiser LR, Kucharczuk JC. Evolving options in the management of esophageal perforation. Ann Thorac Surg. 2004;77(4):1475–83.
5. Okonta KE, Kesieme EB. Is oesophagectomy or conservative treatment for delayed benign oesophageal perforation the better option? Interact Cardiovasc Thorac Surg. 2012;15(3):509–11.
6. Derbes VJ, Mitchell RE. Hermann Boerhaave's Atrocis, nec descripti prius, morbi historia, the first translation of the classic case report of rupture of the esophagus, with annotations. Bull Med Libr Assoc. 1955;43:217–40.
7. Gander JW, Berdon WE, Cowles RA. Iatrogenic esophageal perforation in children. Pediatr Surg Int. 2009;25(5):395–401.
8. Leers JM, Vivaldi C, Schäfer H, Bludau M, Brabender J, Lurje G, et al. Endoscopic therapy for esophageal perforation or anastomotic leak with a self-expandable metallic stent. Surg Endosc. 2009;23(10):2258–62.
9. Blewett CJ, Miller JD, Young JE, Bennett WF, Urschel JD. Anastomotic leaks after esophagectomy for esophageal cancer: a comparison of thoracic and cervical anastomoses. Ann Thorac Cardiovasc Surg. 2001;7:75–8.
10. Hofstetter W, Swisher SG, Correa AM, Hess K, Putnam Jr JB, Ajani JA, et al. Treatment outcomes of resected esophageal cancer. Ann Surg. 2002;236:376–85.
11. Kim-Deobald J, Kozarek RA. Esophageal perforation: an 8-year review of a multispecialty clinic's experience. Am J Gastroenterol. 1992;87:1112–9.
12. Port JL, Kent MS, Korst RJ, Bacchetta M, Altorki NK. Thoracic esophageal perforations: a decade of experience. Ann Thorac Surg. 2003;75(4):1071–4.
13. Jemerin EE. Results of treatment of perforation of the esophagus. Ann Surg. 1948;128:971.
14. Martinez L, Rivas S, Hernández F, Avila LF, Lassaletta L, Murcia J, et al. Aggressive conservative treatment of esophageal perforations in children. J Pediatr Surg. 2003;38(5):685–9.
15. Shepherd RL, Raffensperger JG, Goldstein R. Pediatric esophageal perforation. J Thorac Cardiovasc Surg. 1977;74(2):261–7.
16. van der Zee DC, Festen C, Severijnen RS, van der Staak FH. Management of pediatric esophageal perforation. J Thorac Cardiovasc Surg. 1988;95:692–5.
17. Jones II WG, Ginsberg RJ. Esophageal perforation: a continuing challenge. Ann Thorac Surg. 1992;53:534–43.
18. Attar S, Hankins JR, Suter CM, Coughlin TR, Sequeira A, McLaughlin JS. Esophageal perforation: a therapeutic challenge. Ann Thorac Surg. 1990;50:45–9.
19. Mengoli LR, Klassen KP. Conservative management of esophageal perforation. Arch Surg. 1965;91:232–40.
20. Lyons WS, Seremetis MG. Ruptures and perforations of the esophagus: the case for conservative supportive management. Ann Thorac Surg. 1978;25:346–50.
21. Wesdorp IC, Bartelsman JF. Treatment of instrumental oesophageal perforation. Gut. 1984;25:398–404.
22. Ivatury RR, Moore FA, Biffl W, Leppeniemi A, Ansaloni L, Catena F, et al. Oesophageal injuries: position paper, WSES, 2013. World J Emerg Surg. 2014;9(1):9.
23. Ashcroft GS, Mills SJ, Ashworth JJ. Ageing and wound healing. Biogerontology. 2002;3(6):337–45.
24. Eliçevik M, Alim A, Tekant GT, Sarimurat N, Adaletli I, Kurugoglu S, et al. Management of esophageal perforation secondary to caustic esophageal injury in children. Surg Today. 2008;38(4):311–5.
25. Emil SG. Neonatal esophageal perforation. J Pediatr Surg. 2004;39(8):1296–8.
26. Krasna IH, Rosenfeld D, Benjamin BG, Klein G, Hiatt M, Hegyi T. Esophageal perforation in the neonate: an emerging problem in the newborn nursery. J Pediatr Surg. 1987;22(8):784–90.
27. Santos GH, Frater RW. Transesophageal irrigation for treatment of mediastinitis produced by esophageal rupture. J Thorac Cardiovasc Surg. 1986;91:57–62.
28. Cameron JL, Kieffer RF, Hendrix TR, Mehigan DG, Baker RR. Selective nonoperative management of contained intrathoracic esophageal disruptions. Ann Thorac Surg. 1979;27(5):404–8.
29. Altorjay A, Kiss J, Vörös A, Bohák A. Nonoperative management of esophageal perforations: is it justified? Ann Surg. 1997;225(4):415–21.
30. Freeman RK, Van Woerkom JM, Ascioti AJ. Esophageal stent placement for the treatment of iatrogenic intrathoracic esophageal perforation. Ann Thorac Surg. 2007;83(6):2003–7.
31. Salminen P, Gullichsen R, Laine S. Use of self-expandable metal stents for the treatment of esophageal perforations and anastomotic leaks. Surg Endosc. 2009;23(7):1526–30.
32. van Heel NC, Haringsma J, Spaander MC, Bruno MJ, Kuipers EJ. Short-term esophageal stenting in the management of benign perforations. Am J Gastroenterol. 2010;105(7):1515–20.
33. Kiev J, Amendola M, Bouhaidar D, Sandhu BS, Zhao X, Maher J. A management algorithm for esophageal perforation. Am J Surg. 2007;194(1):103–6.
34. Hamza AF, Abdelhay S, Sherif H, Hasan T, Soliman H, Kabesh A, et al. Caustic esophageal strictures in children: 30 years' experience. J Pediatr Surg. 2003;38:828–33.
35. Mutaf O. Treatment of corrosive esophageal strictures by longterm stenting. J Pediatr Surg. 1996;85:681–5.
36. Peppo FD, Zaccara A, Dall' Oglio L, FedericidiAbriola G, Ponticelli A, Marchetti P, et al. Stenting for caustic strictures: esophageal replacement replaced. J Pediatr Surg. 1998;133:54–7.
37. Tekant GT, Eliçevik M, Sarımurat N, Senyuz OF, Erdogan E. Management of pediatric esophageal strictures with poliflex stents. Dallas: IPEG's 15th Annual Congress for Endosurgery in Children; 2006. April 26–29.
38. Soreidel JA, Asgaust V. Scand J trauma Esophageal perforation: diagnostic work-up and clinical decision-making in the first 24 hours. Resusc Emerg Med. 2011;19:66.
39. Griffiths EA, Yap N, Poulter J, Hendrickse MT, Khurshid M. Thirty-four cases of esophageal perforation: the experience of a district general hospital in the UK. Dis Esophagus. 2009;22(7):616–25.

27

Geriatric trauma hip fractures: is there a difference in outcomes based on fracture patterns?

Alicia Mangram[1]*, Phillip Moeser[1,2], Michael G Corneille[1], Laura J Prokuski[1], Nicolas Zhou[1,3], Jacqueline Sohn[1,3], Shalini Chaliki[1,4], Olakunle F Oguntodu[1] and James K Dzandu[1]

Abstract

Background: Annually in the US, there are over 300,000 hospital admissions due to hip fractures in geriatric patients. Consequently, there have been several large observational studies, which continue to provide new insights into differences in outcomes among hip fracture patients. However, few hip fracture studies have specifically examined the relationship between hip fracture patterns, sex, and short-term outcomes including hospital length of stay and discharge disposition in geriatric trauma patients.

Methods: We performed a retrospective study of hip fractures in geriatric trauma patients. Hip fracture patterns were based on ICD −9 CM diagnostic codes for hip fractures (820.00-820.9). Patient variables were patient demographics, mechanism of injury, injury severity score, hospital and ICU length of stay, co-morbidities, injury location, discharge disposition, and in-patient mortality.

Results: A total of 325 patient records met the inclusion criteria. The mean age of the patients was 82.2 years, and the majority of the patients were white (94%) and female (70%). Hip fractures patterns were categorized as two fracture classes and three fracture types. We observed a difference in the proportion of males to females within each fracture class (Femoral neck fractures Z-score = −8.86, p < 0.001, trochanteric fractures Z-score = −5.63, p < 0.001). Hip fractures were fixed based on fracture pattern and patient characteristics. Hip fracture class or fracture type did not predict short-term outcomes such as in-hospital or ICU length of stay, death, or patient discharge disposition. The majority of patients (73%) were injured at home. However, 84% of the patients were discharged to skilled nursing facility, rehabilitation, or long-term care while only 16% were discharged home. There was no evidence of significant association between fracture pattern, injury severity score, diabetes mellitus, hypertension or dementia.

Conclusions: Hip fracture patterns differ between geriatric male and female trauma patients. However, there was no significant association between fracture patterns and short-term patient outcomes. Further studies are planned to investigate the effect of fracture pattern and long-term outcomes including 90-day mortality, return to previous levels of activity, and other quality of life measures.

Keywords: Femoral neck fractures, Hip fractures, Length of stay, Hip fracture patterns, Geriatric G-60

Introduction

Geriatric trauma in the US is on the rise and at our level-I trauma center we have seen a dramatic increase in our "G-60" geriatric trauma mechanism of injury. There has also been a shift from motor vehicle collision to falls as the new number one mechanism of injury in geriatric trauma. Annually in the US, there are over 300,000 hospital admissions due to hip fractures in geriatric patients. [1] Patients who sustain hip fractures are exposed to significant morbidity [1] and high mortality [2] at a treatment cost between 10.3 to 15.2 billion dollars per year in the US [3,4]. These observations illustrate that hip fractures, especially in the elderly, represent significant health and economic challenges in need of focused attention. Thus, trauma centers across the country are trying to develop ways to improve the quality of care given to elderly trauma patients, which includes a better understanding of hip fracture patterns.

* Correspondence: Alicia.Mangram@jcl.com
[1]John C. Lincoln North Mountain Hospital, Phoenix, USA
Full list of author information is available at the end of the article

The National Hip Fracture Database (NHFD) the largest UK-based national hip fracture audit with 180 contributing hospitals in England, Wales and Northern Ireland has reported differences in outcomes among patients with hip fractures [5]. Similar large observational studies from the US [6] have recently been published which underscore the

A Two major classes of femur fractures.

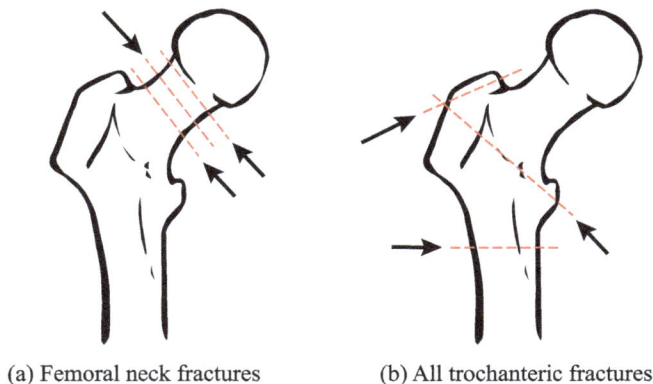

(a) Femoral neck fractures   (b) All trochanteric fractures

B Five categories of femur fracture types.

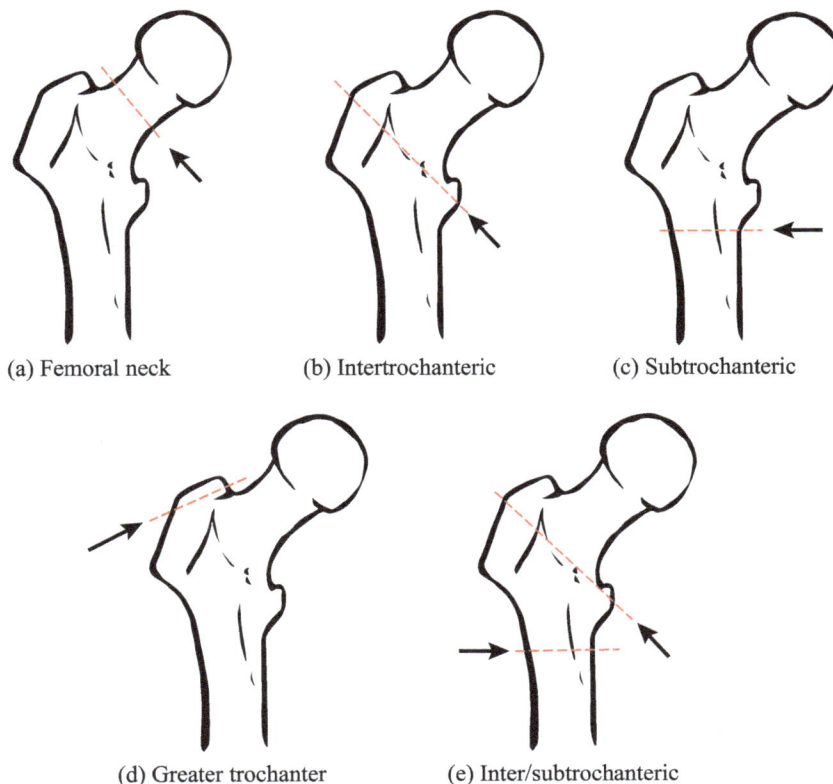

(a) Femoral neck   (b) Intertrochanteric   (c) Subtrochanteric

(d) Greater trochanter   (e) Inter/subtrochanteric

Figure 1 Major classes of femur fractures (A) and categories of femur fracture types (B). A. Femur fracture classes: (a) Femoral neck and (b) All trochanteric fractures. Red lines indicate fracture locations, as indicated by arrows. **B**. Femur Fracture Patterns: (a) Femoral neck (b) Intertrochanteric (c) Subtrochanteric (d) Greater trochanter (e) Combined inter & subtrochanteric. Red lines indicate fracture location, as indicated by arrows. For purposes of statistical analysis, patients with fractures corresponding to figures (c), (d), and (e) were grouped as "other". However, such grouping may not represent homogenous clinical category.

importance of anesthesia technique on mortality and length of stay among patients who underwent surgery for hip fractures.

The term "hip fracture" most commonly refers to fractures of the proximal femur and are generally categorized as (a) femoral neck fractures and (b) trochanteric fractures including intertrochanteric fractures, greater trochanteric fractures and subtrochanteric fractures, and combined inter- and subtrochanteric fractures. Most epidemiologic studies consider only 2 categories, femoral neck and intertrochanteric. Although there are reports showing some decline in the incidence of femur fractures among patients who stopped smoking and drinking alcohol or have been treated for osteoporosis with vitamin D [7-9], mortality and morbidity due to hip fracture remains rather high [7,9,10]. Thus, models have been developed to predict hip fracture mortality [11,12]. However, it remains unclear whether there is a difference in femur fracture pattern distribution (femoral neck vs. trochanteric) in geriatric trauma patients. It is also unknown if there is any association between geriatric G60 trauma patients' fracture pattern and outcomes. The purpose of this study was to determine if there is a difference in patient characteristics or patient outcomes as a function of fracture patterns in geriatric trauma patients age 60 years and older.

Methods

This retrospective study was reviewed and approved by Western Institutional Review Board. Patients were identified by query of the institutional trauma registry at our American College of Surgeons (ACS) verified level-I trauma center for all hip fractures by ICD 9 CM code 820–820.9. Patients with no femur fracture, those with acetabular fracture, or penetrating injuries were excluded. The study period was from August 2012 to February 2014.

Data were collected both from the trauma registry and the electronic medical record. Data recorded included patient variables: age, gender, race/ethnicity, mechanism of injury, hospital and ICU length of stay, discharge disposition and mortality. Data captured were entered into Excel spreadsheets and an Access database. A trauma surgeon reviewed X-ray reports for each femur fracture, and if any ambiguity remained, a radiologist reviewed them. All fractures were described according to fracture class: (a) Femoral neck and (b) trochanteric fractures (Figure 1A). These classes were further categorized into following fracture types: (a) femoral neck, (b) intertrochanteric, (c) subtrochanteric, (d) greater trochanter, and (e) combined inter & subtrochanteric (Figure 1B). Trochanteric fracture class was a combination of intertrochanteric, trochanteric, and subtrochanteric fractures. Patient outcomes variables reviewed included: (a) hospital length of stay (HLOS) days, (b) ICU days (ICU LOS), and (c) discharge disposition including in-patient mortality.

We examined the data for evidence of association between femur fracture type or fracture class and specific outcomes of interest. Covariates were age, gender, ethnicity/race, and injury severity score.

Statistical analysis

Continuous variables were reported as means ± SD and categorical variables as percentages. Comparisons between groups were performed using analysis of variance (ANOVA) or Student's t-test for continuous variables. Pearson's Chi-square test, Fisher's exact test, or two-proportion Z-test was used for categorical variables. Two-sided p-values were used and $p < 0.05$ was considered statistically significant.

Results

Demographics

There were 325 patients, who met all of the study inclusion criteria and none of the exclusion criteria. The mean age (years) was 82.2 ± 9.3 with range of 60 to 101 years. There were 70.2% (n = 228) female and 29.8% (n = 97) male patients. Falls accounted for 95% of mechanism of injury for these patients. Females were older (83.3 ± 8.8 years) than males (79.5 ± 9.8 years) on average (p = 0.001). The majority of subjects (94.2%, n = 306) were white, and all other ethnic groups composed the remaining 5.8% (n = 19) of the patient population. In reviewing patients' co-morbidities, 191 (58.8%) patients had hypertension, 65 (20%) patients had diabetes mellitus, 51 (16%) patients had dementia, 49 (15%) patients had respiratory disease, 20 (6.2%) patients had chronic heart failure, and 20 (6.2%) patients were current smokers. We also studied the fall locations and discharge dispositions of the patients. There were 239 patients (73.5%) who fell at home, 18 patients (5.5%) who fell at nursing home, and 68 patients (21%) who fell at other

Table 1 Description of discharge disposition in relation to their injury locations

Injury locations	Discharge disposition	N	Percent
Home	Home	25	7.7%
	SNF/Rehab/LTC	200	61.7%
	Hospice/Died	13	4.0%
Nursing home	Home	4	1.2%
	SNF/Rehab/LTC	12	3.7%
	Hospice/Died	2	0.6%
Other	Home	11	3.4%
	SNF/Rehab/LTC	52	16.1%
	Hospice/Died	5	1.5%

SNF/Rehab/LTC represents skilled nursing facility, rehabilitation, and long term care. This table represents demographic description of the patients' discharge disposition in relation to their injury locations. There was no statistical analysis performed on this data due to low numbers in some of the sub-groups.

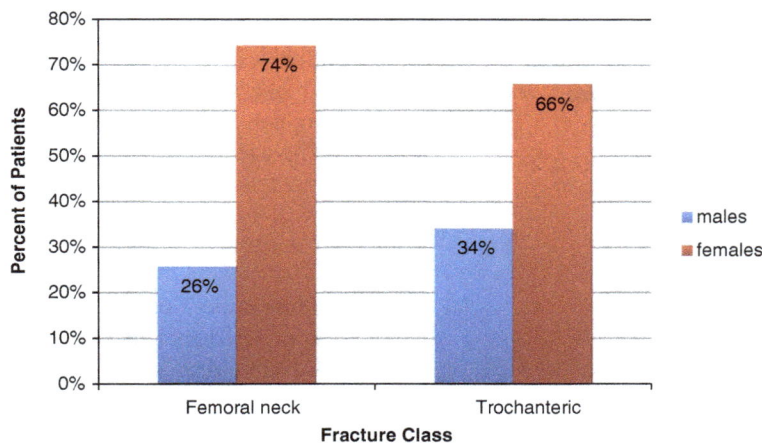

Figure 2 A comparison of proportions of males and females for femoral neck and trochanteric fractures. Femoral neck fractures for males is 43/97 and for females 124/228. Trochanteric fractures for males is 54/97 and for females 104/228, Z-score = −5.63, p < 0.001.

locations. There were 40 patients (12.4%) who were discharged to home, 265 (81.4%) patients who were discharged to SNF, rehabilitation centers, or acute care centers, and 20 patients (6.2%) who either died or were discharged to hospice. The majority of patients fell from home, but the majority of patients were discharged to SNF, rehabilitation center, or acute care facility as it is shown in Table 1.

Fracture class (femoral neck and trochanteric fractures) among elderly G-60 patients

Among our study subjects, 51.4% (n = 167) had femoral neck fractures, and 48.6% (n = 158) had trochanteric fractures. The mean (SD) age of patients with femoral neck fracture was 82.7 ± 8.5 years, and the average age of patients with trochanteric fractures was 82.5 ± 9.6 years (p = 0.84). The difference in age was not statistically significant, (251df) = −0.149, p = 0.881. Patients' mean (SD) injury severity scores (ISS) for femoral neck and trochanteric fractures were 9.4 ± 2.0 and 9.8 ± 3.1, respectively (p = 0.20). We also determined the distribution of femoral neck and trochanteric fractures among the patients based on their gender, and the proportion of males and females with trochanteric fractures and femoral neck fractures showed significantl differences as shown in Figure 2. The HLOS and ICU LOS for each fracture class were also examined. The patients with femoral neck fractures stayed on average (SD) 5.1 ± 2.6 days in hospital, and the patients with trochanteric femur fractures stayed on average 5.4 ± 2.7 days (p = 0.341). The ICU LOS for patients with femoral neck and trochanteric fractures were on average (SD) 3.7 ± 3.6 and 3.3 ± 2.2 days (p = 0.662), respectively. The fall locations and the discharge dispositions were also studied and compared between two fracture classes, and the distribution

of each fracture class was similar in various locations. Table 2.

Femoral fracture types in elderly G-60 patients

When the patients' fracture types were compared, there were 167 patients (51.4%) with femoral neck fractures, and 129 patients (39.7%) with intertrochanteric fractures. The remaining 29 patients (8.9%) had subtrochanteric, greater trochanter only, or combined inter- and subtrochanteric fractures, and were considered as "other" for the purpose of meaningful statistical analysis. The fracture types for females, males, and both sexes were explored, and are shown in Table 3. There were higher proportions of femoral neck and intertrochanteric fractures in females compared to males. The average age was the highest in patients with intertrochanteric fractures (83.1 ± 9.4 years). The average age of patients who had femoral neck fracture was 82.1 ± 8.7 years, and other fracture was 78.5 ± 10.9 years (p = 0.044). The

Table 2 Fracture class, fall locations and discharge dispositions

		Femoral neck (N, %)	Trochanteric (N, %)
Fall locations	Home	124 (74.3)	115 (72.8)
	Nursing home	9 (5.4)	9 (5.7)
	Other	34 (20.4)	34 (21.5)
	Total	167 (100)	158 (100)
Discharge disposition	Home	21 (12.6)	19 (12.1)
	SNF/Rehab/LTC	138 (82.6)	126 (80.3)
	Died/hospice	8 (4.8)	12 (7.6)
	Total	167 (100)	158 (100)

SNF/Rehab/LTC represents skilled nursing facility, rehabilitation and long-term care. Pearson's chi-square (2 df) = 0.09, p = 0.979 for fall locations. Pearson's chi-square (2 df) = 1.14, p = 0.566 for discharge disposition.

Table 3 Hip fracture type distribution for males and females

Fracture types		Gender		Total
		Female	Male	
Femoral neck	Count (N)	124	43	167
	% within fracture pattern	74.3%	25.7%	100.0%
	% within gender	54.4%	44.3%	51.4%
Intertrochanteric	Count (N)	87	42	129
	% within fracture pattern	67.4%	32.6%	100.0%
	% within gender	38.2%	43.3%	39.7%
Other	Count (N)	17	12	29
	% within fracture pattern	58.6%	41.4%	100.0%
	% within gender	7.5%	12.4%	8.9%
Total	Count (N)	228	97	325
	% within fracture pattern	70.2%	29.8%	100.0%
	% within gender	100.0%	100.0%	100.0%

The table shows the number of patients (n) and associated percentage (%) for gender and hip fracture types. Pearson's Chi-Square (2df) = 3.63, p = 0.162.

HLOS for each fracture type was analyzed using one-way analysis of variance (ANOVA), and the average HLOS were similar across the fracture types as shown in Figure 3. There were total of 35 ICU admissions among the patient population. Some of the patients with hip fracture were admitted to ICU due to following reasons including, but not limited to: patients with or on anticoagulation (e.g. Coumadin), significant cardiac history (e.g. pace-makers), hemodynamic instability, arrhythmia, confusion, concussion, mechanical ventilation, or renal dialysis. The average ICU days for patients with femoral neck fractures were 3.7 ± 3.6 days (n = 15), intertrochanteric fractures were 2.8 ± 1.9 days (n = 16), and other fractures were 5.5 ± 2.4 days (n = 4).

Discharge disposition

We completed analysis of the effect of femur fracture class on discharge disposition as shown in Table 2. There were no significant associations between fracture class and discharge disposition, (2 df) = 1.14, p = 0.566.

The effect of age on fracture type

We examined the relationship between patient age in deciles and femoral fracture type in males (Figure 4A) and females (Figure 4B). Males had the highest number of patients with femoral neck fracture in "90 and above" age group and the highest number of patients with intertrochanteric fractures in "80-89" age group. On the other hand, females had the highest number of patients with both femoral neck and intertrochanteric fractures in "80-89" age group. There were significant differences

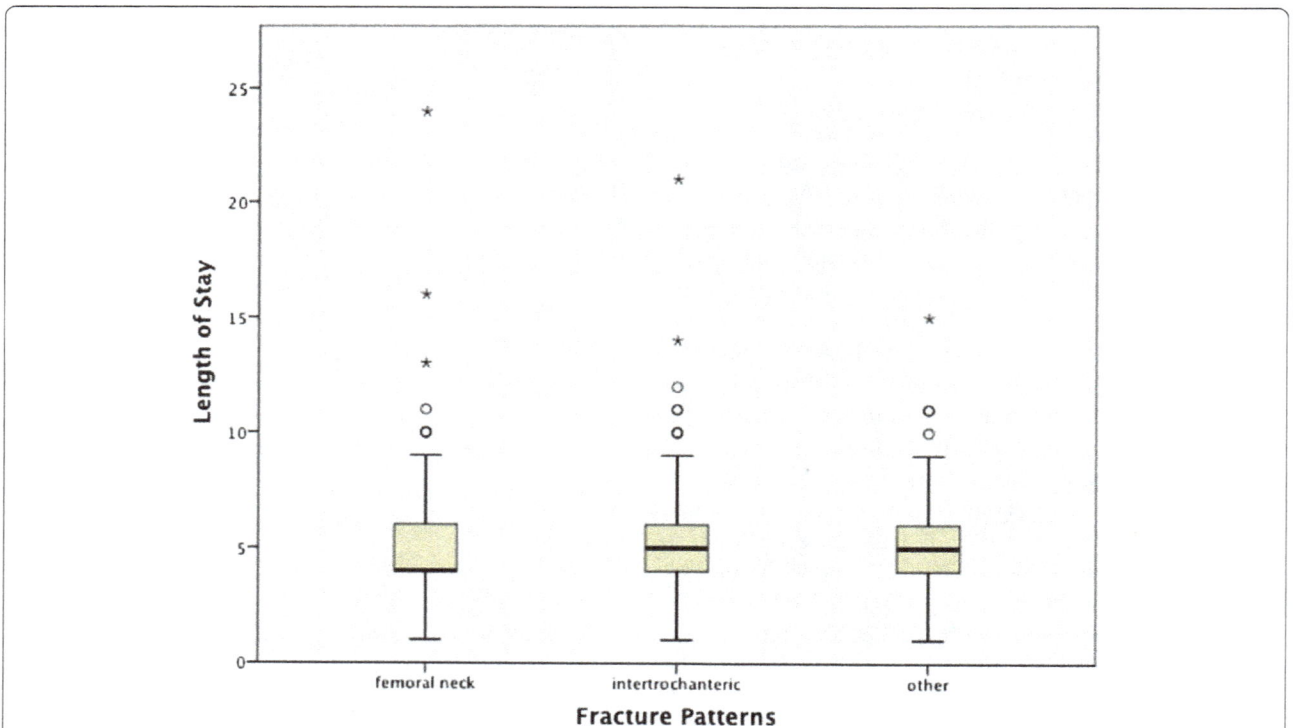

Figure 3 Box plot of HLOS and femur fracture patterns: Femoral Neck, Intertrochanteric, and Other. Results show variations in hospital length of stay among different types of fracture patterns. Using a one-way analysis of variance (ANOVA), there was not a significant effect of fracture patterns on hospital length of stay among the three fracture patterns (femoral neck, intertrochanteric, and other). F (2, 321) = 0.841, p = 0.432.

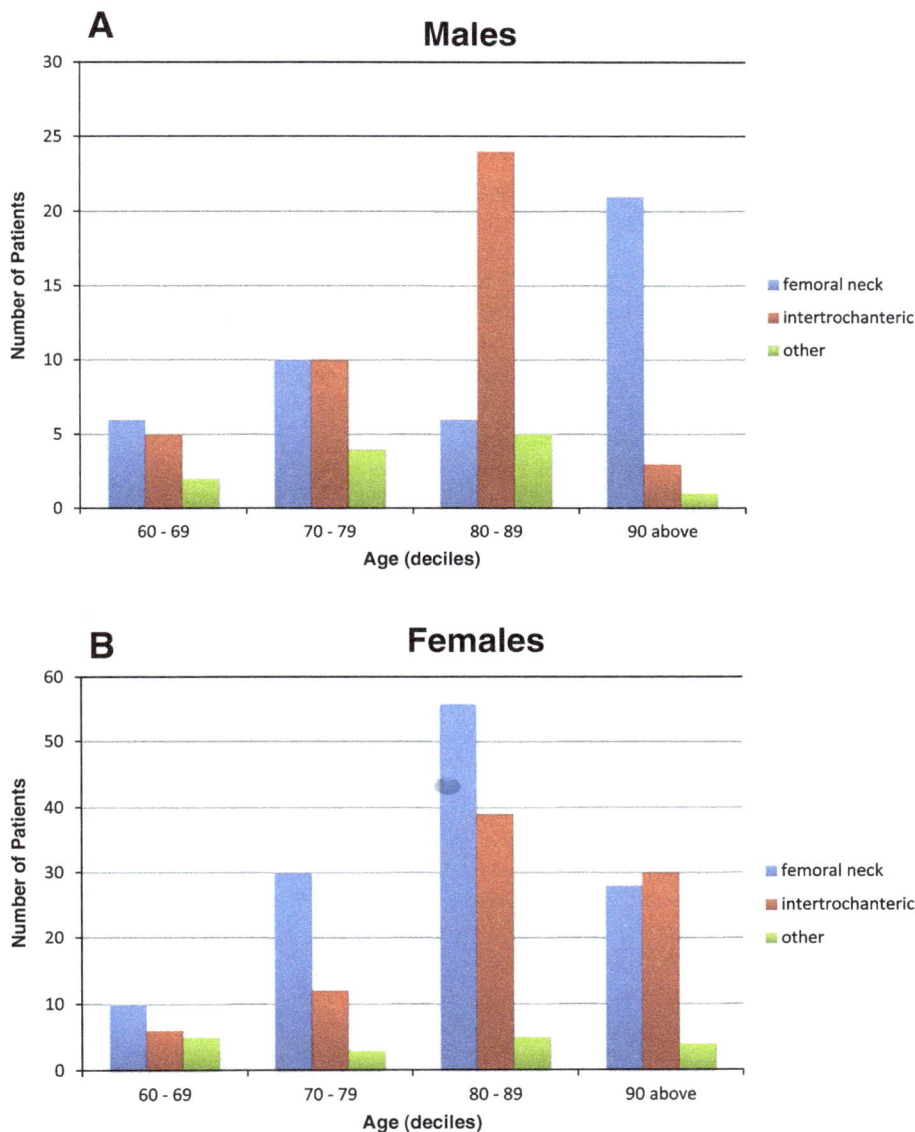

Figure 4 Femur fracture patterns and age in deciles for male (A) and female (B) patients. A. Age group (decile years) and femoral fracture patterns in males. The frequency of different fracture patterns (Femoral neck, Intertrochanteric, and Other) in adult males (decile years) aged 60 and above. Pearson's Chi-square (6 df) = 27.6, p < 0.0001. **B**: Age group (decile years) and femoral fracture patterns in females. The frequency of different fracture patterns (Femoral neck, Intertrochanteric, and Other) in adult females (decile years) aged 60 and above. Pearson's chi-square (6 df) = 14.5, p = 0.023.

between the patient age in deciles and femoral fracture type in males (p < 0.0001) and females (p = 0.023). We also performed an Analysis of variance (ANOVA) using patient age as continuous variables. The result showed that hip fracture types used as categorical variables were not associated with patient age as a continuous variable, $F (4, 248) = 0.600$, p = 0.66.

Surgical treatment

Hip fractures were fixed by orthopedic surgeons based on standard of care. Among the 325 patients with hip

fractures 25 had total hip replacement, 80 had partial hip replacement, 9 had internal fixation without reduction, 207 had open reduction with internal fixation and 2 patients had closed reduction of dislocation of the hip.

Discussion

The primary findings of this study described femur fracture patterns in a group of elderly trauma patients with hip fractures. The study group was predominantly white (94%), female (70%) and in their 8th decade of life. As reported in previous studies [13] and confirmed in this study, about half (51.4%) of the study subjects were diagnosed with femoral neck fractures, whereas 48.6% had trochanteric fractures. Patients in the two fracture groups did not differ in age or injury severity scores. The prevalence of femoral neck fractures was higher in females than in males. Similarly, The prevalence of trochanteric fractures was higher in females than in males. The ratio of male to female in femoral neck fracture was 1:3 and the ratio of male to female in intertrochanteric fracture was 1:2. This is confirmatory of previous study done by Brunner et al. [14], although gender alone was not a significant predictive factor for femoral neck or trochanteric fractures (p = 0.097). The observed higher prevalence of femoral neck fractures in females was not explained by the older age of females. We concluded from our observations that the higher prevalence of femoral neck fractures may be a characteristic of white geriatric females in our service area.

The key question we raised in the introduction to this study was whether there were any connections between hip fracture pattern (class or type) and short-term inpatient outcomes. As reported in the results section, femoral neck or trochanter fractures classes had no effect on HLOS (p = 0.706), ICU-LOS (p = 0 .712), or patient discharge disposition including the number of inpatient deaths (Pearson Chi-Square (2df) = 0.313, p = 0.855). Similarly, fracture types had no effect on HLOS (p = 0.814).

In regards to the classification scheme, certainly AO/OTA classification provides more detail. However, use of this scheme would produce many subgroups, which would need to be grouped as we did for the purpose of analysis. Therefore, for the purpose of this study, we classified the fracture patterns in groups consistent with ICD-9 CM codes. This is also well described in other publications [7,15,16] as a method of categorizing the different types of hip fractures.

There are several factors that influence HLOS and complications such as surgical technique and whether arthroplasty was cemented or uncemented. The majority of hip fracture patients in our study (207/325) or 64% underwent open reduction with internal fixation. The influence of this group relative to patients who underwent total hip replacement (7.7%) internal fixation without reduction (2.7%), closed reduction of dislocation of hip (0.6%) on outcomes, and partial hip replacement (24.8%) needs to be taken into account when interpreting outcomes. We also suspect a higher proportion of patients with hip fractures were admitted to the ICU at our level-I trauma center than would be the case in UK and Europe.

Study limitations

This was a retrospective chart review limited to a single level-I trauma center.

Conclusion

Our examination of fracture pattern in geriatric trauma patients showed no association between fracture patterns and outcomes including hospital length of stay, ICU length of stay, and discharge disposition. Males and females did differ in fracture patterns, but these differences were not associated with different outcomes. Further studies should include greater diversity in demographics, and linkage of fracture patterns to outcomes such as pain scores, infection rate, hospital readmission and patient experience. As elderly population continues to rise and trauma centers are seeing more elderly patients with fall and associated hip fractures, we must continue to explore ways to decrease mortality and morbidity related to hip fractures.

Abbreviations

ICD-9 CM: International Classification of Diseases, Ninth Revision, Clinical Modification; ISS: Injury severity score; ICU: Intensive Care Unit; G-60: Geriatric trauma service; LOS: Length of stay; SNF: Skilled nursing facility; Rehab: Rehabilitation; LTC: Long term care.

Competing interest

The authors declare that they have no competing interests.

Authors' contributions

AM conceived the study and its design and wrote the manuscript. MC collected and reviewed chest x-rays. PM independently reviewed x-rays and performed adjudication of cases where there were differences in classifying hip fracture patterns. LP reviewed several drafts of the manuscript. NZ also reviewed x-rays, CT scans, and prepared illustrations of the fractures. JS performed literature review and collected patient outcomes data. SC performed literature review, provided assistance in writing the manuscript, and prepared the manuscript for submission. OO reviewed manuscripts and made editorial changes. JD participated in the initial design of the study, collected data, performed statistical analysis, and assisted in preparing the final manuscript for submission. All authors have read and approved the manuscript.

Acknowledgements

The authors would like to thank Kalyan Chaliki, Shaun M Stienstra, and Melissa M Moyer for their clerical assistance.

Author details

[1]John C. Lincoln North Mountain Hospital, Phoenix, USA. [2]North Mountain Radiology Group Hospital, Phoenix, USA. [3]Midwestern University – Arizona College of Osteopathic Medicine, Arizona, USA. [4]University of Missouri – Kansas City, School of Medicine, Kansas, USA.

References

1. Bentler SE, Liu L, Obrizan M, Cook EA, Wright KB, Geweke JF, Chrischilles EA, Pavlik CE, Wallace RB, Ohsfeldt RL, Jones MP, Rosenthal GE, Wolinsky FD: The aftermath of hip fracture: discharge placement, functional status change, and mortality. Am J Epidemiol 2009, 170:1290–1299.
2. Wolinsky FD, Fitzgerald JF, Stump TE: The effect of hip fracture on mortality, hospitalization, and functional status: a prospective study. Am J Public Health 1997, 87:398–403.
3. Dy CJ, McCollister KE, Lubarsky DA, Lane JM: An economic evaluation of a systems-based strategy to expedite surgical treatment of hip fractures. J Bone Joint Surg 2011, 93:1326–1334.
4. Cummings SR, Rubin SM, Black D: The future of hip fractures in the United States. Numbers, costs, and potential effects of postmenopausal estrogen. Clin Orthop Relat Res 1990, 252:163–166.

Geriatric trauma hip fractures: is there a difference in outcomes based on fracture...

183

5   White SM, Moppett IK, Griffiths R: Outcome by mode of anesthesia for hip fracture surgery. An observational audit of 65,535 patients in a national dataset. *Anaesthesia* 2014, **69**:224–230.

6.   Neuman MD, Rosenbaum PR, Ludwig JM, Zubizarreta JR, Silber JH: Anesthesia technique, mortality, and length of stay after hip fracture surgery. *JAMA* 2014, **311**:2508–517.

7.   Stevens JA, Rudd RA: The impact of decreasing U.S. hip fracture rates on future hip fracture estimates. *Osteoporis Int* 2013, **24**:2725–2728.

8.   Stevens JA, Rudd RA: Declining hip fracture rates in the United States. *Age Ageing* 2010, **39**:500–503.

9.   Brauer CA, Coca-Perraillon M, Cutler DM, Rosen AB: Incidence and Mortality of Hip Fractures in the United States. *JAMA* 2009, **302**:1573–1579.

10. Michelson JD, Myers A, Jinnah R, Cox Q, Van Natta M: Epidemiology of hip fractures among the elderly. *Risk factors for fracture type Clin Orthop Relat Res* 1995, **311**:129–135.

11. Frost SA, Nguyen ND, Black DA, Eisman JA, Nguyen TV: Risk factors for in-hospital post-hip fracture mortality. *Bone* 2011, **49**:553–558.

12. Hu F, Jiang C, Shen J, Tang P, Wang Y: Preoperative predictors for mortality following hip fracture surgery: A systematic review and meta-analysis Injury. *Int J Care Inj* 2012, **43**:676–685.

13. Karagas MR, Lu-Yao GL, Barrett JA, Beach ML, Baron JA: Heterogeneity of hip fracture: age, race, sex, and geographic patterns of femoral neck and trochanteric fractures among the us elderly. *Am J Epidemiol* 1996, **143**:667–682.

14. Brunner LC, Ehilian-Oates L: Hip fractures in adults. *Am Fam Physician* 2003, **67**:537–543.

15. Katz JN, Wright EA, Polaris JJZ, Harris MB, Losina E: Prevalence and risk factors for periprosthetic fracture in older recipients of total hip replacement: a cohort study. *BMC Musculoskelet Disord* 2014, **15**:168.

16. Adams AL, Shi J, Takayanagi M, Dell RM, Funahashi TT, Jacobsen SJ: Ten-year hip fracture incidence rate trends in a large California population, 1997–2006. *Osteoporos Int* 2012, **24**:373–376.

28

The complications associated with Resuscitative Endovascular Balloon Occlusion of the Aorta (REBOA)

Marcelo A. F. Ribeiro Junior[1*], Celia Y. D. Feng[2], Alexander T. M. Nguyen[2], Vinicius C. Rodrigues[1], Giovana E. K. Bechara[1], Raíssa Reis de-Moura[1] and Megan Brenner[3]

Abstract

Non-compressible torso hemorrhage (NCTH) remains a significant cause of morbidity and mortality in the field of trauma and emergency medicine. In recent times, there has been a resurgence in the adoption of Resuscitative Endovascular Balloon Occlusion of the Aorta (REBOA) for patients who present with NCTH. Like all medical procedures, there are benefits and risks associated with the REBOA technique. However, in the case of REBOA, these complications are not unanimously agreed upon with varying viewpoints and studies. This article aims to review the current knowledge surrounding the complications of the REBOA technique at each step of its application.

Keywords: Complications, Radiology, Interventional, Multiple trauma, Abdomen, Shock, Hemorrhagic, REBOA

Background

Non-compressible torso hemorrhage (NCTH) is a major cause of morbidity and mortality in the trauma setting [1]. The difficulty in controlling NCTH arises from the fact that the bleeding cannot be managed like other types of traumatic hemorrhage, such as the use of tourniquets or direct pressure in limb hemorrhage [2, 3]. Instead, highly invasive techniques such as resuscitative thoracotomies (RT) are used to control thoracic bleeding. RT has low rates of patient survival as well as increased exposure of health care workers to blood-borne pathogens [4, 5]. Resuscitative Endovascular Balloon Occlusion of the Aorta (REBOA) is an old technique that has been receiving renewed interest in recent years [1, 6]. As the name suggests, the technique involves the introduction of a balloon occlusion catheter via the femoral artery into the aorta and inflating the balloon at one of two aortic zones (zone I or zone III) depending on the circumstances [7, 8]. The aorta can be divided into three zones (Fig. 1): with zone I being the aorta between the let subclavian artery and the celiac trunk, zone II being the aorta between the celiac trunk and the lowest renal artery, and zone III

being the area between the lowest renal artery and the aortic bifurcation [8]. Zone II is not for occlusion [8]. The balloon is then inflated to stem the flow of blood and later deflated and removed [8]. Renewed interest particularly in the USA in REBOA has led to its introduction in many trauma centers, as well as increased levels of research and analysis regarding the technique [9].

REBOA shows promise in improving the outcomes for patients with NCTH in comparison to RT. In a recent prospective study, there was no significant difference in overall mortality between patients undergoing RT and those undergoing REBOA for NCTH (REBOA, 71.7 vs. RT, 83.8%; $p = 0.120$) [9]. However, there are also complications associated with the procedure. Excessive ischemia during aortic occlusion, post-operative thrombosis, and limb amputation are among some of the reported complications of the procedure [10].

Methods

Considering the increasing number of cases treated using the REBOA technique, the aim of this paper is to review complications of REBOA at each stage of the procedure using a combination of literature review and clinical experience. PubMed online searches were used including search words such as REBOA, resuscitation,

* Correspondence: drmribeiro@gmail.com
[1]Disciplina de Cirurgia Geral e Trauma, Universidade Santo Amaro, São Paulo, São Paulo, Brazil
Full list of author information is available at the end of the article

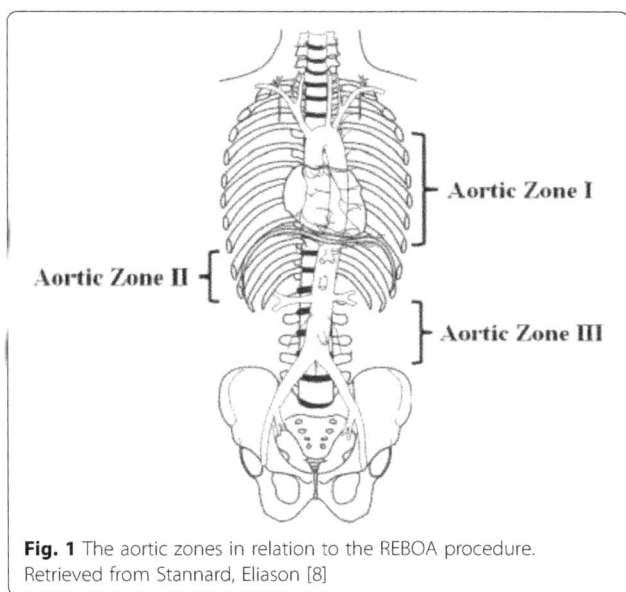

Fig. 1 The aortic zones in relation to the REBOA procedure. Retrieved from Stannard, Eliason [8]

hemorrhage, and shock. We also highlight key areas for further investigation and research.

Results

Arterial access and balloon positioning

Complications of REBOA are numerous and can be caused by the insertion of the intra-aortic balloon occlusion catheter and femoral artery sheath. The major complications of REBOA catheter insertion are vessel injuries (aortic dissection, rupture, and perforation), embolization, air emboli, and peripheral ischemia [11].

The greatest limitation to REBOA is the ischemia caused by total aortic occlusion [12]. Prolonged ischemia followed by reperfusion can result in multiple organ failure including acute kidney injury, liver failure, spinal cord infarction, intestinal ischemia, myonecrosis, limb loss, and death [12, 13].

The severe ischemic complication of the lower extremities can be associated with sheath placement for REBOA, and the use of large-sized sheaths for REBOA can be a critical risk factor for lower extremity ischemia [13].

As blood flow is inversely proportional to the vessel cross-sectional area, it is acceptable that large-sized sheaths may decrease blood flow to the extremities [13]. Some experts recommend first accessing the artery with a 4–5 Fr micropuncture catheter, suggesting that the smaller sheath can be used proactively in patients who may deteriorate, allowing for arterial blood pressure monitoring and collection of blood samples. Then, the micropuncture catheter should be rapidly exchanged for a 7–8 Fr sheath via the Seldinger technique for REBOA access with a relatively low risk of serious complications [14].

REBOA has been used routinely in endovascular management of abdominal aortic aneurysms (EVAR) via large diameter sheaths, typically 12–14 Fr or larger. The development of balloon catheters deliverable via 7 Fr sheaths have led to new enthusiasm for the technique for trauma patients. However, the evidence for its efficacy is limited [12]. Smaller sheaths appear to have fewer complications despite relatively prolonged placement and require external compression on removal [15].

Although these complications are related to sheath insertion and are not specific to REBOA, it is important for surgeons performing REBOA to be aware of these potential access site consequences and address them at time of sheath removal to avoid limb-threatening vascular complications [16]. Moreover, REBOA should be performed by an acute care surgeon or an interventionalist (vascular surgeon or interventional radiologist) trained in REBOA and, in order to resolve possible vascular complications, a vascular surgeon must be available [17]. When performed by an emergency medicine physician, an acute care surgeon or interventionalist should be immediately available to perform definitive hemorrhage control.

An additional challenge of REBOA is the need for rapid and accurate placement. This technique can provide total occlusion of the aorta either just above the diaphragm (zone I), to control intra-abdominal bleeding, or above the aorto-iliac bifurcation (zone III), to control bleeding in the pelvis or proximal extremities [12, 18].

Animal studies suggest that zone I REBOA is survivable for 60 min and zone III for 90 min. However, the Norii registry study shows that zone I occlusion for 45 min was uniformly lethal and there were only two survivors after 90 min of REBOA occlusion in the Inoue registry study. Once the REBOA catheter is inflated, the time to obtain definitive control of bleeding is limited and the need is absolute [12].

Balloon inflation

Balloon inflation is an integral part of the procedure and must be executed carefully. The balloon should be inflated until the blood pressure is augmented and contralateral femoral pulse is stopped, approximately 8 mL for zone I or 3 mL for zone III [19].

It is crucial that the practitioner performing REBOA is aware of the complications related to the inflation level and duration of the inflation in this step of the procedure. The physician should be careful to not over-inflate the balloon, as an over-inflation will rupture the balloon or the blood vessel [19]. A systematic review conducted by Morrison JJ et al. in 2016 identified a total of 83 studies which reported three deaths directly associated with balloon-related complications [20]. All patients were being treated for ruptured abdominal aortic aneurysm (rAAA) and had transbrachial aortic occlusion performed. Two balloons ruptured, resulting in precipitous cardiovascular collapse and death. The aortic injury occurred in the setting of postpartum hemorrhage (PPH) and was promptly recognized because of hypotension after hysterectomy and balloon deflation. It was suspected that balloon over-inflation had caused injury to the aorta [20]. As previously mentioned, in order to avoid balloon rupture, the physician must be attentive to the blood pressure and contralateral femoral pulse checking if the first one augmented and the second one stopped [19].

Another complication that must be avoided is the profound ischemia related to a long-term occlusion. Animal data suggests that prolonged occlusion of the aorta is associated with ischemia-reperfusion injury and potentially an increased risk of death [21]. The profound distal ischemia means that there is a maximal duration of use for REBOA that cannot be extended [22]. Periods of occlusion exceeding 40 min can result in irreversible organ injury and death. Additionally, supraphysiologic increases in blood pressure proximal to the occlusion balloon during REBOA can contribute to cardiac failure and exacerbation of traumatic brain injury [23].

Reinforcing the idea that the duration of the occlusion must be minimal, Saito N et al. reported that the time from inflation to deflation of the aortic balloon in 24-h survivors was shorter than in non-survivors. It was suspected that reperfusion injuries caused by systemic ischemia would lead to death. In experiments with swine, Morrison et al. reported that a longer aortic inflation time increased the release of interleukin-6, incidence of adult respiratory distress syndrome, and use of vasopressors [24].

In an attempt to minimize distal ischemia and extend the duration of use of REBOA, studies have led to the development of partial REBOA (pREBOA), whereby the balloon is deflated slightly, allowing a degree of flow beyond the balloon [21]. Several clinical and translational reports suggest that partial aortic flow restoration via partial aortic occlusion may serve to simultaneously mitigate the adverse effects of aortic occlusion on both proximal and distal vascular beds, whilst aiming to limit ongoing hemorrhage in the bleeding patient [25].

Although the REBOA technique continues to be studied, some studies demonstrate that a partial approach maintained normal physiology better than the complete one, minimized the systemic impact of distal organ ischemia, and reduced hemodynamic instability, allowing the potential for longer periods of intervention [23].

Management during balloon occlusion

During balloon occlusion, specific complications can occur such as accessing the wrong vascular tree, misplacement of the wire or balloon within the arterial system, the creation of dissection flaps or other arterial injury, retroperitoneal hemorrhage, the development of lactic acidosis and organ dysfunction, and the development of clots which may lead to limb ischemia [1].

REBOA placement in some countries currently requires large arterial sheaths such as 7 to 14 Fr in the common femoral artery. It has been reported that these large sheaths may be associated with severe complications, including lower extremity ischemia and amputations. These complications may be related to the near occlusive diameter of these large sheaths, the length of time they remain in the artery, the location of insertion, and potential damage that can be caused during the insertion.

These problems related to the management of REBOA has led physicians to hypothesize that one of the causes associated with the rate of complications could be the diameter of the sheaths. A prospective observational study by Walter L. et al. proposed that the use of new low-profile devices could decrease vascular complications associated with REBOA [6].

A retrospective review of patients receiving REBOA through a 7 Fr sheath for refractory traumatic hemorrhagic shock performed from January 2014 to June 2015 at five tertiary-care hospitals in Japan reported that 7 Fr introducer device for REBOA may be a safe and effective alternative to large-bore sheaths and may remain in place during the post-procedure resuscitative phase without sequelae. The main benefits of a 7 Fr system include tolerance of a prolonged indwelling sheath time and the ability to remove the sheath successfully with only manual compression [5].

Balloon deflation

REBOA balloon deflation and subsequent reperfusion is an integral stage in the procedure and can lead to potential cardiovascular complications. Previously, clinical guidelines have recommended the controlled deflation of the balloon to minimize sudden physiologic derangements. However, a study conducted on use of REBOA in 13 patients with pelvic fractures found six patients experienced hemodynamic shock upon balloon deflation. Of these six patients, three were resuscitated, one recovered after reinflation of the balloon, and the remaining two died from the shock [26]. This is thought to be due to the rapid release of ischemic metabolites such as nitric oxide and pro-inflammatory mediators after deflating the REBOA balloon, resulting in vasodilation and refractory hypotension, which ultimately leads to hemodynamic collapse [10]. Furthermore, adequate communication within the resuscitation team and with the anesthesia team is vital to ensure that preparations are in place for immediate reinflation of the balloon if needed. This approach attempts to prevent the rapid decrease in afterload and subsequent hypotension that can lead to hemodynamic instability [8]. However, an animal study conducted on eight swine models of hemorrhage found that graded balloon deflation still led to a rapid increase in aortic flow followed by a decrease in proximal mean arterial pressure. Furthermore, the time required for return of distal aortic flow was variable and inconsistent across the subjects [27].

Sheath removal and post-operative management

After completion of the procedure and deflation of the balloon, both the REBOA balloon catheter (and wire if used) may be removed and various techniques may be employed to remove the device, ensuring there is no clot in the sheath or distal extremity of the sheath. The sheath can then be removed through a surgical longitudinal incision through the groin, exposing both distal and proximal areas to the sheath, before adequate closure of the artery [8]. In a 5-year retrospective study of 48 patients that underwent REBOA, the development of distal thrombus and arterial dissection was a common occurrence, due to the extended periods of occlusion after insertion of the sheath. Five patients required additional vascular procedures; two required thrombectomy with repair of the dissection flap and patch angioplasty; one required thrombectomy with patch angioplasty; one required thrombectomy, interposition graft, and prophylactic fasciotomy; and one required thrombectomy with repair of dissection flaps. None of these patients experienced any complications from the procedures [16]. Lower limb ischemia resulting in amputation has also been a reported complication following sheath removal. In a 6-year retrospective study conducted in Tokyo, Japan ($n = 24$), two patients experienced lower limb ischemia following sheath removal, both of which required amputation below the knee. This is resultant from the prolonged systemic ischemia [24]. The study also reported other major systemic complications, including nine patients who experienced acute kidney injury and nine patients with multi-organ failure; also complications of systemic ischemia [24]. The inflammatory sequelae of REBOA is not well understood, but these results mandate the need for aggressive and pre-emptive diagnosis and treatment of ischemic metabolites, clinical consequences of prolonged aortic occlusion, and unrecognized procedural vascular complications. Vigilant assessment of abdominal end organ and distal extremity perfusion is critical, and imaging access sites within 24–48 h of sheath removal is prudent.

Areas for future research

The exact indications for REBOA remain uncertain [9]. Future studies should focus on which patient populations are suitable for receiving REBOA, as well as identifying the timeframe at which REBOA is most effective. Before the medical community seeks to widen the indications of REBOA, all of its complications should be understood first [1]. One of the current challenges to the widespread adoption of REBOA is a lack of data. More solid, prospective evidence of the complications at each stage of the REBOA is needed. A stronger evidence base for the complications at each stage of the procedure are needed to fully understand when and where REBOA is most effective as well as the conditions in which it should not be performed. With increasing use worldwide, more research and data will hopefully realize the great potential of REBOA not only for NCTH but also among a wider range of torso hemorrhage in trauma medicine.

Discussion
REBOA or no REBOA?

The use of endovascular aortic occlusion is an adjunct for resuscitation in patients with severe hemorrhage. In the setting of traumatic arrest from hemorrhage below the diaphragm, RT with cross-clamp may be used instead of REBOA for the purpose of aortic occlusion. In patients with physiologic decompensation, the advantage of REBOA is the ability to place the catheter at the intended level of occlusion, monitor the intra-aortic pressure with high-fidelity (if using the ER-REBOA catheter), and rapidly inflate the balloon prior to arrest is less invasive and committal than a RT. In the setting of severe pelvic hemorrhage, traditional control with pelvic packing and/or internal iliac ligation can be augmented by REBOA placed prior to these measures as a bridge to hemostasis. The benefits of using REBOA are largely based on the nature of it being a less invasive procedure and being able to intervene earlier in the downward spiral of exsanguinating hemorrhage: REBOA offers immediate, early temporization of hemorrhage prior to cardiovascular collapse. Consequences of early temporization may include decreased blood product transfusions with their inherent risks and sequela, less stress on cardiac function, decreased secondary brain injury for those with significant TBI, and the chance for survival beyond the ED. Significant research including the role of partial REBOA will help refine its use for a wide variety of clinical scenarios.

Conclusion

REBOA is an emergent and increasingly accepted technique used as a less invasive alternative for controlling bleeding in patients with NTCH. However, for this procedure to be used in widespread practice, a better understanding of the potential complications that can arise in all stages must be well recognized. Complications can arise in arterial access, balloon positioning, inflation, during occlusion, deflation, and removal of the sheath. Comprehensive investigation and studies conducted into each of these stages of REBOA can allow identification of specific complications and adequate measures to be taken to avoid these complications and reduce potential morbidity and mortality associated with REBOA.

Abbreviations
EVAR: Endovascular Management of Abdominal Aortic Aneurysms; NCTH: Non-compressible torso hemorrhage; pREBOA: Partial REBOA; rAAA: Ruptured abdominal aortic aneurysm; REBOA: Resuscitative Endovascular Balloon Occlusion of the Aorta; RT: Resuscitative thoracotomies

Acknowledgements
We would like to thank Dr. Marcelo Ribeiro and Dr. Megan Brenner for their advice, review, and feedback.

Authors' contributions
MR was the main editor and leader of the project group. CF and AN contributed to the research and the writing process as well as the majority of the editing and submission of the manuscript. VR, GB, and RM contributed to the research and writing of the manuscript. MB provided expert feedback and guidance to the team. All authors read and approved the final manuscript.

Competing interests
Dr. Megan Brenner is a Clinical Advisory Board Member––Prytime Medical Inc. All other authors declare that they have no competing interests.

Author details
[1]Disciplina de Cirurgia Geral e Trauma, Universidade Santo Amaro, São Paulo, São Paulo, Brazil. [2]School of Medicine, University of New South Wales, Sydney, New South Wales, Australia. [3]RA Cowley Shock Trauma Center, University of Maryland, Baltimore, MD, USA.

References
1. Qasim Z, Brenner M, Menaker J, Scalea T. Resuscitative Endovascular Balloon Occlusion of the Aorta. Resuscitation. 2015;96:275–9.
2. Kragh Jr JF, Jones JA, Walters TJ, Baer DG, Wade CE, Holcomb JB, et al. Battle casualty survival with emergency tourniquet use to stop limb bleeding. J Emerg Med. 2011;41(6):590–7.
3. Morrison JJ, Rasmussen TE. Noncompressible torso hemorrhage: a review with contemporary definitions and management strategies. Surg Clin North Am. 2012;92(4):843–58.
4. Seamon JM, Haut RE, Van Arendonk RK, Barbosa CR, Chiu JW, Dente SC, et al. An evidence-based approach to patient selection for emergency department thoracotomy: a practice management guideline from the Eastern Association for the Surgery of Trauma. J Trauma Acute Care Surg. 2015;79(1):159–73.
5. Teeter WA, Matsumoto J, Idoguchi K, Kon Y, Orita T, Funabiki T, et al. Smaller introducer sheaths for REBOA may be associated with fewer complications. J Trauma Acute Care Surg. 2016;81(6):1039–45.

6. Biffl WL, Fox CJ, Moore EE. The role of REBOA in the control of exsanguinating torso hemorrhage. J Trauma Acute Care Surg. 2015;78(5): 1054–8.
7. Gamberini E, Coccolini F, Tamagnini B, Martino C, Albarello V, Benni M, et al. Resuscitative endovascular balloon occlusion of the aorta in trauma: a systematic review of the literature. World J Emerg Surg. 2017;12:42.
8. Stannard A, Eliason JL, Rasmussen TE. Resuscitative Endovascular Balloon Occlusion of the Aorta (REBOA) as an adjunct for hemorrhagic shock. J Trauma. 2011;71(6):1869.
9. Dubose JJ, Scalea TM, Brenner M, Skiada D, Inaba K, Cannon J, et al. The AAST prospective Aortic Occlusion for Resuscitation in Trauma and Acute Care Surgery (AORTA) registry: data on contemporary utilization and outcomes of aortic occlusion and Resuscitative Balloon Occlusion of the Aorta (REBOA). J Trauma Acute Care Surg. 2016;81(3):409.
10. Davidson AJ, Russo RM, Reva VA, Brenner ML, Moore LJ, Ball C, et al. The pitfalls of resuscitative endovascular balloon occlusion of the aorta: risk factors and mitigation strategies. J Trauma Acute Care Surg. 2018; 84(1):192.
11. Tsurukiri J, Akamine I, Sato T, Sakurai M, Okumura E, Moriya M, et al. Resuscitative endovascular balloon occlusion of the aorta for uncontrolled haemorrahgic shock as an adjunct to haemostatic procedures in the acute care setting. Scand J Trauma Resusc Emerg Med. 2016;24:13.
12. Doucet J, Coimbra R. REBOA: is it ready for prime time? J Vasc Bras. 2017; 16(1):1–3.
13. Okada Y, Narumiya H, Ishi W, Ryoji I. Lower limb ischemia caused by resuscitative balloon occlusion of aorta. J Surg Case Rep. 2016;2(1):1–4.
14. Ribeiro Junior MAF, Brenner M, Nguyen ATM, Feng CYD, de-Moura RR, Rodrigues VC, etal. Resuscitative endovascular balloon occlusion of the aorta (REBOA): an updated review. Rev Col Bras Cir. 2018;45(1):e1709.
15. Matsumura Y, Matsumoto J, Kondo H, Idoguchi K, Ishida T, Kon Y, et al. Fewer REBOA complications with smaller devices and partial occlusion: evidence from a multicentre registry in Japan. Emerg Med J. 2017; 34(12):793.
16. Taylor JR, Harvin JA, Martin C, Holcomb JB, Moore LJ. Vascular complications from resuscitative endovascular balloon occlusion of the aorta: life over limb? J Trauma Acute Care Surg. 2017;83(1 Suppl 1):S120.
17. Brenner M, Bulger EM, Perina DG, Henry S, Kang CS, Rotondo MF, et al. Joint statement from the American College of Surgeons Committee on Trauma (ACS COT) and the American College of Emergency Physicians (ACEP) regarding the clinical use of Resuscitative Endovascular Balloon Occlusion of the Aorta (REBOA). Trauma Surg Acute Care Open. 2018;3(1):1–3.
18. Ordoñez CA, Manzano-Nunez R, del Valle AM, Rodriguez F, Burbano P, Naranjo MP, et al. Uso actual del balón de resucitación aórtico endovascular (REBOA) en trauma. Rev Colomb Anestesiol. 2017;45(Supplement 2):30–8.
19. Pasley J, Cannon J, Glaser J, Polk T, Morrison J, Brocker J, et al. Resuscitative Endovascular Balloon Occlusion of the Aorta (REBOA) for hemorrhagic shock (CPG ID: 38). JTS CPG. 2017:1–21.
20. Morrison JJ, Galgon RE, Jansen JO, Cannon JW, Rasmussen TE, Eliason JL. A systematic review of the use of resuscitative endovascular balloon occlusion of the aorta in the management of hemorrhagic shock. J Trauma Acute Care Surg. 2016;80(2):324–34.
21. Madurska MJ, Jansen JO, Reva VA, Mirghani M, Morrison JJ. The compatibility of computed tomography scanning and partial REBOA: a large animal pilot study. J Trauma Acute Care Surg. 2017;83(3):557–61.
22. Johnson AM, Davidson JA, Russo MR, Ferencz ES-A, Gotlib EO, Rasmussen PT, et al. Small changes, big effects: the hemodynamics of partial and complete aortic occlusion to inform next generation resuscitation techniques and technologies. J Trauma Acute Care Surg. 2017;82(6):1106–11.
23. Russo RM, Neff LP, Lamb CM, Cannon JW, Galante JM, Clement NF, et al. Partial Resuscitative Endovascular Balloon Occlusion of the Aorta in swine model of hemorrhagic shock. J Am Coll Sur. 2016;223(2):359–68.
24. Saito N, Matsumoto H, Yagi T, Hara Y, Hayashida K, Motomura T, et al. Evaluation of the safety and feasibility of resuscitative endovascular balloon occlusion of the aorta. J Trauma Acute Care Surg. 2015;78(5):897–903.
25. Williams TK, Johnson A, Neff L, Hörer TM, Moore L, Brenner M, et al. "What's in a Name?" A Consensus Proposal for a Common Nomenclature in the Endovascular Resuscitative Management and REBOA Literature. JEVTM. 2017; 1(1):9–12.

29

Liver trauma: WSES position paper

Federico Coccolini[1*], Giulia Montori[1], Fausto Catena[2], Salomone Di Saverio[3], Walter Biffl[4], Ernest E. Moore[4], Andrew B. Peitzman[5], Sandro Rizoli[6], Gregorio Tugnoli[3], Massimo Sartelli[7], Roberto Manfredi[7] and Luca Ansaloni[1]

Abstract

The liver is the most injured organ in abdominal trauma. Road traffic crashes and antisocial, violent behavior account for the majority of liver injuries. The present position paper represents the position of the World Society of Emergency Surgery (WSES) about the management of liver injuries.

Keywords: Liver trauma, Surgery, Hemorrage, Operative management, Non-operative management

Background

The liver is the most injured organ in abdominal trauma [1–3]. Road traffic crashes and antisocial, violent behavior account for the majority of liver injuries [2]. As demonstrated by several studies the management of liver trauma has deeply changed through the last three decades with a significant improvement in outcomes, especially in blunt trauma [1, 2, 4]. Most liver injuries are grade I, II or III and are successfully treated by observation only (Non-Operative Management, NOM). In contrast two-thirds of grade IV or V injuries necessitate laparotomy (Operative Management, OM) [3]. These operations are generally challenging and difficult. Richardson et al. proposed as the main reasons for improvement in survival: 1) improved results with packing and reoperation, 2) use of arteriography and embolization, 3) advances in operative techniques for major hepatic injuries, and 4) decrease in hepatic venous injuries undergoing operation [1, 3]. The severity of traumatic liver injuries is universally classified according to the AAST classification system (Table 1) [5]. The present paper represents the position of the World Society of Emergency Surgery (WSES) about the treatment of liver trauma. This paper results from the Second World Congress of WSES that has been held in Bergamo (Italy) on July 2013. Levels of evidence have been evaluated in agreement with the Oxford guidelines [6]. As the WSES includes surgeons from the whole world, this position paper aims to give the state of the art of the management of liver trauma, maintaining into account the secondary different possibilities in its management. In actuality, not all trauma surgeons work in the same conditions and have the same facilities and technologies.

Classification

Hepatic traumatic lesions can be classified as minor (grade I, II), moderate (grade III) or major/severe (grade IV, V) injuries (Fig. 1a, b) [3, 7–9]. This classification is not well defined in the literature, but aims to define the type of management that can be adopted and the related outcome [8]. Frequently low-grade American Association for the Surgery of Trauma (AAST) lesions (i.e., grade I-III) are considered as minor or moderate and treated with NOM [8, 9]. However some patients with high-grade lesions (i.e., grade IV-V laceration with parenchymal disruption involving more than 75 % of the hepatic lobe or more than 3 Couinaud segments within a single lobe) may be hemodynamically stable and treated with NOM [3]. This demonstrates that the classification of liver injuries as minor or major ones must consider not only the anatomic AAST classification but more importantly, the hemodynamic status of the patient, the ISS and the associated injuries.

A few studies considered as minor injuries those lesions with hemodynamic stability, a low AAST organ injuries scale and a low ISS [8, 9]. These patients can be safely managed non-operatively with good results in term of morbidity and mortality. On the other hand major injuries are those with a higher AAST organ injuries scale, high ISS and a higher transfusions rate and are often associated with the worst outcome in terms of morbidity and mortality [8, 9]. For all the aforementioned reasons major injuries are associated with a higher necessity of OM.

* Correspondence: federico.coccolini@gmail.com
[1]General, Emergency and Trauma Surgery, Papa Giovanni XXIII Hospital, P.zza OMS 1, 24128 Bergamo, Italy
Full list of author information is available at the end of the article

Table 1 AAST organ injury scale – liver injury

Grade	Injury type	Injury description
I	Haematoma	Subcapsular < 10 % surface
	Laceration	Capsular tear < 1 cm parenchymal depth
II	Haematoma	Subcapsular 10–50 % surface area; intraparenchymal, < 10 cm diameter
	Laceration	1–3 cm parenchymal depth, < 10 cm in length
III	Haematoma	Subcapsular > 50 % surface area or expanding, ruptured subcapsular or parenchymal haematoma. Intraparenchymal haematoma > 10 cm
	Laceration	> 3 cm parenchymal depth
IV	Laceration	Parenchymal disruption 25–75 % of hepatic lobe
V	Laceration	Parenchymal disruption involving > 75 % of hepatic lobe
	Vascular	Juxtavenous hepatic injuries i.e., retrohepatic vena cav/central major hepatic veins
VI	Vascular	Hepatic avulsion

Advance one grade for multiple injuries up to grade III
AAST liver injury scale (1994 revision)

Fig. 1 a b CT immages of Grade V liver injury

Diagnostic procedures in liver trauma (blunt and penetrating)

Focused abdominal sonography for trauma (FAST) has superseded the diagnostic peritoneal lavage (DPL) or diagnostic peritoneal aspirate (DPA) in many centers to evaluate the presence/absence of intra-abdominal fluid in unstable patients with blunt trauma [7]. DPL however remains valuable in patients in shock without an overt source of blood loss. The greatest advantages of FAST are that it is an economic, non-invasive, rapid, repeatable procedure, with sensitivity between 80–85 % and a specificity of 97–100 % [10]. The procedure has some limitations: reduced sensitivity and specificity in obese patients, in case of ileus, or subcutaneous emphysema, and that it is operator dependent [10]. Richards et al. [11] reported a 98 % of sensitivity in grade III to V liver injuries, but there are demonstrated differences between groups with different expertise [12]. FAST will generally document 400 ml or more of intra-peritoneal fluid, and for this reason is a useful exam in unstable patients to decide for OM or not [7]. As a counterpart if positive FAST is absolutely helpful in deciding for OM or not, an apparent negative study does not definitely exclude significant intra-peritoneal bleeding. In penetrating trauma FAST is highly specific (94.1–100 %), however is not able to evaluate the exact lesion grade and is not very sensitive (28–100 %) [7, 13].

CT-scan has over the last years has improved the detection of the abdominal injuries. In patients who are hemodynamically stable, with either penetrating or blunt injuries, CT is the gold standard [7, 14–16]. Triple contrast CT has been shown to have a good sensitivity, except for diaphragm, pancreas and small bowel injuries [7]. Some authors consider CT as a predictive factor, along with systolic blood pressure (SBP), to determine the risk of failure of non-operative management (NOM) and to predict the patient outcome, particularly in grade IV lesions or higher [17]. In fact, in the setting of involvement by one or more hepatic veins, liver surgery is 6.5 times more common, and there is a 3.5 times higher risk of arterial bleeding. As a counterpart, the risk of false negative for vascular injuries at CT can delay proper intervention. For this reason some authors suggested angiography in all patients with grade 3–5, irrespective of hemodynamic stability or blush on CT-scan, particularly when there is associated major hepatic venous involvement [17–19]. On the other hand hepatic angiography does not appear to be warranted in the absence of active bleeding on CT among patients with CT grade II or grade III injuries, because in these patients the principal risk appears to be venous bleeding [17].

Diagnostic peritoneal lavage (DPL) or diagnostic peritoneal aspirate (DPA) has been commonly used since its introduction in 1965. It has been the technique of choice in ATLS until being replaced by the FAST. It is a diagnostic approach to evaluate the presence of hemoperitoneum or free bowel contents in unstable patients [10]. DPL is considered rapid, accurate, and sensitive tool to identify intra-abdominal injuries, but it is an invasive procedure [10]. Contraindications for DPL are obesity, previous laparotomy, coagulopathy and advanced pregnancy [10]. Despite being replaced by FAST over the last few years, in a recent randomized controlled trial DPL was consider superior to FAST in identifying intra-abdominal injuries, even though it required significantly more time to be performed [10].

Recommendations for Non Operative Management (NOM) in blunt liver trauma (BLT)

Patients should undergo an initial attempt of NOM in a scenario of blunt trauma, hemodynamic stability, and isolated liver injury, irrespective of injury grade (GoR 2 A).

NOM is not indicated in case of hemodynamic instability or peritonitis (GoR 2 A).

NOM should be considered only in an environment that provides capability for patient intensive monitoring, angiography and an always available operating room (GoR 2 A).

Abdominal CT with intravenous contrast should be always performed to identify the liver injuries and provides critical information for consideration of NOM (GoR 2 A).

Angiography with embolization may be considered the first-line intervention in patients with hemodynamic stability and arterial blush on CT-scan (GoR 2 B).

NOM for liver injury, has increased during the last century due to its high success rates (82–100 %) [14, 8, 20–28]. This non-operative approach was at first applied to pediatric patients and has rapidly been extended to adults. In blunt trauma, NOM is the standard of care in hemodynamically stable patients, without other associated injuries requiring an OM [29]. It is contraindicated in case of hemodynamic instability or peritonitis [14]. Croce et al. in a prospective case–control trial, reported a lower rate of complications and a lower number of transfusions in stable patients treated non-operatively, regardless of the liver injury severity [8].

The advantages of NOM include: lower hospital cost, earlier discharge, avoiding non-therapeutic laparotomy and unnecessary liver resection, fewer intra-abdominal complications and reduced number of transfusions [20]. However, in patients with severe head injuries and in the elderly, hypotension may be deleterious, and an OM can be suggested as safer [7].

The definition of 'hemodynamic instability' is not well established [14]. The Advanced Trauma Life Support (ATLS) definition [30] consider as "unstable" the patient with: blood pressure < 90 mmHg and heart rate > 120 bpm, with evidence of skin vasoconstriction (cool,

clammy, decreased capillary refill), altered level of consciousness and/or shortness of breath.

After hemodynamic status, the American Association for the Surgery of Trauma (AAST) grade of injury and the presence of multiple organs lesions seem to be the principal predictors of failure [31]. However there is no consensus about the NOM failure risk factors. For this reason NOM should only be attempted in centers capable of a precise diagnosis of the severity of liver injuries and capable of intensive management (frequent hemoglobin controls, frequent clinical monitoring and 24-h CT-scan, angiography and operating room availability) [20, 32–34]. At present, no studies report the optimal type and duration of monitoring. Velmahos et al. considered as predictors of NOM failure hypotension on admission, high CT-grade of injury, active contrast extravasation on CT-scan, and the need for blood transfusion [35]. Furthermore others authors add the dimension of the hemoperitoneum (blood around liver, peri-colic gutter, and in pelvis), the age greater than 55 years, the altered neurologic status, associated injuries, lactate level at the admission and drop of the hematocrit >20 % in the first hour, as risk factors for NOM failure [7, 20, 36]. However these criteria were not identified as absolute contraindications to NOM.

The total number of transfusions required, in deciding to opt either for NOM or OM, is still debated [20]. Pachter et al. suggest that more than 2 units transfusion and an intraperitoneal blood estimated quantity of more than 500 mL suggest ongoing bleeding and that an OM is necessary [37]. Carillo et al. suggested no more than 4 units of blood in hepatic-related transfusion [38], and Kozar at al. reported as predictor of liver-related complications the grade of liver injuries and the 24-h transfusion requirement [39].

To improve better use of blood products and hemostatic agents, the use of thromboelastography (TEG) and the thromboelastometry (ROTEM) analysis may be safer and helpful to guide the transfusion strategy [40]. No definitive recommendations actually exist for the use of recombination activated factor VII (rFVIIa) either in prevention or in routinely use in hemorrhage management in trauma [41]. Some authors suggest that rFVIIa has no role [42].

Angioembolization is considered by several studies as an "extension" of resuscitation in patients with ongoing resuscitative needs, but this practice can be applied safely only in selected centers (Fig. 2) [14]. Some papers have reported early angio-embolization can decrease the need for transfusions and surgery [43, 44]. A recent Norwegian prospective trial with historical control, applied NOM to stable patients with blush at the CT-scan or with clinical bleeding without blush with grade 3–5 liver lesions. It demonstrated a decreased number of total laparotomy (24 % vs. 49 %) with a stable NOM failure rate (13 %),

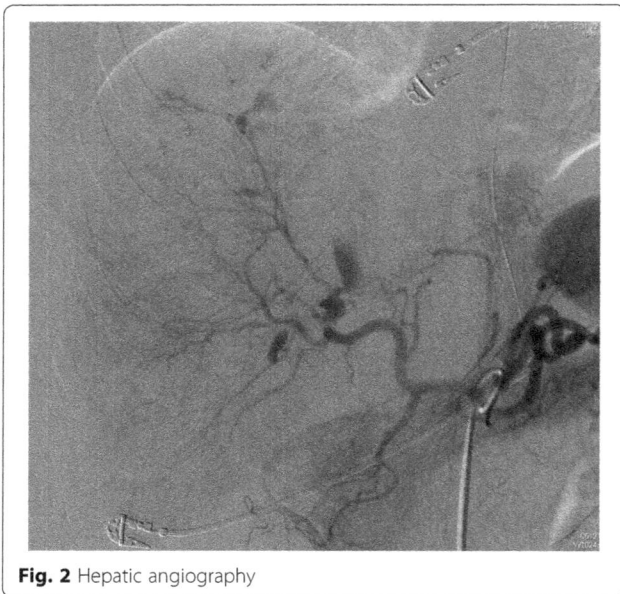

Fig. 2 Hepatic angiography

decreased transfusions and mortality, and a reduced complications rate (44 % vs. 58 %) [18]. In any case the early use of this procedure may be beneficial [31, 45].

In multi-organ injuries, particularly in cases of associated liver and splenic injuries, a recent study by Hsieh et al. reported that NOM is feasible also in case of high-grades hepato-splenic injuries (81.4 % NOM vs. 18.7 % OM) with a failure rate of 3.7 % for liver trauma and 7.1 % failure rate for the spleen trauma [46]. In multi-organ injuries predictors of failure of NOM are: initial low hemoglobin level, increased need for transfusions in ICU [46].

Complications of NOM in blunt hepatic trauma arise particularly in high-grade injury (overall complication rate: 0–7 %, complications in grade III-V injuries: 12.6 % - 14 %) [7, 14]. Clinical examination, blood tests, ultrasound and CT-scan can help in the diagnosis, but a routine follow-up with CT-scan is not necessary [3, 7, 14]. However control CT-scan is required in case of persistent inflammatory response at laboratory tests, fever, abdominal pain, jaundice and drop of hemoglobin level [14]. The most frequent complications of NOM are: biliary (bile leak, hemobilia, bilioma, biliary peritonitis, biliary fistula), bleeding, abdominal compartment syndrome, infections (abscesses and other infections) and liver necrosis [7, 20]. Ultra-sound evaluation is useful in liver trauma NOM follow-up, especially in the assessment of bile leak/biloma in grade IV-V injuries, especially with a central laceration.

The main complication that can occur is re-bleeding or secondary hemorrhage (as in the rupture of a capsulate hematoma or a pseudo-aneurysm) [7, 14]. "Late" bleedings generally occur within 72 h after trauma, and the overall incidence is 0 % to 14 %. Fortunately the majority of cases (69 %) can be treated non-operatively [7, 14]. Unlike the splenic injuries, liver lesions behave predominantly in two ways: either with a copious hemorrhage at the beginning requiring an OM, or with no active bleeding that can be safely managed with NOM [47]. Post-traumatic hepatic artery pseudo-aneurysms are rare (1.2 %, with the 70–80 % extra-hepatic and 17–25 % intra-hepatic) and they can usually be managed with selective embolization [48].

Biliary complications can occur in 1/3 of cases and can be controlled with endoscopic retrograde cholangio-pancreatography (ERCP) and eventual stenting, percutaneous drainage and lastly with surgical intervention (open or laparoscopic) [14]. Bile leaks can occur in 3–20 % of NOM [7, 14]. In case of minor bile leaks a conservative approach can be safely attempted, however high-output biliary fistula (greater than 300–400 mL/d or when bilious drainage was at least 50 mL/d continuing after 2 weeks) will benefit from an early ERCP [49]. Also intrahepatic bilio-venus fistula (frequent associated with bilemia) can be treated with ERCP [50].

Peri-hepatic abscesses have a low incidence (0 %–7 %) and can be managed with CT-scan or ultrasound-guided drainage [7, 14, 31]. Necrosis and devascularization of hepatic segments may occur and clinically may produce elevation of transaminases, coagulopathy, bile leak, abdominal pain, feeding intolerance and sepsis if more severe [7]. In these cases surgical management would be indicated [7]. Hemobilia is uncomomon (less than 3 %), but is frequently associated with pseudo-aneurysm [3, 7]. Embolization is safe and is the first approach in hemodynamically stable and non-septic patients; otherwise surgical management is mandatory [7]. Another infrequent complication is the liver compartment syndrome that may occur with the presence of large sub-capsular hematomas [7]. The decompression of the hematoma with percutaneous drainage can be safe [7]. A valid option to manage these complications could be the delayed laparotomy or laparoscopy that should be considered as a part of therapeutic strategy, and not a failure for NOM [51]. Some authors reported that delayed surgery can occur in 24 % of patients treated non-operatively, and up to 67 % in those patients with major hepatic lesions (grade IV-V) [52]. Letoublon et al. [51] considered a laparoscopic abdominal exploration between the second and fifth day safer and useful particularly in case of significant hemoperitoneum, or peritoneal inflammation or in case of any kind of clinically relevant abdominal hypertension. The simple laparoscopic or laparotomic lavage-drainage can be sufficient in the majority of the cases [51].

The trauma-related thromboembolic diseases are considered the third cause of death in patients who survive the first 24-h after trauma [53]. Deep venous thrombosis is found in 58 % of cases and the risk of pulmonary embolism ranges from 2 to 22 %. Concern of hemorrhage may delay the initiation of deep venous thrombosis prophylaxis (DVTP) in hepatic trauma is often delayed, particularly in NOM. Datta et al. in a multicenter review shows that DVTP is safe and effective if initiated within 48 h from hospital admission [54]. Also Joseph et al. confirmed data about the safety and efficacy of early DVTP in blunt solid abdominal injuries [55]. Delay in starting DVTP results in increased venous thrombo-embolic events without increasing the NOM failure rate [20, 54]. In NOM patients after liver trauma, Parks et al. [29] suggested an initial treatment with sequential compression devices and as soon as possible (when the hemoglobin level variations are ≤ 0.5 g from the previous draw) the introduction of DVTP in addition to the compression device.

The post-injury follow-up is an issue that remains unclear in NOM. There is no standard follow-up and monitoring protocol to evaluate patients with NOM liver injuries. Parks and coll. reviewed NOM guidelines for patient safety and optimal length of stay based solely on clinical criteria [29]. They suggested a serial hemoglobin measurements every 6 h for the first 24 h in stable patients with I-II grade before the discharge if patient remain stable, and every 6 h during the first 12 h and subsequently after every 12 h in grade III-IV-V injuries; the patients were allowed to walk after 24 h [29].

Recommendations for NOM in penetrating liver trauma (PLT)

NOM in penetrating liver trauma could be considered only in case of hemodynamic stability, absence of peritonitis and or evisceration and or impalement (GoR 2 A).

NOM in penetrating liver trauma should be considered only in an environment that provides capability for intensive monitoring of the patients, angiography and an operating room always viable (GoR 2 A).

Serial clinical examinations and local wound exploration must be always performed in case of stab wounds (GoR 2 A).

CT scan must be always performed to identify penetrating liver injuries suitable for NOM (GoR 2 A).

Angioembolisation is to be considered in case of arterial bleeding in a hemodynamic stable patient without signs of peritonitis, evisceration or impalement (GoR 2 A).

Until past years NOM has not been considered feasible in case of penetrating trauma both in stab wounds and in gunshot wounds [7, 14, 56–62]. In fact, in these cases, the majority of surgeons considered the OM as the standard or, at least, laparoscopic exploration is considered a viable option. However, particularly for stab wounds in 70 % of patients it can be unnecessary [61]. Recent studies reviewed the conservative approach, showing a high success rate (50 % of stab wounds (SW)

in the anterior abdomen and about 85 % in the posterior abdomen) [57]. This concept has been applied also in gunshot wounds (GSWs) [58]. However to decide either for NOM or for OM in these cases should be kept in mind the distinction between low and high energy penetrating trauma. Only in case of low energy, both SW and GSW, NOM can be safe. In fact high energy GSW and other ballistic injuries are perceived to be less amenable to NOM because of the high-energy transfer, and in 90 % of cases an OM is required [60, 63]. Despite that some studies reported a 25 % non-therapeutic laparotomies rate in abdominal GSWs, confirming that in selective cases NOM could be pursued [63].

10 trials and case series reported about the NOM of penetrating liver injuries with a success rate ranging from 69 % to 100 %. Some of these studies also suggested an algorithm for the management of penetrating abdominal trauma [56–60]. The key points for NOM remain: hemodynamic stability, absence of peritonitis, and an evaluable abdomen. In hemodynamic instability, in presence of peritonitis or evisceration and or impalement OM should be pursued [58–60]. These findings are particularly important in cases of gunshot injuries. Navsaria et al. suggested as predictive criteria of NOM failure in abdominal GSWs are: associated head and spinal cord injuries (that preclude regular clinical examination) and significant reduction in hemoglobin requiring more than 2–4 units of blood transfusion in 24 h [57].

The role of CT scan in the evaluation of patients with SWs has not been proven, and local wound exploration (LWE) is considered more accurate than CT-scan [58]. Some papers showed an emergency laparotomy was necessary even in presence of a negative CT-scan [59]. Biffl et al. considered CT-scan necessary particularly in NOM in obese and when the wound tract is long, tangential and difficult to determine the trajectory [59]. Particularly in case of GSWs the CT-scan can help in determining the trajectory, but not all authors consider it mandatory in all patients undergoing to NOM. Some authors did not use CT-scan at all in their algorithm, and others used CT-scan only in selected patients but without explaining selection criteria [57, 63]. Velmahos et al. reported that in GSWs the CT-scan has a specificity of 96 % and a sensibility of 90.5 % for injuries requiring laparotomy [64]. The potential benefit of CT should be to reduce the rates of non-therapeutic laparotomies and consequently to increase the patients underwent to NOM [63]. However the serial clinical examination remains the gold standard to decide for OM or NOM [63].

In case of CT scan detection of free intra- or retroperitoneal air, free intra-peritoneal fluid in the absence of solid organ injury, localized bowel wall thickening, bullet tract close to hollow viscus with surrounding hematoma, NOM is contraindicated [56]. A strict clinical and hemoglobin evaluation should be done (4-hourly for at least 48 h, once stabilized the patient could be transferred to the ward) [57, 59, 61].

Demetriades et al. [65] reported a 27.6 % of cases in which no significant intra-abdominal injuries are found at the exploration. Thus suggests the possibility for a safe NOM in selected cases. In case of liver injuries Demetriades et al. showed a 28.8 % of patients treated non-operatively, a 24.3 % treated with simple surgical techniques, and a 22.5 % of patients treated with damage-control procedures, with an overall NOM success rate (in all organ injuries) between 60 % and 90 % [56]. In liver penetrating injuries angio-embolization may be a valuable tool to stop the hemorrhage or to treat a pseudo-aneurysm when a CT-scan blush is present [56, 57].

The main reluctance of surgeons to approach non-operatively a penetrating trauma is related to the doubt to miss others abdominal lesions, especially hollow viscus perforation [56]. However on one hand, in patients without peritonitis at the admission, no increase in mortality rates in case of missed hollow viscus perforation has been reported [66]. On the other hand non-therapeutic and routine laparotomy has been demonstrated to increase the complication rate [66]. Nevertheless OM in penetrating liver injuries has a higher liver-related complication rate (50–52 %) than in blunt ones [56].

Follow-up after successful NOM

No definitive indications exist for post-injury follow-up and normal activity resumption in patients underwent to NOM. Some authors suggest a post discharge CT-scan and an outpatient visit after 4–6 weeks in case of grade II-V lesions [7]. In patients with uncomplicated hospital course the activity can be resumed after 3–4 months (because of the majority of lesions heal in 4 months) [7, 29]. Therefore the activity can be restarted 1 month after trauma, if the CT-scan follow-up (in grade III-V lesions) has shown a significant healing [7].

The patients have to be counseled to not remain alone for long periods and to return to the hospital immediately if they experience and increasing abdominal pain, lightheadedness, nausea or vomiting [29].

Recommendations for Operative Management (OM) in liver trauma (blunt and penetrating)

Patients should undergo to OM in liver trauma (blunt and penetrating) in case of hemodynamic instability, concomitant internal organs injury, evisceration or impalement (GoR 2 A)

Primary surgical intention should be to control the hemorrhage, to control bile leak and to allow for an intensive resuscitation as soon as possible (GoR 2 B)

Major hepatic resections should be avoided at first, and considered subsequently (delayed fashion) only in case of large devitalized liver portions and in centers with the necessary expertise (GoR 3 B).

Angioembolisation is a useful tool in case of persistent arterial bleeding (GoR 2 A).

The leading cause of death in liver injuries is exsanguination. The decision for an OM in liver trauma mainly depends from the hemodynamics patient's status and from the concomitant internal organ injury.

For minor (grade I-II) and moderate (grade III) liver injuries, and in favorable cases (no major bleeding at the laparotomy) minimal bleeding may be controlled by packing alone or with electrocautery, bipolar devices, or argon beam coagulation, topical hemostatic agents, omental packing [7, 9, 67, 68].

In case of severe liver injuries (grade IV-V) (Fig. 1a, b) and in not favorable cases (when the risk of "lethal triad" is high or it is already present) more aggressive procedures can be necessary (first of all hepatic manual compression and hepatic packing, with eventually vessels ligation, hepatic debridement, balloon tamponade up to shunting procedures or hepatic exclusion) associated with an intraoperative intensive resuscitation aiming to revert the lethal triad [9, 68].

In all cases of Damage Control Surgery (DCS) for liver trauma when the risk to develop abdominal compartment syndrome is high and when a second look after patients hemodynamic stabilization would be needed, a temporary abdominal closure can be safely considered [9, 67, 68].

Hepatic packing is the first maneuver in severe hepatic injury (Fig. 3). It could be manual at first and pads compression subsequently both aiming to stop the bleeding [7, 9, 67–72]. Do not pack excessively with resultant compression of the inferior cava vein [7, 67]. Packing must be removed or changed within 48–72 h to avoid the risk of intra-abdominal sepsis [7].

The Pringle maneuver (with the purpose to temporarily stop the portal and arterial flow into the injured liver) is either the second option, particularly in case of

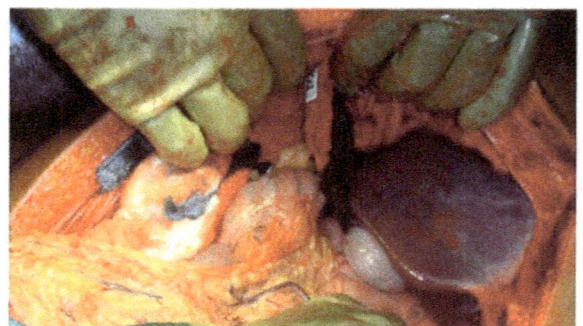

Fig. 3 Liver packing

persistent bleeding after hepatic packing, or to be done concurrently with packing in the patient dying of a massive liver injury (Fig. 4) (many authors advocated that clamping periods of 20 min with 5 min left for liver reperfusion decreases ischemia-reperfusion) [7, 9, 67].

In case of deep tracts into the liver parenchyma balloon tamponade, using a Foley or a Sengstaken-Blakemore catheter to control the hemorrhage is a viable option in patients not responding to packing alone (Fig. 5) [73]. The catheter is brought out through the skin, and can be removed after deflation 3–4 days after when the bleeding has stopped.

Fibrin sealants can be use in trauma patients and are apparently safe. These agents combine fibrin glue with thrombin, calcium chloride and aprotinin to form a stable clot [74]. However at present not many studies on human have been published, but in animal models these materials have been found to improve the bleeding control in high-grade liver lesions [75, 76].

In high-grade liver trauma, anatomic hepatic resection can be considered as a surgical option. Polanco et al. in a 15-years series of 1049 patients with liver injuries showed a decrease of mortality (9–24 % compared to 46–80 % at the beginning of the last century) and low complication rate (morbidity related to liver resection was 30 %) [3, 77, 78]. Two-thirds of 216 patients with high grade injury (with blunt and penetrating trauma) underwent surgery, and 56 underwent liver resection: 21 segmentectomies, 8 right lobectomy, 3 left lobectomies, 23 non-anatomic resections, and 1 total hepatectomy with liver transplantation. The authors reported a mortality rate from liver injury of 9 %, and an overall mortality near to 18 % [78]. However, the role of liver resection in trauma patients remains controversial and the published

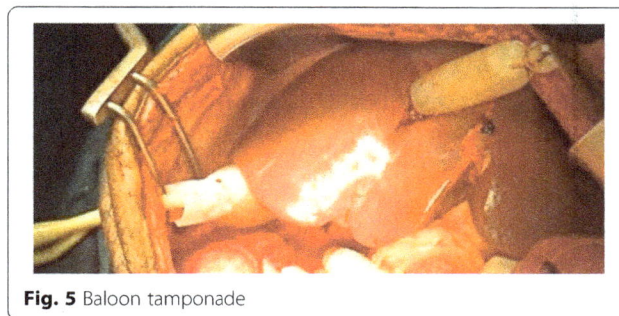
Fig. 4 Pringle maneuver

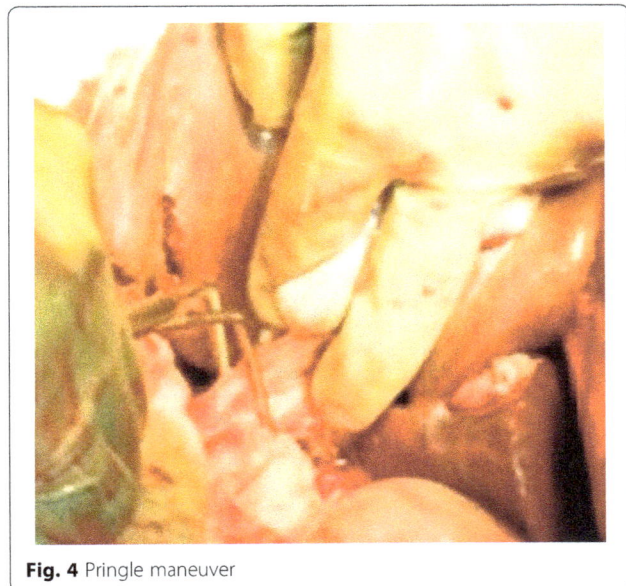
Fig. 5 Baloon tamponade

series demonstrate the frequency of liver resections in trauma ranges between 2 % and 5 % [3]. In unstable patients and during damage control surgery a non-anatomic resection is safer and easier [7, 9, 79]. Either anatomic or non-anatomic liver resection can be safely made with stapling device in experienced hands [79].

If bleeding persists despite the initial maneuver (hepatic packing, Pringle maneuver), and an evident hepatic artery lesion is found during operation, the artery should be repaired. If it's impossible, a selective hepatic artery ligation can be considered as a viable option. In this case cholecystectomy (for right or common hepatic artery ligation) should be performed to avoid gallbladder necrosis [79]. This procedure is used in 1 % of patients with severe liver trauma [80]. In fact post-operative angio-embolization is a viable option, when possible, allowing hemorrhage control while reducing the complications (Fig. 2) [7, 9, 81]. In fact, after artery ligation, the risk of hepatic necrosis, biloma and abscesses increases.

Portal vein injuries should be repair primarily, and a vein ligation is to be avoided because of liver necrosis or massive bowel edema may occur. Liver Packing and a second look or liver resection are preferable to portal ligation [79].

When the Pringle maneuver or arterial control is fails to control bleeding, and bleeding persists from behind the liver, a retro-hepatic caval or hepatic vein injury is present [81]. These lesions often occur when the suspensory ligaments, diaphragm, or liver parenchyma are disrupted [7]. Therapeutic options are 3: 1) tamponade with hepatic packing, 2) direct repair (with or without vascular isolation), and 3) lobar resection [7]. Actually the most successful method of managing severe venous injuries is liver packing [7, 82–84]. Direct venous repair is less safe in non-experienced hands, with a high mortality rate [7]. However, in the past, venous repair cases with or without shunting were described. However the most of these descriptions still anecdotal; these lesions require a planned surgical intervention when suspected [7]. Pacher and Feliciano proposed direct venous repair without shunting [7]. When hepatic vascular exclusion is necessary, different types of shunting procedures have been described. The most frequent type of shunt used is the veno-veno bypass (femoral to axillary or jugular by pass) or fenestrated stent grafts by surgeons familiar with their use [7, 9, 79, 85]. The atrio-caval shunt, introduced by Schrock in 1968, by pass the retro-hepatic cava blood with a chest tube put into the inferior cava vein, up the liver, through the right atrium. Mortality rates are high, due to the complexity of the lesions and the difficulty of the procedure [9]. Liver exclusion consists to stop the blood flow to the liver and out of the liver, clamping inferior vein cave (supra-hepatic and sub-hepatic cava), the hepatic hilum (Pringle maneuver), associated or not with intra-abdominal aorta clamping [68]. This is generally poorly tolerated in the unstable patient with major blood loss.

In emergency setting, hepatic transplantation has been described in case of liver avulsion or total crush injury, when a total hepatic resection must be done. In these cases portal and systemic venous systems must be decompressed with a porto-caval shunt. During the anhepatic phase (which should last no more than 36 h) the patient will require constant intra-venous fresh-frozen plasma and glucose [79]. This procedure is also called 2-step transplantation. However the majority of patients who underwent to liver transplantation in trauma setting are transplanted during the 1st week after the injury, due to liver failure in almost 50 % of cases [86]. Survivorship has been reported at 60 %.

At the moment, the exact role of post-operative angio-embolization is not well defined. Some authors reported high rate of patients who require angiography to control arterial bleeding post DCS (52–62 %) [87, 88] and others reported low mortality (12 % vs 36 %) in patients with grade IV-V hepatic injuries who underwent angio-embolization [89]. A French retrospective study has reported two principal indications in the acute post-injury phase for this procedure after high-grade liver injuries: 1) after primary operative hemostatic control in hemodynamically stable or stabilized patients, with CT-scan evidence of active bleeding, and 2) as adjunctive hemostatic control in patients with uncontrolled suspect arterial bleeding despite emergency laparotomy [90]. However not all authors agree about angiography use, and a high rate of post-procedure complications (parenchymal necrosis, bile leak, abscess and liver failure) are reported [91, 92].

Competing interests
The authors declare that they have no competing interests.

Authors' contributions
FC, GM contributed equally to this work, manuscript conception and draft. FC, SDS, WB, EEM, ABP, SR, GT, MS, RM and LA critically revised the manuscript and contribute with important scientific knowledge giving the final approval.

Author details
[1]General, Emergency and Trauma Surgery, Papa Giovanni XXIII Hospital, P.zza OMS 1, 24128 Bergamo, Italy. [2]Emergency and Trauma Surgery, Maggiore Hospital, Parma, Italy. [3]General, Emergency and Trauma Surgery, Maggiore Hospital, Bologna, Italy. [4]Trauma Surgery, Denver Health, Denver, CO, USA. [5]Surgery Department, University of Pittsburgh, Pittsburgh, Pensylvania, USA. [6]Trauma & Acute Care Service, St Michael's Hospital, Toronto, ON, Canada. [7]General and Emergency Surgery, Macerata Hospital, Macerata, Italy.

References
1. Richardson JD, Franklin GA, Lukan JK, Carrillo EH, Spain DA, Miller FB, et al. Evolution in the management of hepatic trauma: a 25-years perspective. Ann Surg. 2000;232:324–30.
2. Badger SA, Barclay R, Campbell P, Mole DJ, Diamond T. Management of liver trauma. World J Surg. 2009;33:2522–37.
3. Piper GL, Peitzman AB. Current management of hepatic trauma. Surg Clin N Am. 2010;90:775–85.
4. Peitzman AB, Richardson JD. Surgical treatment of injuries to the solid abdominal organs: a 50-years perspective from the Journal of Trauma. J of Trauma. 2010;69:1011–21.
5. Moore EE, Cogbill TH, Jurkovich GJ, Shackford SR, Malangoni MA, Champion HR. Organ injury scaling: spleen and liver (1994 revision). J Trauma. 1995;38:323–4.
6. Phillips B, Ball C, Sackett D, Badenoch D, Straus S, Haynes B, et al. Oxford Centre for Evidence-based Medicine Levels of Evidence. 2009.
7. Fabian TC, Bee TK. Ch.32 Liver and biliary tract. In: Feliciano DV, Mattox KL, Moore EE, editors. Trauma. 7th ed. 870: The McGraw-Hill Companies, Inc; 2013. p. 851.
8. Croce MA, Fabian TC, Menke PG, Waddle-Smith L, Minard G, Kudsk KA, et al. Nonoperative management of blunt hepatic trauma is the treatment of choice for hemodynamically stable patients. Results of a prospective trial. Ann Surg. 1995;221(6):744–53.
9. Kozar RA, Feliciano VD, Moore EE, Moore FA, Cocanour CS, West MA, et al. Western trauma Association/Critical Decision in Trauma: Operative management of blunt Hepatic Trauma. J Trauma. 2011;71(1):1–5.
10. Kumar S, Kumar A, Joshi MK, Rathi V. Comparison of diagnostic peritoneal lavage and focused assessment by sonography in trauma as an adjunct to primary survey in torso trauma: a prospective randomized clinical trial. Ulus Travma Acil Cerr Derg. 2014;20(2):101–6.
11. Richards JR, McGahan JP, Pali MJ, Bohnen PA. Sonographic detection of blunt hepatic trauma : hemoperitoneum and parenchymal patterns of injury. J Trauma. 1999;47:1092.
12. Sato M, Yoshii H. Reevaluation for ultrasonography for solid-organ injury in blunt abdominal trauma. J Ultrasound Med. 2004;23:158.
13. Quinn AC, Sinert R. What is the utility of the Focused Assessment with Sonography in Trauma (FAST) exam in penetrating torso trauma? Injury. 2011;42(5):482–7.
14. Kozar RA, Moore FA, Moore EE, West M, Cocanour CS, Davis J, et al. Western Trauma Association critical decisions in trauma: Nonoperative Management of adult blunt hepatic trauma. J Trauma. 2009;67:1144–49.
15. Moore EE, Shackford SR, Pachter HL, McAninch JW, Browner BD, Champion HR et al. Organ injury scaling: spleen, liver, and kidney. J Trauma. 1989 Dec;29(12):1664-6.
16. Chatoupis K, Papadopoulou G, Kaskarelis I. New technology in the management of liver trauma. Ann Gastroenterol. 2013;26(1):41–4.
17. Poletti PA, Mirvis SE, Shanmuganathan K, Killeen KL, Coldwell D. CT criteria for management of blunt liver trauma : correlation with angiography and surgical findings. Radiology. 2000;216:418–27.
18. Gaarder C, Naess PA, Eken T, Skaga NO, Pillgram-Larsen J, Klow NE, et al. Liver injuries-Improved results with a formal protocol including angiography. Injury. 2007;38:1075–83.
19. Hagiwara AT, Yukioka T, Ohta S, Tokunaga T, Ohta S, Matsuda H, et al. Nonsurgical management of patients with blunt hepatic injury: efficacy of transcatheter arterial embolization. AJR Am J Roentgenol. 1997;169:1151–6.
20. Stassen NA, Bhullar I, Cheng JD, Crandall M, Friese R, Guillamondegui O, et al. Kerwin A; Eastern Association for the Surgery of Trauma. Non operative management of blunt hepatic injury: an Eastern association for the surgery of trauma practice management guideline. J Trauma Acute Care Surgery. 2012;73(5 Suppl 4):S288–93.
21. Tinkoff G, Esposito T, Reed J, Kilgo P, Fildes J, Pasquale M, et al. American Association for the Surgery of Trauma Organ Injury Scale I: spleen, liver, and

kidney, validation based on the National Trauma Data Bank. J Am Coll Surg. 2008;207:646–55.

22. Velmahos GC, Toutouzas K, Radin R, Chan L, Rhee P, Tillou A, et al. High success with non-operative management of blunt hepatic trauma : the live ris a sturdy organ. Arch Surg. 2003;138:475–80.

23. Helling TS, Morse G, McNabney WK, Beggs CW, Behrends SH, Hutton-Rotert K, et al. Treatement of liver injuries at Level I and II centers in a multi-istitutional metropolitan trauma system. J Trauma. 1997;42:1091–96.

24. Carrillo EH, Platz A, Miller FB, Richardson JD, Polk Jr HC. Non-operative management of blunt hepatic trauma. Br J Surg. 1998;85:461–68.

25. Brasel KJ, DeLisle CM, Olson CJ, Borgstrom DC. Trends in the management of hepatic injury. Am J Surg. 1997;174:674–77.

26. Coimbra R, Hoyt DB, Engelhart S, Fortlage D. Non-operative management reduces the overall mortality of Grade 3 and 4 of blunt liver injuries. Int Surg. 2006;91:251–57.

27. Di Saverio S, Sibilio A, Coniglio C, Bianchi E, Biscardi A, Villani S, et al. A proposed algorithm for multimodal liver trauma management from a surgical trauma audit in a western European trauma center. Minerva Anestesiol. 2014;80(11):1205–16.

28. Di Saverio S, Moore EE, Tugnoli G, Naidoo N, Ansaloni L, Bonilauri S, et al. Non operative management of liver and spleen traumatic injuries: a giant with clay feet. World J Emerg Surg. 2012;7(1):3.

29. Parks NA, Davis JW, Forman D, Lemaster D. Observation for Nonoperative management of blunt liver injuries: how long is long enough? J Trauma. 2011;70(3):626–9.

30. American College of Surgeons. Advanced Trauma Life Support for Doctors (ATLS) Student Manual. 8th ed. 2008.

31. Stein DM, Scalea TM. Nonoperative management of spleen and liver injuries. J Int Care Med. 2006;21:296.

32. Fang JF, Wong YC, Lin BC, Hsu YP, Chen MF. The CT risk factors for the need of operative treatment on initially stable patients after blunt hepatic trauma. J Trauma. 2006;61:547–53.

33. Fang JF, Chen RJ, Wong YC, Lin BC, Hsu YB, Kao JL, et al. Pooling of contrast material on computed tomography mandates aggressive management of blunt hepatic injury. Am J Surg. 1998;176:315–9.

34. Poletti AP, Mirvis SE, Shanmuganathan K, Takada T, Killeen KL, Perlmutter D, et al. Blunt abdominal trauma patients: can organ injury be excluded without performing computer tomography? J Trauma. 2004;57:1072–81.

35. Velmhaos GC, Toutouzas KG, Radin R, Chan L, Demetriades D. Nonoperative treatment of blunt injury to solid abdominal organs. Arch Surg. 2003;138:844.

36. Yanar H, Ertekin C, Taviloglu K, Kabay B, Bakkaloglu H, Guloglu R. Nonoperative treatment of multiple intra-abdominal solid organ injury after blunt abdominal trauma. J Trauma. 2008;64(4):943–8.

37. Pachter HL, Hofstetter SR. The current status of nonoperative management of adult blunt hepatic injuries. Am J Surg. 1995;169(4):442–54.

38. Carillo E, Spain D, Wohltmann CD, Schmieg RE, Boaz PW, Miller FB, et al. Interventional techniques are useful adjuncts in nonoperative management of hepatic injuries. J Trauma. 1999;46:619.

39. Kozar RA, Moore FA, Grade M, Szöke R, Liersch T, Becker H, et al. Risks factors for hepatic morbidity following nonoperative management. Arch Surg. 2006;141:451–8.

40. Afshari A, Wikkelso A, Brok J, Møller AM, Wetterslev J. Thromboelatography (TEG) or thromboelastometry (ROTEM) to monitor haemotherapy versus usual care in patients with massive transfusion (Review). Cochrane Database Syst Rev. 2011;3:CD007871.

41. Zatta A, Mcquilten Z, Kandane-Rathnayake R, Isbister J, Dunkley S, Mcneil J, et al. The Australian and New Zealand Haemostasis Registry: ten years of data on off-licence use of recombinant activated factor VII. Blood Transfus. 2015;13(1):86–99.

42. Hauser CJ, Boffard K, Dutton R, Bernard GR, Croce MA, Holcomb JB et al. Results of the CONTROL trial: efficacy and safety of recombinant activated Factor VII in the management of refractory traumatic hemorrhage. J Trauma. 2010 Sep;69(3):489–500.

43. Wahl WL, Ahrns KS, Brandt MM, Franklin GA, Taheri PA. The need for early angiographic embolization in blunt hepatic injuries. J Trauma. 2002;52:1097–101.

44. Mohr AM, Lavery RF, Barone A, Bahramipour P, Magnotti LJ, Osband AJ, et al. Angioembolization for liver injuries: low mortality, high morbidity. J Trauma. 2003;55(5):1077–81.

45. Ward J, Alarcon L, Peitzman AB. Management of blunt liver injury: what is new? Eur J Trauma Emerg Surg. 2015 Jun;41(3):229-37.

46. Hsieh TM, Tsai TC, Liang JL, Che LC. Non-operative management attempted for selective high grade blunt hepatosplenic trauma is a feasible strategy. WJES. 2014;9:51.

47. Van der Wilden GM, Velmhaos GC, Emhoff T, Brancato S, Adams C, Georgakis G, et al. Successful Nonoperative management of the most severe blunt liver injuries. Arch Surg. 2012;147(5):423–8.

48. Marcheix B, Dambrin C, Cron C, Sledzianowski JF, Aguirre J, Suc B, et al. Transhepatic percutaneous embolisation of a post-traumatic pseudoaneurysm of hepatic artery. Ann Chir. 2004;129(10):603–6.

49. Hommes M, Nicol AJ, Navsaria PH, Reinders Folmer E, Edu S, Krige JE. Management of biliary complications in 412 patients with liver injuries. J Trauma Acute Care Surg. 2014;77(3):448–51.

50. Harrell DJ, Vitale GC, Larson GM. Selective role for endoscopic retrograde cholangiopancreatography in abdominal trauma. Surg Endosc. 1998;12(5):400–4.

51. Letoublon C, Chen Y, Arvieux C, Voirin D, Morra I, Broux C, et al. Delayed celiotomy or laparoscopy as part of the nonoperative management of blunt hepatic trauma. Worls J Surg. 2008;32:1189–93.

52. Carrillo EH, Wohltmann C, Richardson JD, Polk Jr HC. Evolution in the treatment of complex blunt liver injuries. Curr Probl Surg. 2001;38:1–60.

53. Geerts WH, Jay RM, Code KI, Chen E, Szalai JP, Saibil EA, et al. A comparison of low-dose heparin with low-molecular-weight heparin as prophylaxis against venous thromboembolism after major trauma. NEJM. 1996;335(10):701–7.

54. Datta I, Ball CG, Rudmik LR, Paton-Gay D, Bhayana D, Salat P, et al. A multicenter review of deep venous thrombosis prophylaxis practice patterns for blunt hepatic trauma. J Trauma Manag Outcomes. 2009;3:7.

55. Joseph B, Pandit V, Harrison C, Lubin D, Kulvatunyou N, Zangbar B, et al. Early thromboembolic prophylaxis in patients with blunt solid abdomen organ injuries undergoing nonoperative management: is it safe? Am J Surg. 2015;209(1):194–8.

56. Demetriades D, Hadjizacharia P, Constantinou C, Brown C, Inaba K, Rhee P, et al. Selective nonoperative management of penetrating abdominal solid organ injuries. Ann Surg. 2006;244(4):620–8.

57. Navsaria PH, Nicol AJ, Krige JE, Edu S. Selective Nonoperative management of liver gunshot injuries. Ann Surg. 2009;249(4):653.

58. Biffl WL, Leppaniemi A. Management Guidelines for Penetrating Abdominal Trauma. World J Surg. 2015;39(6):1373–80.

59. Biffl WL, Kaups LK, Pham TN, Rowell SE, Jurkovich GJ, Burlew CC, et al. Validating the western trauma association algorithm managing patients with anterior abdominal stable wounds: a western trauma association multi center trial. J Trauma. 2011;71(6):1494–502.

60. Biffl WL, Moore EE. Management guidelines for penetrating abdominal trauma. Curr Opin Crit Care. 2010;16(6):609–17.

61. Biffl WL, Kaups KL, Cothren CC, Brasel KJ, Dicker RA, Bullard MK, et al. Management of patients with anterior abdominal stab wounds: a Western Trauma Association multicenter trial. J Trauma. 2009;66(5):1294–301.

62. Sugrue M, Balogh Z, Lynch J, Bardsley J, Sisson G, Weigelt J. Guidelines for the management of haemodynamically stable patients with stab wounds to the anterior abdomen. ANZ J Surg. 2007;77(8):614–20.

63. Lamb CM, Garner JP. Selective non-operative management of civilian gunshot wounds to the abdomen: a systematic review of the evidence. Injury. 2014;45(4):659–66.

64. Velmahos GC, Constantinou C, Tillou A, Brown CV, Salim A, Demetriades D. Abdominal computed tomographic scan for patients with gunshot wounds to the abdomen selected for non-operative management. J Trauma. 2005;59(5):1155–60.

65. Demetriades D, Rabinowitz B. Indications for operation in abdominal stab wounds. A prospective study of 651 patients. Ann Surg. 1987;205(2):129–32.

66. Demetriades D, Velmahos G. Indication for and technique of Laparotomy. In: Moore E, Feliciano D, Mattox K, editors. Trauma. 6th ed. New York: McGraw-Hill; 2006.

67. Letoublon C, Arvieux C. Traumatisme fermés du foie, Principes de technique et de tactique chirurgicales. EMC. Techniques chirurgicales – Appareil digestif, 40–785, 2003, 20 p.

68. Letoublon C, Reche F, Abba J, Arvieux C. Damage control laparotomy. J Visc Surg. 2011;148(5):e366–70.

69. Nicol AJ, Hommes M, Primrose R, Navsaria PH, Krige JE. Packing for control oh hemorrhage in major liver trauma. World J Surg. 2007;31:569–74.

70. Di Saverio S, Catena F, Filicori F, Ansaloni L, Coccolini F, Keutgen XM, et al. Predictive factors of morbidity and mortality in grade IV and V liver trauma undergoing perihepatic packing: single institution 14 years experience at European trauma centre. Injury. 2012;43(9):1347–54.

71. Baldoni F, Di Saverio S, Antonacci N, Coniglio C, Giugni A, Montanari N, et al. Refinement in the technique of peri-hepatic packing: a safe and effective surgical hemostasis and multidisciplinary approach can improve the outcome in severe liver trauma. Am J Surg. 2011;201(1):e5–e14.

72. Filicori F, Di Saverio S, Casali M, Biscardi A, Baldoni F, Tugnoli G. Packing for damage control of nontraumatic intra-abdominal massive hemorrhages. World J Surg. 2010;34(9):2064–8.

73. Letoublon C, Morra I, Chen Y, Monnin V, Voirin D, Arvieux C. Hepatic arterial embolization in the management of blunt hepatic trauma: indications and complications. J Trauma. 2011;70(5):1032–6.

74. Poggetti RS, Moore EE, Moore FA, Mitchell MB, Read RA. Balloon tamponade for bilobar transfixing hepatic gunshot wounds. J Trauma. 1992;33(5):694–7.

75. Kram HB, Reuben BI, Fleming AW, Shoemaker WC. Use of Fibrin glue in hepatic trauma. J Trauma. 1988;45:1195.

76. Holcomb JB, Pusateri AE, Harris RA, Charles NC, Gomez RR, Cole JP, et al. Effect of dry fibrin sealant dressing versus gauze packing on blood loss in grade V liver injuries in resuscitated swine. J Trauma. 1999;46:49.

77. Sena MJ, Douglas G, Gerlach T, Grayson JK, Pichakron KO, Zierold D. A pilot study of the use of Kaolin-impregnated gauze (Combat Gauze) for packing high-grade hepatic injuries in a hypothermic coagulopathic swine model. J Surg Res. 2013;183(2):704–9.

78. Strong RW, Lynch SV, Wall DR, Liu CL. Anatomic resection for severe liver trauma. Surgery. 1998;123:251–7.

79. Polanco P, Stuart L, Pineda J, Puyana JC, Ochoa JB, Alarcon L, et al. Hepatic resection in the management of complex injury to the liver. J Trauma. 2008;65(6):1264–9.

80. Peitzman AB, Marsh JW. Advanced operative techniques in management of complex liver injury. J Trauma Acute Care Surg. 2012;73(3):765–70.

81. Richardson JD. Changes in the management of injuries to the liver and spleen. J Am Coll Surg. 2005 May;200(5):648–69.

82. Frenklin GA, Casos SR. Current advances in the surgical approach to abdominal trauma. Injury. 2006;37:1143–56.

83. Beal SL. Fatal hepatic hemorrhage: an unresolved problem in the management of complex liver injuries. J Trauma. 1990;30:163.

84. Fabian TC, Croce MA, Stanford GG, Payne LW, Mangiante EC, Voeller GR, et al. Factors affecting morbidity following hepatic trauma. A prospective analysis od 482 injuries. Ann Surg. 1991;213:540.

85. Cue JI, Cryer HG, Miller FB, Richardson JD, Polk Jr HC. Packing and planned re-exploration for hepatic and retroperitoneal hemorrhage: critical refinements of a useful technique. J Trauma. 1990;30(8):1007.

86. Biffl WL, Moore EE, Franciose RJ. Venovenous bypass and hepatic vascular isolation as adjuncts in the repair of destructive wounds to the retrohepatic inferior vena cava. J Trauma. 1998;45:400–3.

87. Plackett TP, Barmparas G, Inaba K, Demetriades D. Transplantation for severe hepatic trauma. J Trauma. 2011;71(6):1880–4.

88. Misselbeck TS, Teicher E, Cipolle MD, Pasquale MD, Shah KT, Dangleben DA, et al. Hepatic angioembolization in trauma patients:indications and complications. J Trauma. 2009;67:769–73.

89. Johnson JW, Gracias VH, Gupta R, Guillamondegui O, Reilly PM, Shapiro MB, et al. Hepatic angiography in patients undergoing damage control laparotomy. J Trauma. 2002;52:1102–6.

90. Asensio JA, Petrone P, García-Núñez L, Kimbrell B, Kuncir E. Multidisciplinary approach for the management of complex hepatic injuries AAST-OIS grades IV-V: a prospective study. Scand J Surg. 2007;96(3):214–20.

91. Dabbs DN, Stein DM, Scalea TM. Major hepatic necrosis: a common complication after angioembolization for treatement of high grade injuries. J Trauma. 2009;66:621–7.

92. Dabbs DN, Stein DM, Scalea TM. Major hepatic necrosis: a common complication after angioembolization for treatment of high-grade liver injuries. J Trauma. 2009 Mar;66(3):621-7; discussion 627-9.

Permissions

The contributors of this book come from diverse backgrounds, making this book a truly international effort. This book will bring forth new frontiers with its revolutionizing research information and detailed analysis of the nascent developments around the world.

We would like to thank all the contributing authors for lending their expertise to make the book truly unique. They have played a crucial role in the development of this book. Without their invaluable contributions this book wouldn't have been possible. They have made vital efforts to compile up to date information on the varied aspects of this subject to make this book a valuable addition to the collection of many professionals and students.

This book was conceptualized with the vision of imparting up-to-date information and advanced data in this field. To ensure the same, a matchless editorial board was set up. Every individual on the board went through rigorous rounds of assessment to prove their worth. After which they invested a large part of their time researching and compiling the most relevant data for our readers.

The editorial board has been involved in producing this book since its inception. They have spent rigorous hours researching and exploring the diverse topics which have resulted in the successful publishing of this book. They have passed on their knowledge of decades through this book. To expedite this challenging task, the publisher supported the team at every step. A small team of assistant editors was also appointed to further simplify the editing procedure and attain best results for the readers.

Apart from the editorial board, the designing team has also invested a significant amount of their time in understanding the subject and creating the most relevant covers. They scrutinized every image to scout for the most suitable representation of the subject and create an appropriate cover for the book.

The publishing team has been an ardent support to the editorial, designing and production team. Their endless efforts to recruit the best for this project, has resulted in the accomplishment of this book. They are a veteran in the field of academics and their pool of knowledge is as vast as their experience in printing. Their expertise and guidance has proved useful at every step. Their uncompromising quality standards have made this book an exceptional effort. Their encouragement from time to time has been an inspiration for everyone.

The publisher and the editorial board hope that this book will prove to be a valuable piece of knowledge for researchers, students, practitioners and scholars across the globe.

List of Contributors

Mark R Harrigan and Beverly C Walters
Division of Neurosurgery, University of Alabama, Birmingham, Birmingham, Alabama, USA

Jordan A Weinberg
Division of Trauma and Critical Care Surgery, University of Tennessee Health Science Center, Memphis, Tennessee, USA

Ya-Sin Peaks
University of Alabama, Birmingham School of Medicine, Birmingham, Alabama, USA

Steven M Taylor
Division of Vascular Surgery, University of Alabama, Birmingham, Birmingham, Alabama, USA

Luis P Cava
Department of Neurology, University of Alabama, Birmingham, Birmingham, Alabama, USA

Joshua Richman
Division of Preventative Medicine, University of Alabama, Birmingham, Birmingham, Alabama, USA

Michael Cudworth, Angelo Fulle and Juan P Ramos
Adult Emergency Services, Surgery, Hospital Dr. Sotero del Rio, Concha y Toro, 3459 Puente Alto, Santiago, Chile

Ivette Arriagada
Vascular Surgery, Hospital Dr. Sotero del Rio, Concha y Toro, 3459 Puente Alto, Santiago, Chile

Antonio Marttos, Fernanda M Kuchkarian, Emmanouil Palaios, Daniel Rojas and Carl Schulman
University of Miami Miller School of Medicine Surgery Department (D40), Miami, FL 33101, USA

Phillipe Abreu-Reis
Universidade Federal do Parana, Rua XV de Novembro, 1299, CEP 80.060-000. Curitiba, PR Brasil

Alma Rados, Corina Tiruta and Zhengwen Xiao
Regional Trauma Services, Foothills Medical Centre, University of Calgary, 29 Street, Calgary, NW 1403, Alberta

Chad G Ball
Departments of Surgery, Foothills Medical Centre, University of Calgary, Calgary, Alberta

John B Kortbeek and Andrew W Kirkpatrick
Critical Care Medicine, Foothills Medical Centre, University of Calgary, Calgary, Alberta
Departments of Surgery, Foothills Medical Centre, University of Calgary, Calgary, Alberta

Paul Tourigny
Radiology, Foothills Medical Centre, University of Calgary, Calgary, Alberta
Emergency Medicine, Foothills Medical Centre, University of Calgary, Calgary, Alberta

Andrea Melo Alexandre Fraga and Marcelo Conrado Reis
Pediatric Emergency Division, Hospital de Clinicas, University of Campinas, Campinas, SP, Brazil

Joaquim Murray Bustorff-Silva
Division of Pediatric Surgery, Department of Surgery, School of Medical Sciences, University of Campinas (Unicamp), Campinas, SP, Brazil

Thais Marconi Fernandez
School of Medical Sciences, University of Campinas (Unicamp), Rua Alexander Fleming, 181, Cidade Universitária "Prof. Zeferino Vaz", Barão Geraldo, Campinas, SP, Brazil

Gustavo Pereira Fraga
Division of Trauma Surgery, School of Medical Sciences, University of Campinas (Unicamp), Campinas, SP, Brazil

Emilio Carlos Elias Baracat
Pediatric Emergency Division, Department of Pediatrician, School of Medical Sciences, University of Campinas (Unicamp), Campinas, SP, Brazil

Raul Coimbra
The Monroe E. Trout Professor of Surgery, Department of Surgery, Division of Trauma, Surgical Critical Care, and Burns, University of California San Diego, 200 West Arbor Dr, #8896, San Diego, CA 92103-8896, USA

Rishi Mamtani
Sunnybrook Health Sciences Centre, 2075 Bayview Avenue, Room H113, Toronto, ON M4N 3M5, Canada

Bartolomeu Nascimento
Trauma Program, Department of Surgery, Sunnybrook Health Sciences Centre, 2075 Bayview Avenue, Room B5 12, Toronto, ON M4N 3M5, Canada

Sandro Rizoli
Departments of Surgery and Critical Care Medicine, Sunnybrook Health Sciences Centre, University of Toronto, Canada

Ruxandra Pinto
Sunnybrook Health Sciences Centre, 2075 Bayview Avenue, Room K3W-25, Toronto, ON M4N 3M5, Canada

Yulia Lin
Sunnybrook Health Sciences Centre, 2075 Bayview Avenue, Room B2 04, Toronto, ON M4N 3M5, Canada

Homer Tien
Trauma Services, Division of General Surgery, Sunnybrook Health Sciences Centre and Canadian Forces Health Services, 2075 Bayview Avenue, Room H1 86, Toronto, ON M4N 3M5, USA

Antonino Agrusa, Giorgio Romano, Daniela Chianetta, Giovanni De Vita, Giuseppe Frazzetta, Giuseppe Di Buono, Vincenzo Sorce and Gaspare Gulotta
Department of General Surgery, Urgency and Organ Transplantation, University of Palermo, Via L. Giuffrè, Palermo 5 90127, Italy

Antonio Krüger, Carla Florido, Amelie Braunisch and Eric Walther
Department of Trauma-, Hand- and Reconstructive Surgery, Philipps-University, Baldingerstr. 1, Marburg, Germany

Dietrich Doll
Department of Visceral, Thoracic and Vascular Surgery, Philipps-University of Marburg, Marburg, Germany
Department of Trauma, Chris Hani Baragwanath Academic Hospital, Johannesburg, Soweto, South Africa
Department of Surgery, St.-Marien-Hospital Vechta, Teaching Hospital of the MHH Hannover University, Vechta, Germany

Tugba Han Yilmaz
Department of Surgery, Izmir, Turkey, Baskent University, Ankara, Turkey

Yukihiro Ikegami, Tsuyoshi Suzuki, Chiaki Nemoto, Yasuhiko Tsukada, Arifumi Hasegawa, Jiro Shimada and Choichiro Tase
Department of Emergency and Critical Care Medicine, School of Medicine, Fukushima Medical University, 1 Hikarigaoka, Fukushima 960-1295, Japan

Gustavo Pereira Fraga
Division of Trauma Surgery, Department of Surgery, School of Medical Sciences, University of Campinas (Unicamp), Rua Alexander Fleming, 181 Cidade Universitária "Prof. Zeferino Vaz" - Barão Geraldo, Campinas - SP, Brazil

Vitor Augusto de Andrade, Ricardo Schwingel and Jamil Pastori Neto
School of Medical Sciences, University of Campinas (Unicamp), Campinas - SP, Brazil

Sizenando Vieira Starling
Hospital João XXIII, Belo Horizonte - MG, Brazil

Sandro Rizoli
Departments of Surgery and Critical Care Medicine, Sunnybrook Health Sciences Centre, University of Toronto, Canada

Carlos Eduardo Carrasco
Faculty of Medical Sciences, University of Campinas (FCM / UNICAMP) Campinas, SP, Brazil

Mauricio Godinho
Division of Trauma Surgery, Department of Surgery, Faculty of Medical Sciences, University of Campinas (FCM/UNICAMP), Campinas, SP, Brazil

Marilisa Berti de Azevedo Barros
Department of Public Health, Faculty of Medical Sciences, University of Campinas (FCM/UNICAMP), Campinas, SP, Brazil

Sandro Rizoli
Departments of Surgery and Critical Care Medicine, Sunnybrook Health Sciences Centre, University of Toronto, Canada

Suleyman Ersoy
Emergency Department, Ahi Evran Univercity Training and Research Hospital, Kırsehir (40100), Turkey

Bedriye Müge Sonmez, Fevzi Yilmaz and Fatma Cesur
Emergency Department, Ankara Numune Training and Research Hospital, Talatpaşa Bulvarı, Ankara (06100), Turkey

Cemil Kavalci
Emergency Department, Baskent Univecity, Taşkent caddesi, Ankara (06490), Turkey

Derya Ozturk and Ertugrul Altinbilek
Emergency Department, Şişli Etfal Training and Research Hospital, Halaskargazi caddesi, İstanbul (34371), Turkey

Ali Erdem Yildirim, Ozhan Merzuk Uckun and Fatih Alagöz
Neurosurgery Department, Ankara Numune Training and Research Hospital, Talatpaşa Bulvarı, Ankara (06100), Turkey

Tezcan Akin
General Surgery Department, Ankara Numune Training and Research Hospital, Talatpaşa Bulvarı, Ankara (06100), Turkey

Kenneth N Ozoilo, Simon J Yiltok and Hyacinth C Nwadiaro
Surgery Department, Jos University Teaching Hospital, Jos, Nigeria

Ishaya C Pam
Obstetrics and Gynaecology Department, Jos University Teaching Hospital, Jos, Nigeria

Alice V Ramyil
Ophthalmology Department, Jos University Teaching Hospital, Jos, Nigeria

Thiago Messias Zago, Bruno Monteiro Tavares Pereira, Thiago Rodrigues Araujo Calderan, Mauricio Godinho and Gustavo Pereira Fraga
Rua Alexander Fleming, 181 Zip code: 13.083-970, Cidade Universitaria "Prof. Zeferino Vaz, Campinas – SP, Brazil

Bartolomeu Nascimento
2075 Bayview Ave., Room B5 12, Toronto, Ontario, M4N 3M5 Canada

Kaan Celik, Fevzi Yilmaz, Miray Ozlem, Ali Demir, Tamer Durdu, Bedriye Müge Sonmez, Muhittin Serkan Yilmaz, Muhammed Evvah Karakilic, Engin Deniz Arslan and Cihat Yel
Numune Training and Research Hospital, Emergency department, Ankara, Turkey

Cemil Kavalci
Baskent University Faculty of Medicine, Emergency department, Ankara, Turkey

Pedro Henrique Alves de Morais, Vinícius Lacerda Ribeiro, Igor Eduardo Caetano de Farias, Luiz Eduardo Almeida Silva and João Batista de Sousa
Medical School, Academic League of Emergency and Trauma, University of Brasilia, Brasilia, Brazil

Fabiana Pirani Carneiro and Joel Paulo Russomano Veiga
Medical School, University of Brasilia, Brasilia, Brazil

João Batista de Sousa
Campus Universitário Darcy Ribeiro, Prédio da Reitoria, 2° pavimento, sala B2-16, 70910-900 Brasília – DF Brasil, Brazil

Ting-Min Hsieh
Division of Trauma Surgery, Kaohsiung Chang Gung Memorial Hospital and Chang Gung University College of Medicine, 123 Ta Pei Road, Niao-Sung District, Kaohsiung, Taiwan

Tsung Cheng Tsai
Department of Emergency, Kaohsiung Chang Gung Memorial Hospital and Chang Gung University College of Medicine, 123 Ta Pei Road, Niao-Sung District, Kaohsiung, Taiwan

Jiun-Lung Liang
Department of Radiology, Kaohsiung Chang Gung Memorial Hospital and Chang Gung University College of Medicine, 123 Ta Pei Road, Niao-Sung District, Kaohsiung, Taiwan

Chih Che Lin
Division of General Surgery, Kaohsiung Chang Gung Memorial Hospital and Chang Gung University College of Medicine, 123 Ta Pei Road, Niao-Sung District, Kaohsiung, Taiwan

Carolina Prevaldi
Emergency Department, Hospital of San Donà di Piave VE, Parma, Italy

Ciro Paolillo
Emergency Department, Academic Hospital of Udine, Parma, Italy

Carlo Locatelli
Institute of Toxicology, IRCCS Fondazione Maugeri Pavia, Parma, Italy

Giorgio Ricci
Emergency Deparment, Academic Hospital of Verona, Parma, Italy

Fausto Catena
Emergency Surgery, Academic Hospital of Parma, Parma, Italy

Luca Ansaloni
Emergency surgery, Hospital of Bergamo, Parma, Italy

Gianfranco Cervellin
Emergency Department, Academic Hospital of Parma, Parma, Italy

Bahadir Danisman, Bahattin Isik and M Evvah Karakilic
Emergency Department, Dıskapi Yıldırım Beyazit Training and Research Hospital, Ankara, Turkey

Muhittin Serkan Yilmaz, Cihat Yel, Alper Gorkem Solakoglu, Burak Demirci and Selim Inan
Emergency Department, Numune Training and Research Hospital, Ankara, Turkey

Cemil Kavalci
Emergency Department, Baskent University Faculty of Medicine, Ankara, Turkey

Manuel Burggraf, Arzu Payas and Max Daniel Kauther
Department for Orthopaedics and Emergency Surgery, University Hospital Essen, University Duisburg-Essen, Hufelandstr. 55, 45147 Essen, Germany

Carsten Schoeneberg and Sven Lendemans
Clinic for Accident Surgery and Orthopaedics, Alfried Krupp Hospital Steele, Hellweg 100, 45276 Essen, Germany

Jeffry Nahmias, Andrew Doben, Shiva Poola, Samuel Korntner, Karen Carrens and Ronald Gross
Baystate Medical Center, affiliate of Tufts University School of Medicine, 759 Chestnut Street, Springfield, MA 01199, USA

Carlos A. Ordoñez, Ramiro Manzano-Nunez, Maria Paula Naranjo, Alvaro I. Sanchez Ortiz and Alberto F. García
Division of Trauma and Acute Care Surgery, Fundación Valle del Lili, Cali, Colombia
Clinical Research Center, Fundación Valle del Lili, Cali, Colombia

Cecibel Cevallos
Department of Surgery, Universidad del Valle, Cali, Colombia

Maria Alejandra Londoño
School of Medicine, Universidad ICESI, Cali, Colombia

Ernest E. Moore
Department of Surgery, Trauma Research Center, University of Colorado, Denver, CO, USA

Esteban Foianini
Department of Surgery, Clinica Foianini, Santacruz de la Sierra, Bolivia

Federico Coccolini
General Emergency and Trauma Surgery Department, Papa Giovanni XXIII Hospital, Piazza OMS 1, 24127 Bergamo, Italy

Fausto Catena
Emergency and Trauma Surgery, Parma Maggiore Hospital, Parma, Italy

Ernest E. Moore
Trauma Surgery, Denver Health, Denver, CO, USA

Rao Ivatury
Virginia Commonwealth University, Richmond, VA, USA

Sandro Rizoli
Trauma & Acute Care Service, St Michael's Hospital, Toronto, ON, Canada

Yoram Kluger
Division of General Surgery Rambam Health Care Campus, Haifa, Israel

Fikri M. Abu-Zidan
Department of Surgery, College of Medicine and Health Sciences, UAE University, Al-Ain, United Arab Emirates

Noel Naidoo
Department of Surgery, University of KwaZulu-Natal, Durban, South Africa

Frederick A. Moore
Department of Surgery, University of Florida, Gainesville, FL, USA

Nicola Zanini
General Surgery Department, Infermi Hospital, Rimini, Italy

Makoto Aoki, Minoru Kaneko, Masato Murata, Jun Nakajima, Shuichi Hagiwara, Masahiko Kanbe and Kiyohiro Oshima
Department of Emergency Medicine, Gunma University Graduate School of Medicine, Maebashi, Gunma, Japan

Kei Shibuya, Ayana Koizumi, Yoshinori Koyama and Yoshito Tsushima
Department of Diagnostic and Interventional Radiology, Gunma University Graduate School of Medicine, Maebashi, Gunma, Japan

Federico Coccolini and Giulia Montori
General, Emergency and Trauma Surgery, Papa Giovanni XXIII Hospital, P.zza OMS 1, 24128 Bergamo, Italy

Philip F. Stahel
Department of Orthopedic Surgery and Department of Neurosurgery, Denver Health Medical Center and University of Colorado School of Medicine, Denver, CO, USA

Walter Biffl
Acute Care Surgery, The Queen's Medical Center, Honolulu, HI, USA

Tal M Horer
Dept. of Cardiothoracic and Vascular Surgery & Dept. Of Surgery Örebro University Hospital and Örebro University, Örebro, Sweden

Sandro Rizoli
Trauma & Acute Care Service, St Michael's Hospital, Toronto, ON, Canada

Andrew Kirkpatrick
General, Acute Care, Abdominal Wall Reconstruction, and Trauma Surgery Foothills Medical Centre, Calgary, AB, Canada

Ari Leppaniemi
Abdominal Center, University Hospital Meilahti, Helsinki, Finland

Noel Naidoo
Department of Surgery, University of KwaZulu-Natal, Durban, South Africa

Dieter Weber
Department of General Surgery, Royal Perth Hospital, Perth, Australia

Fikri Abu-Zidan
Department of Surgery, College of Medicine and Health Sciences, UAE University, Al-Ain, United Arab Emirates

Massimo Sartelli
General and Emergency Surgery, Macerata Hospital, Macerata, Italy

Biplab Mishra and Subodh Kumar
Jai Prakash Narayan Apex Trauma Center, All India Institute of Medical Sciences, New Delhi, India

Saurabh Singhal and Nitesh Kumar
All India Institute of Medical Sciences, New Delhi, India

Divya Aggarwal
University College of Medical Sciences, New Delhi, India

Alicia Mangram, Phillip Moeser, Michael G Corneille, Laura J Prokuski, Nicolas Zhou, Jacqueline Sohn, Shalini Chaliki, Olakunle F Oguntodu and James K Dzandu
John C. Lincoln North Mountain Hospital, Phoenix, USA

Phillip Moeser
North Mountain Radiology Group Hospital, Phoenix, USA

Nicolas Zhou and Jacqueline Sohn
Midwestern University – Arizona College of Osteopathic Medicine, Arizona, USA

Shalini Chaliki
University of Missouri – Kansas City, School of Medicine, Kansas, USA

Marcelo A. F. Ribeiro Junior, Vinicius C. Rodrigues, Giovana E. K. Bechara and Raíssa Reis de-Moura
Disciplina de Cirurgia Geral e Trauma, Universidade Santo Amaro, São Paulo, São Paulo, Brazil

Celia Y. D. Feng and Alexander T. M. Nguyen
School of Medicine, University of New South Wales, Sydney, New South Wales, Australia

Megan Brenner
RA Cowley Shock Trauma Center, University of Maryland, Baltimore, MD, USA

Federico Coccolini, Giulia Montori and Luca Ansaloni
General, Emergency and Trauma Surgery, Papa Giovanni XXIII Hospital, P.zza OMS 1, 24128 Bergamo, Italy

Fausto Catena
Emergency and Trauma Surgery, Maggiore Hospital, Parma, Italy

Salomone Di Saverio and Gregorio Tugnoli
General, Emergency and Trauma Surgery, Maggiore Hospital, Bologna, Italy

Walter Biffl and Ernest E. Moore
Trauma Surgery, Denver Health, Denver, CO, USA

Andrew B. Peitzman
Surgery Department, University of Pittsburgh, Pittsburgh, Pensylvania, USA

Sandro Rizoli
Trauma & Acute Care Service, St Michael's Hospital, Toronto, ON, Canada

Massimo Sartelli and Roberto Manfredi
General and Emergency Surgery, Macerata Hospital, Macerata, Italy

Index

www.ingramcontent.com/pod-product-compliance
Lightning Source LLC
Chambersburg PA
CBHW082030190326
41458CB00010B/3327